YOUR
NATURAL
MEDICINE
CHEST

YOUR
NATURAL
MEDICINE
CHEST

Natural Remedies
for 101 Ailments

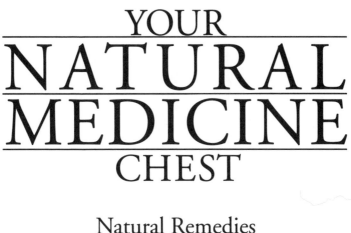

JEANNE MARIE MARTIN

Macmillan Canada

Toronto

First published in Canada in 2001 by
Macmillan Canada, an imprint of CDG Books Canada

Canadian Cataloguing in Publication Data
Martin, Jeanne Marie, 1951–
    Your natural medicine chest: natural remedies for 101 ailments

ISBN: 1-55335-003-0

1. Alternative medicine—Handbooks, manuals, etc. I. Title.

R733.M375 2001   615.5   C2001-930526-5

This book is available at special discounts for bulk purchases by your group or organization for
sales promotions, premiums, fundraising and seminars. For details, contact: CDG Books
Canada Inc., 99 Yorkville Avenue, Suite 400, Toronto, ON, M5R 3K5. Tel: 416-963-8830.
Toll Free: 1-877-963-8830. Fax: 416-923-4821.
Web site: cdgbooks.com.

1 2 3 4 5 TRANS 05 04 03 02 01

Cover and text design by Susan Thomas / Digital Zone
Cartoons by Graham Harrap. Copyright © Graham Harrap, 2001

Macmillan Canada
An imprint of CDG Books Canada Inc.
Toronto

Printed in Canada

To God
This book is dedicated to
my truest friend,
my dearest love,
my constant companion,
the light of my life,
my guiding force
and inspiration.

CONTENTS

ACKNOWLEDGMENTS

Thanks to dear ones who believe in me: Ross Seidel, Graham Harrop, Lillian Hanner, Lucienne and Gerard Barthe, Betty Toohey, and special thanks to my computer teacher: Glade Thomas.

FOREWORD

Your Natural Medicine Chest is a treasure of healing pearls of wisdom. Jeanne Marie Martin has done a truly admirable job of drawing from a wide variety of healing modalities and traditions that are sure to appeal to readers of every health and healing persuasion.

Her treatment of the most current health concerns, such as allergies, toxin-overload, wrinkles, viruses and yeast infection, is not only user-friendly, but also timely and based upon the most current research. The reader will especially appreciate Jeanne Marie's detailed discussion of each health condition's cause, modern natural treatment and helpful supplementation—complete with dosages.

I particularly enjoyed the section "Natural Remedies from Your Refrigerator and Cupboard"; her "Fantastic Foods for Healing" and "Remedy Recipes for Health" parts make this book eminently practical and convenient. In addition, for those of us whose time is at a premium, the section "Healing Aids: Natural Ways to Speed Healing" introduces us to the many different and powerful ways that healing can be achieved, be it in body, mind or spirit.

I highly recommend Jeanne Marie Martin's latest offering, which is her 13th health book. She is well qualified and is to be congratulated for this fine addition to your natural healing library.

ANN LOUISE GITTLEMAN,
N.D., M.S., C.N.S.,
author of *The Living Beauty Detox Program*

THE NATURAL APPROACH TO HEALTH

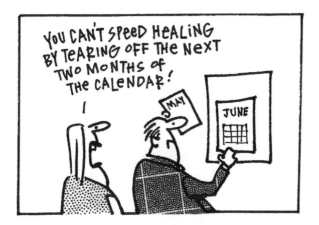

"The doctor of the future will give no medicine but will interest patients in the care of the human frame, in proper diet, and in the cause and prevention of disease."

— Thomas A. Edison

BEFORE YOU USE THIS BOOK

Read all of the following information in this section to ensure proper use of this book and to receive the maximum benefits of the natural remedies and foods described in the remainder of the book. This section explains where to look for everything from remedy usage to buying information. Most important, this section gives safety guidelines and practical advice on when to use this book and when to call a doctor. Be sure to read: "How to Use This Book."

WHY USE NATURAL REMEDIES?

Have you wondered about, or perhaps already explored, alternatives to drug therapy in order to avoid overusing drugs and suffering unneeded side effects? Or have you just been determined to find and utilize a more natural approach to healing? If so, this book was written for you.

The ancient Greek physician Hippocrates, who is known as "the father of medicine," practiced natural medicine and explored the uses of herbs and natural healing treatments. Up until the middle of the 16th century, foods, herbs and natural remedies were used as medicines throughout Europe and the rest of the world.

In the early 1500s, a German physician named Theophratus von Hohemhein, who called himself "Paracelsus," witnessed the process of crude minerals being purified by other minerals in the mines of Tyrol and decided to try similar processes in the healing of his patients. He is considered to be the first doctor to give mercury to his patients in small and large amounts.

There are no exact records of his experiments. History states that he burned the books of Hippocrates and disavowed Hippocrates's ideals. Paracelsus's practices of discontinuing the use of herbs for medicine and purifying the body with chemicals did little to help him. He died at 50 years of age. However, he transformed medical practice, and foods, herbs—leaves, flowers, roots, barks—and natural treatments were replaced by minerals used to purge the body and eventually led to giving drugs of all kinds, as medicine.

Herbalogy, the study and use of herbs for healing, also called herbalism, is still alive and well in Great Britain, most of Europe, Asia, Africa, South America and many other parts of the world. Herbalists are still making a comeback in North America, where herbalism was lost along with many of the Indian tribes.

The use of herbs for medicine is thousands of years old. Using crude minerals for purging/healing and the use of drugs for medicines is less than 500 years old. Deaths from herb use worldwide are rarely more than a few per year, usually less! Deaths from drug misuse are hundreds of thousands per year, in North America alone!

This is not meant to advocate the complete dismissal of drugs from our society. They have their places and purposes. However, use of herbs, natural remedies and treatments could be used as an alternative to overactive drug use, especially for common, everyday ailments such as: headaches, earaches, minor burns, constipation, diarrhea, colds, flu, coughs, indigestion and other health concerns mentioned in this book. These are safe, non-toxic, potent yet gentle, natural methods of healing when used correctly, according to the guidelines given in this book.

My years of personal herbal studies with Dr. John Christopher and roaming the hills of Thunder Bay, Ontario and the backyards and bush of Manitoba, Iowa, Illinois and British Columbia, studying herbs, along with 30 years' experience as a natural cook, nutrition expert and clinical nutritionist have prepared me for the preparation and creation of this book's food and herb recommendations and recipes.

Ill health and a "3 months to live" death sentence from doctors nearly 30 years ago led me to explore and discover the realm of healthy possibilities. This book is the thirteenth in a line of natural health and cookbooks, authored and co-authored—three written with doctors, that I was inspired to write to help heal myself and the many individuals who came to me on their own to search for answers to health questions and problems.

Here is simple, natural wisdom from personal experience, hundreds of source books, articles, doctors and other health experts. Sift through these pages and see what you can use to assist your own quest for health solutions. Be sure to read: "How to Use This Book" before using these remedies, for more effective and successful treatments and optimum healing.

Important Note: Remember, no book or non-personalized health advice can replace your doctor's years of experience. Your personal physician's medical advice supercedes all information given here for your own individualized health care. Consult your doctor, or holistic doctor for all severe health problems, side effects and emergencies.

How to Use This Book

Be sure you know how to use this book before proceeding with the use and application of recipes and natural remedies for maintaining health and for healing ailments. Take some time to skim through the book and become familiar with the various sections.

Even after reading about the treatments in the "Ailments and Remedies" section, it is important to read about any products you plan to utilize in the "Natural Remedies Glossary," to see if there are any cautions, exceptions—contraindications, or special considerations for each supplement, herb, remedy or natural product that you need to be concerned about. Special instructions were given for those who are sensitive, allergic, pregnant, and for children and those in a weakened state of health.

Before you prepare *any* teas, tinctures, compresses or poultices, be sure to follow, *completely*, the instructions for preparing these properly in the "Herbal Teas, Tinctures and Treatments" section.

"Remedies from Your Refrigerator or Cupboard" gives detailed information on special foods for healing—contraindications and considerations, just like the "Natural Remedies Glossary" gives for products.

If side effects occur, or are anticipated, see the "Healing Aids" section for ways to help minimize symptoms and discomfort. When help with fasting and cleansing, or special therapies like chiropractic or acupressure are required, see the "Healing Aids" section as well.

Before you proceed with any of the suggestions in the aforementioned sections, you will need to see: "Stocking Your Natural Medicine Chest" for guidelines on what to buy. There are several different ways provided to select items for your own personalized, natural medicine chest.

Do not attempt to incorporate too many new foods, supplements, remedies and cleansing treatments into your life, too soon. Give yourself time to get acquainted with the book and healing foods first. Then slowly integrate a few new natural remedies into your daily routine, one by one, in a way that is comfortable for your intellect and body.

Enjoy the thousands of facts, folklore stories and researched properties and uses given for these marvelous natural remedies and refer to the "Bibliography and Recommended Reading" section for more sources of information on vitamins and minerals, natural remedies, herbs, healing foods, health and cookbooks.

WHY I WROTE THIS BOOK

The motivation and inspiration for this book came from an inward urge to share more of the knowledge I gained over the last 30 years in the health industry, managing health food stores, working in wholesale vitamin and herb sales, teaching and consulting. After fighting for my life for years, struggling to grasp health principles and learning to apply them, I wanted to share what I found with so many individuals who are searching for answers and solutions to health problems.

This is the only part of the book where I allow myself to get up on a little soap box and state plainly my personal beliefs on health, healing and holistic medicines.

One of the most important things I learned while my ex-husband was attending chiropractic college was that the body heals itself. The old joke goes: "Try putting drugs or even herbal remedies on a piece of steak and you'll never get it to come back to life." Medicines can only assist a *living* body to heal itself. Health is our natural state and comes from within us. It is our birthright, our natural heritage. Poisons and chemicals in our environment—in our food, water, land, air and medicines—build up in our bodies and create blockages to our health with the help of: heredity factors, stress, unhappiness, anger, depression, exhaustion, laziness, and lack of: proper exercise, sunshine, rest and love, along with poor cleanliness habits, ignorance and a host of other attitudes and actions that rob us of our natural birthright—good health. It is up to us to uncover and recover our inner state of health that exists under layers of body toxins, like layers of an onion. First, begin with making up your mind to make diet and lifestyle changes: "Intention is everything."

Once you have the sincere desire and intention to change, nothing can get in your way, except stopping. Secondly, we can discover the exceptionally delicious flavor of wholesome natural foods, properly prepared (see my cookbooks), and experience the tremendous boost of energy and the feeling of well-being that comes from eating these delightful foods daily, in balanced meals. Experiment with new, wholesome foods and good recipes and see for yourself.

Thirdly, we can stop putting poisonous and toxic substances, foods, water and medicines, into our bodies. Quit smoking and drinking alcohol and reduce or eliminate excessive meat and sugar intake. Enjoy some vegetarian meals. Try sugar substitutes like honey and maple syrup. Decades ago, I gave up smoking 2½ packs of cigarettes a day. More than 15 years ago I gave up alcoholic beverages. I used to love the taste. Now they are foreign to me and undesirable. Can anyone claim they really enjoyed their first drink of straight whiskey or hard liquor, or did you drink it, at first, to be "grown up"? And how about that first cigarette? Was there anyone who did not turn green? Many holistic health experts now believe alcohol, as well as smoking, interferes with longevity and good health.

This book avoids the use of most remedies that contain alcohol, as it is my personal preference not to use it in healing, however, you may choose differently. The main focus of this book's healing remedies is on food, herbs, natural remedies, vitamins and minerals. There are some homeopathic and aromatherapy remedies included as well. "Food First" is my motto for healing, then cleansing, fasting, remedies, supplements and treatments.

To be fair, some individuals can be healthy even though they drink alcohol and/or consume meat—in proper balance with other foods. Let's face it: Meat eaters can be healthy and vegetarians can be sickly or the reverse can be true. It is a matter of balance. Life and health are said to be juggling acts. We succeed (and live) if we don't drop all the balls at one time. Balance is the key word when it comes to good health, happiness and longevity.

Fourth, we can use cleansing and fasting—safely and wisely—to slowly rid our bodies of the poisons we collected earlier in our lives. This book provides a number of food and remedy cleanses and fasts. Information on varied methods are provided from the simple to complex. Improving the diet is the "first cleanse," then individual food cleanses, remedy and supplement cleanses and finally fasting can be integrated into our (healthy) lifestyles. Then we can—little by little—reclaim our natural heritage, good health.

There are some impediments to complete healing and good health that cannot be overcome with good foods and natural remedies like: hereditary diseases, birth defects, loss of or severe damage to internal organs or limbs, chemical imbalances and other factors, however, wholesome foods and natural remedies may still help to lessen the discomfort and side effects of these conditions.

The human body was created to live indefinitely, I believe. The body can be regenerated with: proper attitudes, positive thinking, inspirational and uplifting beliefs, creative work, constructive play, vigorous as well as gentle stretching exercises, real foods, pure water, natural medicines, and by slowing down and simplifying our lifestyles and having definite purpose in living.

Why do some people live 120 years and others less than 20? How do some individuals heal so-called incurable diseases while many others do not? Did people really live as long as 900 years in early biblical times? With the use of the aforementioned proper attitudes and wholesome living, and perhaps, if it serves my soul's purpose, I will live another 30 years longer and then some.

Holistic health experts have discovered that health lies within. We create our health each minute of living and we have the power to change it. The knowledge is available from many sources. It is up to us to sift through the available information and create a way to use it that serves our purposes and life goals. We will however, have to work for it! No one gets it handed over on a silver platter. There are actually billions of ways to eat correctly, live healthily or heal a health problem. There are as many solutions as there are problems. For each person alive, I believe there are individual choices and individual ways they can each carve out a healthy life and make it a reality.

If each person reading this book derives even a little of the benefits I have personally obtained from this knowledge, writing this book will have been time well spent.

Raise a glass of vegetable juice and salute mother earth for her bounty.

Then, if you choose, raise a word of thanks to God who made this healing exploration and discovery possible.

To health, long life, and better yet, to a good life!

JEANNE MARIE MARTIN

P.S. While I was writing this book, I took one clove of garlic every other day (not daily, so I would not have any possible cleansing side effects), minced, not chewed (so I never smelled like garlic), and washed down in the middle of a meal. My energy, strength, endurance and mental clarity were consistently more than doubled.

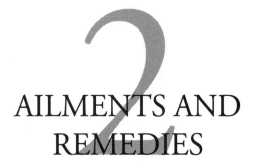

AILMENTS AND REMEDIES

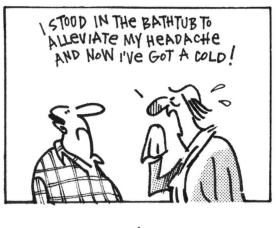

-A-

ACHES

See *Backache, Earache, Headache, Muscle Ache, Stomachache, Toothache*

ACNE

See *Blemishes*

ALLERGIES

1. Condition and Cause

More than 90 percent of what most people call allergies are not true allergies, they are temporary food intolerances or food sensitivities. True allergies are a chemical response to an outside substance within the body that causes severe physical distress, sometimes pain and may even cause death in certain circumstances. According to *Alternative Medicine,* a book compiled by the Burton Goldberg Group, "An allergy is an adverse immune system reaction to a substance that most people find harmless." If a person is sensitive to wheat or dairy products only sometimes, or even most of the time, it is not a true allergy. Only if a person reacts severely to a substance every time is it an allergy rather than a temporary intolerance. In some instances, true allergies can be overcome through natural treatments or a process of desensitization administered by holistic medical doctors or naturopathic physicians.

Food sensitivities or intolerances are usually temporary and can be alleviated or "cured" when the underlying causes of the problem(s) are recognized and healing remedies, treatments or processes are administered and completed. Sensitivities or intolerances are not usually hereditary but may have the same causes as allergies.

While some allergies are hereditary, others can be attributed to environmental factors (i.e. home conditions, neighborhood atmosphere, pollutants), not being breastfed as an infant, childhood health factors, illness, disease complications, nutritional deficiencies, toxic overload in the body, overexposure to a substance, weakened immune system, viruses, Candida albicans (yeast) overgrowth, parasites, digestive disorders and bowel problems. The most common allergies are triggered by environmental substances like: mold, pollen, grass, plants, flowers, dust, fumes, chemicals, smog, pets, synthetic fabrics, perfumes, household cleaners, toxic paint and building materials and hundreds of other items. Allergies can also be aggravated by food substances, especially: wheat, gluten (the high protein part of grains particularly oats, barley, rye and wheat), milk sugar (lactose), dairy products, eggs, chocolate, sugar, alcohol, shrimp or other seafood, meats, nuts, strawberries or other fruits, food additives and preservatives, sulfites, artificial sweeteners such as aspartame, foods that are excessively consumed, and all other foods are possible allergens (substances that can trigger allergies).

For true allergies, the (agitating) substances that trigger the reaction must be completely removed from the immediate environment and diet and/or prescription drugs or natural remedies must be administered to counteract the effects. Diet factors are easier to control than environmental factors, as objectionable foods can be replaced with similar tasting food substitutes.

2. Ailment History, Signs and Early Treatments
Allergies used to be rare. Only in the latter half of the 20th century were food allergies even recognized and began to be treated.

Signs and symptoms of allergies may include: headaches, tiredness, digestive and bowel problems, coughing, sneezing, wheezing, congestion, hyperactivity, anxiety, skin rashes, itching, breathing difficulties and feeling sleepy after eating.

3. Modern Natural Treatments and Remedies
Modern holistic treatments include wholesome diet, herbs, natural remedies, cleansing and homeopathic medicines to lessen symptoms and side effects and in some cases allergies can be healed. A process called desensitization is employed by some holistic doctors. It uses an extremely small dose of the substance that triggers the allergic reaction (known as an "agitating substance" or "allergen") given gradually to the allergic individual (often by sublingual drops). The dose is increased over a period of weeks or months until the individual builds up a tolerance to the offending food or environmental substance. Individuals suspecting allergies may employ the special diets suggested under "1. Condition and Cause" and "6. Nutrition Aids and Recommended Foods," as well as getting allergy tests from a doctor.

4. Helpful Supplements and Dosages
- Vitamin C—especially Allergy C, Ester C or buffered C, can help reduce symptoms, energize and boost the immune system. Take 500-1,000 mg one to four times daily as needed at least three or four hours before sleeping. (Take more if energy is low or when suffering

from allergic reactions. Adjust amounts according to personal needs.) Do not take chewable vitamin C as it may contain sweeteners and other substances that may aggravate allergies. (For children, Vitamin C powder can be mixed in some solid foods.)

- Calcium and magnesium (chelated)—for stress reduction and calming effect. Take 300–500 mg one to four times daily especially at bedtime. (Children can take ¼ to ½ the amount as needed.)
- B50 complex vitamins—for stress reduction and calming effect. Adults and children may take one to four or more daily. More if stressed or during allergic reactions.
- Other supplements that are helpful include: bioflavonoids, acidophilus, echinacea, and digestive aids. See the "Remedies Glossary" for more information.
- Herbs that may be helpful for some and dangerous for others require holistic doctor recommended dosages: cayenne pepper (for circulation, anti-inflammatory and antibacterial effects), goldenseal (for inflammation of the mucus membranes and antibacterial effects), and dandelion or milk thistle (for immune, digestion and liver support and for healing).

5. Cautions and Exceptions

Avoid any foods, substances, drugs, herbs or remedies that may agitate your specific allergies. Do not attempt any herbal remedies or treatments without your holistic physician's approval. Some severe allergies may require drug treatments.

6. Nutrition Aids and Recommended Foods

A wholesome natural diet including a wide range of non-allergic foods supports the immune system, assists healing and lessens allergy symptoms. See my book: *Complete Candida Yeast Guidebook* for a complete list of food substitutions. The Phase II and III diets and recipes in that book are excellent with some additions and changes for most allergies. Also see my *All Natural Allergy Cookbook* for additional allergy recipes and information on Elimination diets (removing offending food(s) from the diet and slowly reintroducing them one by one), rotation diets (eating the same foods only every four days or so) and food families.

7. Beverage and Herbal Tea Suggestions

Peppermint or spearmint tea is a mild digestive aid good for both adults and children. Flower teas like chamomile, lavender, hibiscus and rose hips should be avoided by most allergy sufferers, as they tend to aggravate and increase symptoms. Ginseng tea may be used for energy for those above age 40, during the day. See *Energy, Low* for more teas and supplements that boost energy levels. Burdock tea or the root (cooked as a vegetable in small amounts) helps to counteract some agitating substances and is a mild bowel stimulant. Vegetable juices are particularly beneficial for those with allergies, especially those with carrot and beet juice and the Blood Sugar Balancer (See "Remedies from Your Refrigerator and Cupboard," p. 222.)

ALCOHOL PROBLEMS

1. Condition and Cause

Excessive drinking and related problems are considered to be the result of genetic predisposition by some health experts while other experts claim it is caused by mental, emotional and/or physical environment or both genetics and environment. Alcoholism is considered a disease and is not dealt with in this book. Occasional problems with drinking including: preventing drunkenness and hangover, hangover remedies, nausea and sobering up are covered here. Alcohol depresses the nervous system, affects and may alter perception and memory and may impair speech, reaction time and physical abilities including driving, work functioning and sexual performance.

2. Ailment History, Signs and Early Treatments

Alcohol and drunkenness are included in the histories of many civilizations. Biblical references to wine and drink are recorded in Genesis as early as Noah and the Flood also in the New Testament at the wedding in Cana and the Last Supper. Alcohol has been considered a curse, from Satan, a plague, a remedy and a sacred drink used in spiritual rituals, throughout the ages. In small amounts it is considered by some to be therapeutic, useful for preserving medicines and natural remedies. Alcohol has been used as a stimulant, sedative and a pain reliever. Four to six ounces of red wine, drunk regularly (daily or several times weekly), is reputed to be good for the circulation, digestion (it stimulates the appetite), and long life for certain body types only, usually hardier types without allergies or digestive problems. (For some more sensitive body types it is a definite detriment in any amount.)

Sobering up rituals include drinking massive amounts of coffee, taking a cold shower or splashing cold water on the face and neck, walking, eating cucumber or administering a teaspoon of honey every few minutes until improved (for medicinal neutralizing effects).

Hangovers are traditionally treated with "the hair of the dog that bit you," meaning a tablespoon more or less of the drink that got you drunk taken with tomato juice and sometimes added Tabasco® sauce taken the morning after. An old folk remedy recommends rubbing your underarms with a lemon wedge at night so you don't wake up with a hangover the next morning.

3. Modern Natural Treatments and Remedies

Eating solid meals and taking nutritional supplements, before and after drinking, are the best prevention for drunkenness and hangover. (See "Nutrition Aids and Recommended Foods" and "Helpful Supplements and Dosages" following.) It is important not to drink alcohol on an empty stomach. If a person is predisposed to drinking problems, strict adherence to good diet and taking supplements are required to avoid problems.

For after drinking, see the Hangover Special beverages in the "Refrigerator Remedies." Hangover remedies and sobering up techniques should not be necessary if diet and supplement advice are heeded. However, after a good sleep, energizing supplements like extra vitamin C, B complex, B6, royal jelly and gingko or ginseng can be helpful the next day. Tests done by the U.S. Navy show that B6 in particular helps prevent hangover and nausea. Individual B supplements like B6 should always be taken with B complex to be properly utilized! Also see *Nausea*.

4. Helpful Supplements and Dosages

Preventing Drunkenness and Hangover: (To build up the body,

stabilize it and the blood sugar and help neutralize ill effects of alcohol):

- Take 1,000 to 2,000 mg vitamin C one hour or preferably a few hours before drinking.
- Take two to four B50 complex with the vitamin C an hour or more before or earlier in the day of drinking.
- Take 50 mg extra B6 to help prevent hangover with the B complex and C.
- Optional: Take a green food product sometime during the day, at least four hours or more before drinking. See *Cleansing* for directions on how to take.
- Optional but helpful additional supplements include 15–30 mg of zinc and 200 mcg of chromium taken earlier in the day of drinking.

Day After Recovery and Hangover: (to boost the immune system and help counteract alcohol effects):

- Take 500–2,000 mg vitamin C once or twice during the day.
- Take two to four B50 complex with the vitamin C. You may take the B50 all together or spread throughout the day.
- Take 50 mg extra B6 with the B50 complex and C if there is a hangover.
- Take ginseng in the morning if over 40 or take 60 mg ginkgo or 300–500 mg royal jelly for extra energy.
- Optional: Take a green food product sometime during the day. See *Cleansing* for directions on how to take.
- Optional but helpful additional supplements include 15–30 mg of zinc and 200 mcg chromium.

5. Cautions and Exceptions

Do not take supplements *with* alcoholic beverages. It is best to take supplements at the very least—one hour (or preferably more) before drinking and two or preferably more hours after the last drink. Do not take alcohol with any drugs. Do not drive or attempt to perform work or sports that could endanger a person, with impaired abilities due to drinking any alcohol whatsoever.

6. Nutrition Aids and Recommended Foods

If you usually eat a good, balanced diet, you generally will not want or need to drink that much alcohol. Avoid drinking before noon.

Eat two to three well-balanced meals during the day of drinking and the day after as well. This helps to stabilize the body and blood sugar and "ground" a person so the alcohol does not have an over-powering (or as detrimental) effect. It is best if the last meal before drinking is high in complex carbohydrates like rice, other whole grains, legumes, squash, yams and/or potatoes with skins. Include green vegetables too if possible. If for some reason you are unable to eat supper before drinking, do not drink on an empty stomach! Have at least a complex carbohydrate snack with vegetables if possible. Helpful supplements can be taken with supper or a snack for better absorption. The following day, have steamed yams, baked winter squash, cooked carrots or cooked, warm whole-grain cereal—for breakfast to help neutralize the effects of the alcohol. Avoid fatty foods, refined foods, sugars, pasta and all junk foods.

Have yogurt early in the day as a high enzyme, mild digestive aid if desired to replenish friendly body bacteria that can be destroyed by alcohol, or take 2 acidophilus capsules with four ounces of water one hour away from meals. Be sure to eat two to three wholesome meals the day after drinking as well.

7. Beverage and Herbal Tea Suggestions

A glass of vegetable juice can be wonderful for the body the day of drinking and the day after. Club soda can help sooth nausea, especially when a slice of fresh, peeled ginger is placed in it. (This works better than ginger ale, because it does not contain sugar.) Club soda also helps digestion, unlike sparkling bottled waters, which can be constipating. Dandelion "coffee" can be helpful the day after for its soothing and healing effects on the liver. Peppermint or spearmint tea is a mild stimulant/digestive aid, and can be taken with alfalfa if possible for added green food nutrients. Passion flower tea can help control cravings and has a mild sedative effect. Dandelion herb, globe artichoke extract and milk thistle herb are healing supplements for the liver. See also Hangover Helper 1 and 2 beverages.

ANTI-AGING

See *Wrinkles* and *Memory Problems*

ANXIETY

1. Condition and Cause

Webster's dictionary says anxiety is: "Pain or uneasiness of mind respecting some event, future or uncertain; concern; solicitude; care; disquietude." Anxiety can also be caused by a certain state of health or rather lack of health. Extreme anxiety can lead to hyperactivity, excessive stress, chronic uneasiness or, more severely, panic attacks where the body and mind create an involuntary response that can cause adrenaline rush, rapid heart beat, muscle tension, breathing irregularity, heightened or unrealistic fears and sometimes even more severe consequences.

Non-acute anxiety can be aggravated by: poor diet, sleep deprivation, excessive stress, over-working, family or emotional problems, weakening immune system, ill health, disease, environment and many other factors. It may be helpful to get testing for allergies, Candida, parasites, blood sugar problems, thyroid problems, digestive problems and vitamin/mineral imbalances, as any of these can greatly contribute to anxiety. For acute anxiety and panic attacks, seek a physician's advice immediately. The following information is for occasional anxiety only.

2. Ailment History, Signs and Early Treatments

As long as humans have populated the planet, anxiety has been a part of every life. However, anxiety levels have escalated, especially during the last 50 years due to: poor eating habits, increased substance abuse, increased radiation from excessive use of TVs to microwaves, increasing health and financial problems, our fast-paced and crowded society, as well as other factors recognized by holistic health experts but not necessarily credited by traditional doctors.

People have breathed into paper bags to calm down, stood on their head, exercised, rested, talked out their problems, meditated, taken relaxants and sleep aids and drugs and dozens of other methods to calm down, relax and reduce the anxieties and stresses of life. No one method works every time for every person. The multiple contributing factors of anxiety make it difficult, if not impossible, to discern a simple cure.

3. Modern Natural Treatments and Remedies

Monitoring and limiting stressful situations can help. Avoiding extremes in living—working, playing, thinking and resting—can diminish stress and anxiety. Proper diet and supplements can be an important part of maintaining a stable mental and physical balance. For extreme anxiety, St. John's wort (hypericin) herbal supplement can be quick-acting to calm and reduce anxious thoughts and accompanying body tension. One to three 300 mg capsules (with 0.9 percent hypericin each) can be taken daily for adults. Use less if too much drowsiness or sluggishness occurs. (Capsules are generally more digestible and faster acting than tablets.) Do not use while taking conflicting drugs! Check with your holistic doctor if taking any other prescribed medication. Children should only be given St. John's wort with a doctor's consent. Vitamin C (500 mg or more) or acidophilus capsules (one or two) can be taken with St. John's wort to speed its action. (Do not take with vitamin C if planning to sleep soon after.) B complex vitamins, calcium/magnesium and special herbal teas can be used instead of, or as well as, St. John's wort for mild or moderate anxiety. A few drops of Bach's flower Rescue Remedy® can be a helpful alternative to St. John's wort. Traumeel®, a homeopathic remedy, is another natural anti-anxiety treatment available in health food stores.

Follow package directions or consult a qualified herbalist or naturopathic physician for these or other alternatives. It is generally best to take only one of these products at a time.

See also the sleep aids under *Insomnia*.

4. Helpful Supplements and Dosages

- A daily, high quality, natural, multiple vitamin can help combat stress.
- A daily total of 500–2,000 mg vitamin C, taken in two to four stages through the day, will boost the immune system and help to de-stress.
- Take 500–1,000 mg calcium/magnesium daily as it has a calming effect.
- Take two to four B50 complex daily, spread throughout the day or as needed. If zinc is not included in your multivitamin, take 15–50 mg daily, or when under stress.

5. Cautions and Exceptions

Extreme anxiety with accompanying side effects should be treated by a doctor immediately and not self-treated! Check with your holistic physician before taking St. John's wort while taking any medication or for children's use. Taking too much St. John's wort for your particular body can cause drowsiness or sluggishness. Do not take herbs or products you are allergic to.

6. Nutrition Aids and Recommended Foods

A well balanced, whole-foods diet is a great protection against severe anxiety. Enjoy lots of warm, cooked whole grains, blended or mashed warm beans and cooked vegetables—especially: orange yams, winter squash, carrots, Jerusalem artichokes, leafy greens, broccoli, asparagus and others. See my book *For the Love of Food* or for those with healing problems of any kind, see my *Complete Candida Yeast Guidebook* for detailed information on regular, good eating habits. Eat two to three wholesome meals daily and avoid: excessive wheat or red meats, dairy foods, junk foods, sugar, sugar substitutes and excessive natural sweeteners as well.

Getting allergy testing may be helpful to rule out food and environmental allergies as a source of anxiety and get checked for blood sugar problems, Candida and parasites and other body imbalances such as vitamin and mineral deficiencies as well. Do not eat refined starches or sweets of any kind, including sweet or tropical fruit, on an empty stomach (or consume too much in general) as these upset blood sugar levels and greatly increase stress levels.

7. Beverage and Herbal Tea Suggestions

Chamomile, catnip, skullcap, hops, kava kava, and/or passion flower herbal teas—and sometimes St. John's wort tea—are relaxing and soothing and may induce sleep, provided you are not allergic to any of them. Other helpful teas that are *not* sleep-inducing are: ginger, buchu, black cohosh, red raspberry and spearmint. Do not use sweetening with them if you have blood sugar problems as these may cause more, instead of less anxiety. For children use chamomile or natural catnip herbal teas to relax or induce sleep and ginger, red raspberry or spearmint for daytime. Hawthorn tea can be taken for heart palpitations, for adults. Also see sleep aids under *Insomnia*.

Vegetable juices are very balancing and healing for anxiety as well, especially those that contain carrot juice and green food products.

APHRODISIACS

See *Sexual Energy, Low*

-B-

BACKACHE

1. Condition and Cause

Four out of five North Americans have backaches during their lives. Back pain can be debilitating and may lead to hospitalization. There can be many reasons for upper and/or lower backache or pain: injury, weakened immune system, disease, illness, kidney infection, bowel problems, exhaustion, emotional stress, pregnancy, excessive body toxins, improper or extreme cleansing, damaged or "slipped" disks, muscle strain, improper lifting, obesity, lack of exercise, too strenuous exercise, poor posture, unsupportive footwear, poor diet, constipation, vitamin/mineral deficiencies and many other reasons.

2. Ailment History, Signs and Early Treatments

Quasimodo, the "Hunchback of Notre Dame," must have had one heck of a backache! Traditionally remedies for backache include: peppermint, chamomile, catnip, skullcap and valerian herbal teas and poultices.

3. Modern Natural Treatments and Remedies

The best defense is: proper exercise, a good mattress, a wholesome balanced diet, adequate calcium and other needed minerals and vitamins, using proper lifting methods and not straining. Valuable help can also be derived from regular chiropractic treatments, professional massages, acupressure or acupuncture, and excellent muscle stretching exercising with one or more of the following: yoga, tai chi, qi gong, martial arts, swimming and dancing. Strengthening techniques—tensing and relaxing exercises can be very beneficial for the back. (See the "Healing Aids" section.)

When backache occurs, it helps to already have a good chiropractor and/or acupressurist or acupuncturist. If possible, have someone rub an ice cube(s), moving quickly over the aching or painful area for the first 10–15 minutes, while the person with the backache rests in a prone position. Apply an ice pack during the first 48 hours, for periods of fifteen minutes or less at a time. Do not use blocks of freezing ice, but rather a bag of frozen peas or corn, possibly wrapped in a thin dishtowel so the cold is not extreme. After 48 hours, intermittent hot and cold packs can be most beneficial.

An Epsom salt bath, a bath with a cup of baking soda added, or a bath with several shakes of tea tree oil added can be soothing. Saunas and steam baths can also help expel body poisons that contribute to backaches. Keep the pores of the skin clean, so toxins can exit, by employing these and other skin cleansing methods in the "Healing Aids" section. Poultices like those used in #2 preceding can also be employed. A *gentle* massage using one of the following: warm castor oil, olive oil, warm olive oil with a teaspoon or two of added witch hazel, or room temperature aloe vera gel, may be helpful. Cleansing or fasting can be very beneficial. See also *Joint Aches and Pain.*

4. Helpful Supplements and Dosages

- Take multivitamin and mineral capsule daily containing vitamin A.
- Take 1,000–2,000 mg of calcium (mixed sources are best) daily, and half as much magnesium.
- Take 10,000–15,000 IU beta-carotene daily.
- Take 1000–2000 mg vitamin C two to four times daily for healing.
- Optional: Take digestive aids (especially bromelain) or laxatives if constipation occurs.
- Optional: Take MSM, DMSO, Anti-Flam®, Flammaforce® or Infla-Zyme Forte® for inflammation and healing, as required.
- Optional: Take arnica for pain and inflammation if needed.
- Optional: Take glucosamine sulfate and/or horsetail (silica), for cartilage repair, bone and connective tissue healing.

5. Cautions and Exceptions

If you have pain, numbness and trouble moving after an injury, do not move but call for help in case the spine is injured. If back pain lasts more than three or four days or if it is extreme, if you have a fever, shooting pain down the legs, tingling or other troublesome side effects, call your doctor immediately!

6. Nutrition Aids and Recommended Foods

Meats (which are high in uric acids) and dairy products can contribute to back pain and should be completely avoided during back pains except for fish, yogurt and possibly a little bit of butter. Eat mainly vegetarian/vegan foods especially: warm cooked whole grains, mashed or blended warm beans (especially those high in calcium—pinto, kidney and black beans, soybeans and chickpeas), hot soups, cooked tofu (two or three times weekly), soymilk (used in soups and cooking), cooked green and orange vegetables and fresh vegetable juices, green food products, flaxseed, sesame seeds and tahini. It is best to follow mainly the Phase II diet in my book *Complete Candida Yeast Guidebook*.

7. Beverage and Herbal Tea Suggestions

Drink lots of fresh spring water daily—four to eight glasses at least. Drink a glass of fresh vegetable juice five or six days weekly during backaches, and to provide nutrients that help prevent and heal them. Enjoy some of these herbal teas separately, or in combination: alfalfa, parsley (occasionally), peppermint, spearmint, lemon grass, chamomile, horsetail, slippery elm and white willow bark. For kidney strengthening, drink three or four ounces of unsweetened cranberry juice with the same amount of spring water two or three times daily between meals.

BAD BREATH

1. Condition and Cause

There are several contributing factors for bad breath or halitosis. A body that is overloaded with toxins (chemicals, preservatives and poisons) can be a breeding ground for bacteria and parasites that may contribute to this condition. Also, poor diet and improper digestion can lead to food spoiling in the digestive and elimination tracts. This can result in bad breath and/or body odor. Gum disease, tooth decay and mouth or sinus infections may also be the cause. See also *Oral Hygiene Problems* and *Infections*.

2. Ailment History, Signs and Early Treatments
Bad breath is unmistakable, from "morning mouth" to offensive odor. Folk remedies include people chewing on mint leaves, parsley, peeled gingerroot, lemons and fennel seeds for partial relief. Most recently, mint and cinnamon breath mints, chewing gums and an array of commercial mouthwashes have been employed to mask the problem, however, these are temporary aids that offer little or no lasting solutions.

3. Modern Natural Treatments and Remedies
Be sure to brush and floss the teeth regularly with natural baking soda (and water), mint, peelu or other toothpastes recommended by holistic doctors. Brush or scrape the tongue one or more times each day. Use a variety of natural antibacterial mouthwashes in daily rotation. Options include 1. aloe vera, 2. aerobic oxygen (about 20 drops) in pure (spring or distilled) water, 3. 100 percent tea tree oil (several drops or couple of shakes) in pure water, 4. sea salt in pure water, 5. six to 10 ppm (parts per million) colloidal silver, 6. one to two teaspoons peelu extract in pure water. Do not use commercial mouthwashes!

Improve the diet (See #6 following, the "Nutrition Aids" section) and use digestive aids and flushing agents to assist proper breakdown of foods and to avoid foods spoiling in the digestive and elimination tracts. (See *Indigestion* for digestive aids and flushing agents.) Use bee propolis for the most effective remedy. Take quarter to half a teaspoon propolis powder, or chew one or two tablets or open one to two capsules in the mouth once or twice daily between meals with pure water along with diet changes, until the breath improves. See also *Oral Hygiene Problems*.

4. Helpful Supplements and Dosages
- Take green foods, especially chlorophyll or alfalfa tablets or liquid (one or two teaspoons or six to eight tablets) daily until the condition improves. (Liquid or tablets can

be taken with water or in vegetable juice about an hour or so after meals.)

- Take 1,000 mg vitamin C once or twice daily plus 500 mg bioflavonoids.
- Take two potent acidophilus capsules (including bifidus if possible) twice daily, one hour or more away from all foods with four to six ounces of pure water. (Take before and/or after breakfast and/or lunch, not after supper.)
- Take B50 complex once or twice daily.
- Take digestive aids if needed. See the "Natural Remedies Glossary" or consult your holistic physician for which ones to take.

5. Cautions and Exceptions
One or more 12–30 day bowel cleanses may be necessary if the preceding treatments and supplements do not bring the desired results. Bad breath could also be a sign of another major health problem. If it persists, see your holistic physician. Be sure to get your vitamin and mineral balances checked as bad breath and indigestion could result from major imbalances of these.

6. Nutrition Aids and Recommended Foods
Be sure to include lots of high enzyme foods like yogurt, kefir, miso, citrus and lactic-acid fermented vegetables (like sauerkraut) in the diet to assist digestion. Avoid red meats, spicy foods, alcohol, corn on-the-cob, improperly cooked (over or under cooked or cooked with too many fats, spices or sugars) foods, fried foods, sugars, artificial sweeteners and excessive naturally sweetened foods. Include four to six servings of vegetables daily (raw, cooked and juiced) including at least two green vegetables and one orange vegetable (e.g., carrots, winter squash, and/or orange yams). Fresh parsley and mint leaves (preferably organic) can also be chewed with or right after meals. Food combining is very important for bad breath. See my *Complete Candida Yeast Guidebook* or *For The Love of Food* for detailed information on proper food combining.

7. Beverage and Herbal Tea Suggestions
Herbal teas, two or more cups daily drunk away from meals, can

assist digestion and help bad breath. Enjoy mint, raspberry leaf, ginger, fennel seed, fenugreek seed and alfalfa-mint teas, rotated or as desired one half hour or more before or after meals. Special laxative teas like mild licorice, or senna taken with flax, can also be taken if digestive problems are obvious.

BEE STINGS (and Wasp, Yellow Jacket or Hornet Stings) AND INSECT BITES

1. Condition and Cause
Bees and stinging insects do not sting unless provoked as most of them die within hours of using their stingers. Stings often occur when the insect is stepped on, swatted at, the insect is bumped into while it is on or near a person or if its hive is threatened. Be careful to wear shoes when running through grassy fields with clover or other abundant small flowers in them.

Bites can occur from spiders, ants, mosquitoes, black flies, deer flies, no-see-ums, and other crawling and flying insects. Most bites cause redness and itching but are harmless, however some mosquitoes carry disease, though usually in tropical areas or countries. Only a few spiders are poisonous. Contact your poison control center, tropical disease center or contact your doctor if you suspect a deadly insect may have bitten you and try to capture the insect, alive if possible (very carefully with a jar) or be able to describe it to a health expert.

Stinging and some bites can cause throbbing pain, swelling, itchiness and redness. Those highly allergic to insect stings may experience difficulty swallowing or breathing, weakness, mental confusion or even shock.

2. Ailment History, Signs and Early Treatments
Raw honey was traditionally placed on stings to draw out the poison and soothe the wound. It is still used today quite effectively for many minor stings. Use pasteurized rather than raw honey on children under two years old as they have trouble handling the bacteria in raw honey and it may be harmful to them. Just a mere decade and more ago, people used tweezers to remove insect stingers, however this caused the poison remaining in the sac at the end of the stinger to be pumped into the body and increased inflammation.

In the past centuries as well as today, people used one (or more at different times) of the following items held or packed over stings to ease itchiness and swelling: mud, wet baking soda, potato or onion slices, vinegar, clay, chewed yarrow leaves, comfrey or plantain poultices, papaya skins and ice packs.

3. Modern Natural Treatments and Remedies

It is best to remove the stinger as soon as possible by quickly scratching or flicking it out of wound. Tweezers may be used if most of the stinger remains above the skin and the tweezers grab below the poison sac, pulling straight up and out. Take care not to squeeze the poison sac, or you may squeeze more poison into your body, increasing inflammation.

Stings can be dangerous if a person is allergic to them. A doctor-recommended insect sting emergency treatment kit should be kept close by any person with severe allergies to insect stings or bites. Look for a medical bracelet or necklace on a victim if side effects are extreme. For severe allergies, emergency hospital treatment may be required. Individuals without allergies, and those who experience only minor reactions, can often obtain complete relief by sweating out the poison in a sauna or steam bath within hours of the insect attack, especially if there are multiple stings or bites.

Hydrogen peroxide or alcohol may be used to cleanse the wound(s) if needed. Honey can be used on the wound if nothing else is available. Tea tree oil is most effective to help counteract the poison and speed healing. Place a drop (use a cotton swab if needed) on the sting every hour or so as desired, during the first four hours and every four to six hours the first day—once to four times daily after that for a day or two as long as needed. (Tea tree oil does sting a little as it heals!) Oregano oil and colloidal silver can also be used on stings and bites. A baking soda compress or bath (for multiple stings) can also relieve itching and soreness of insect stings and bites. Epsom salt baths are another alternative. To ease itching after treating bites, use aloe vera gel, calendula or comfrey cream or yarrow tincture.

Excellent insect repellants include: tea tree oil, eucalyptus, cedar, citronella, lemon or lime juice, and calendula. Pennyroyal can also be used, though not during pregnancy. For itching after bites use aloe vera gel, calendula or comfrey cream or yarrow tincture or paste. Avoid wearing bright colors and floral perfumes and essences when outside in insect infested areas.

4. Helpful Supplements and Dosages
- Take 2,000–5,000 mg vitamin C with bioflavonoids daily, until effects of sting(s) subside.
- Take 1,000 mg echinacea once or twice daily to protect the immune system.
- Take two to four vitamin B50 complex daily for healing and calming, spread throughout the day.

5. Cautions and Exceptions
Remember that those highly allergic to insect stings may experience difficulty swallowing or breathing, weakness, mental confusion or even shock. If more than slight discomfort and swelling occur, call a doctor or proceed to a hospital emergency room.

6. Nutrition Aids and Recommended Foods
Unless there are allergies or severe reactions to bee stings, only a few diet changes are required. Avoid refined foods, sugars and sweets and alcohol for at least 24 hours or more after stings occur. A balanced, whole-foods diet is always beneficial to healing.

7. Beverage and Herbal Tea Suggestions
Calming and relaxing herbal teas may include kava kava, passion flower, chamomile or valerian. Vegetable juices and protein energy drinks can give a boost while healing the effects of stings and bites.

BLADDER CONTROL PROBLEMS

Statistics show that more than one in four women in the U.S. and Canada over the age of 40 have problems with incontinence or bladder control. Soft drinks, especially diet colas, can be a big contributing factor, as can overall diet. The coffee, junk food, refined food, sugars, artificial additives, excessive meats and other agitating foods that trigger bladder control problems have to go!

For bladder control problems, follow the tips and diet under *Bladder Infections* that follows for: bacterial cystitis.

BLADDER INFECTIONS (Cystitis)

1. Condition and Cause

Bladder infections are usually caused by bacteria, often from the anus or vagina, that have traveled up the urethra (the tube through which urine is emptied). This infection is more common in women since their urethra is shorter and closer to the rectum and sex organs. Uncleanliness, poor hygiene habits and improper wiping after going to the bathroom may be the cause. Three in ten American and Canadian women get bladder infections each year.

Bladder infections are much less common for men. Elderly men are more susceptible because of blockages in the urinary tract, including an enlarged prostate gland. Infections create a frequent need to urinate, which is sometimes painful or burning. This may occur even if the bladder is not full, due to inflammation. The urine may be cloudy and have a strong, unpleasant smell.

2. Ailment History, Signs and Early Treatments

Folk remedies that are still used today include: eating lots of parsley and drinking parsley tea, eating carrot and celery leaves, drinking corn silk tea from young corn, eating onions and garlic and eating watermelon among the many.

3. Modern Natural Treatments and Remedies

Bladder infections are sometimes treated with antibiotics, though usually they are treated without drugs or remedies but rather with diet.

Alternative Medicine by the Burton Goldberg Group, suggests that it is better for a woman *not* to urinate right after intercourse, but wait until there is a real need to. It is healthier and more preventative of infections to urinate in a steady stream rather than "tinkling drops out." Instead of urinating *after* sex, it is better prevention against bladder infections to urinate *before* sex. When going to the bathroom, wipe from the front to the back to avoid spreading bacteria from the anus to the vagina and urethra. Use light-colored cotton underwear and avoid tampons. Keep the genital area clean and dry.

Take a hot sitz bath for at least 20 minutes, 1–2 times daily with one or two shakes (several drops) of tea tree oil or 2–6 drops oil of oregano. (One teaspoon of fresh squeezed garlic juice can also be used instead of tea tree or oregano oil, however this is unpleasant smelling to many women.)

The most common treatment for bladder infections caused by bacteria (bacterial cystitis) is drinking two or three glasses of unsweetened cranberry juice daily, which helps to acidify the urine and fight bacteria. Some people prefer to take cranberry extract capsules, taken as directed on the package. Citricidal grapefruit seed liquid extract may also be taken once or twice daily, several drops mixed in three to four tablespoons very warm water taken alone. If the taste of the extract is too formidable, take the extract tablets.

For non-bacterial bladder infections (interstitial cystitis), avoid acidic treatments and foods. Instead of cranberry juice or capsules and citricidal, garlic and baking soda can be used (as explained in "Helpful Supplements and Dosages") or colloidal silver may be taken, about one half to one teaspoon 10 ppm taken once daily away from other foods with an ounce or two of water. Another alternative is one or two drops of oil of oregano daily in a tablespoon of water. Take one of these for one or two weeks, or for several days (preferably for at least a week *after* symptoms disappear). Be sure to include the recommended foods and beverages following. (Garlic, colloidal silver and oil of oregano are not acidic.)

4. Helpful Supplements and Dosages
- Take a natural multiple vitamin daily.
- Take 2,000 mg vitamin C once or twice daily to help acidify urine and fight bacteria.
- Take two B50 complex twice daily.
- Take 500 mg calcium/magnesium twice daily.
- For non-bacterial bladder infection, take a teaspoon of baking soda in a glass of water once at the beginning of problem.
- Optional: Take 15–30 mg zinc daily for healing.
- Optional: Take one small clove of chopped garlic daily or every other day (unchewed) for 14 days or longer. See *Toxin Overload* for garlic cleansing how-to.

5. Cautions and Exceptions
Avoid all supplements and foods that you are allergic to. Consult

your doctor if symptoms are severe and/or treatment does not bring some positive results within days.

6. Nutrition Aids and Recommended Foods
Eat mainly whole foods and a natural diet. Enjoy the following foods daily or several times weekly: whole grains, legumes, watermelon, carrots, orange yams, winter squash, green vegetables, a green food product such as spirulina or alfalfa, celery, cucumbers and parsley. Avoid excessive amounts of meats, smoked and pickled foods, cheese, breads of all kinds, pasta, fatty foods, sugars both natural and artificial, sweets, sweet fruits like bananas, pineapple and grapes, sweet tropical fruits, oranges, junk foods, refined foods, chocolate, tomatoes, rhubarb and cooked spinach. If avoiding acid foods (for non-bacteria infections) like cranberries, also exclude all citrus and yogurt, as well as tomatoes and other acidic foods. (Follow mainly the Phase II diet in my *Complete Candida Yeast Guidebook,* if possible.)

7. Beverage and Herbal Tea Suggestions
Drink lots of distilled water or tested spring water (at least 8 glasses daily) for two to three weeks. Avoid alcohol, all soft drinks (especially those with artificial sweeteners), coffee and black tea, instead drink organic green tea or herbal teas. Drink a glass of vegetable juice with carrots, beets and parsley or celery 4–6 days weekly.

Enjoy daily corn silk herbal tea. Also enjoy marshmallow root tea, raspberry leaf tea and dandelion coffee.

BLEEDING, EXCESSIVE

See also *Cuts and Wounds*

1. Condition and Cause
Excessive bleeding can occur due to an external injury, internal health problems or diseases or hemorrhoids, during miscarriage or childbirth, or during the menstrual cycle. A mild nosebleed is not generally serious. Losing more than about one quart or one litre of blood can be life-threatening.

2. Ailment History, Signs and Early Treatments

In many centuries past, "physicians" actually bled people intentionally, as many diseases were thought to be the result of "bad blood." Even during the American Civil War, leeches—a type of bloodsucking worms were applied to wounded solders for the purpose of "bloodletting." This was thought to purify the blood and promote healing. This seemingly antiquated treatment is now making a comeback in some "modern" medical treatments for plastic and reconstructive surgery.

Garlic and onion slices were placed on wounds to disinfect them and help them heal, up to and including the First World War, when medical supplies ran out.

Some North American Indians chewed yarrow leaf herb and applied it to small wounds to help stop bleeding. Enzymes from the person's own saliva mixed with the herbal ingredients and stopped blood flow and speeded up healing. This is still a helpful method to use if out in the woods and far from medical supplies and doctors, for small wounds only. Comfrey and witch hazel were, and still are, also applied (not chewed) to some small wounds.

Cobwebs are an ancient remedy used on wounds to bind them and dry up the bleeding faster. It actually works and is still recommended by some holistic practitioners and herbalists today, for use in a pinch, when medical supplies and doctors are unavailable.

3. Modern Natural Treatments and Remedies

SMALL WOUNDS If bleeding occurs from a small cut or wound, let it bleed a little to clean it out. Wash the wound with cool, clean water and apply a natural antiseptic, like tea tree oil, colloidal silver, oregano oil or rubbing alcohol. (Some herbalists recommend a bit of cayenne pepper be placed on the wound, however be sure the person is not allergic to cayenne and is willing, as it may burn. Place a bandage or gauze wrapping over the wound while applying firm pressure. Wrap snugly, but not too tightly, to keep pressure on the wound and help stop the bleeding. Usually, if bleeding continues, not enough pressure was applied and the bandage was not wrapped snugly enough. Do *not* remove the first bandage, but apply a second one on top with firmer pressure, and wrap a little more tightly. If bleeding continues, get the person to a doctor or hospital immediately.

Apply tea tree oil, oregano oil, or aloe vera externally, daily until the wound heals. Use shark oil for final healing of the scar.

LARGE WOUNDS   If a wound is large, cover it and apply pressure with your hand until a clean cloth or gauze can be applied and held in place or wrapped while proceeding immediately to a hospital emergency room or doctor if no hospital is available. *Do not* attempt to clean or put antiseptic on large wounds. Let an experienced health professional tend larger wounds. Some stitches (and/or a tetanus shot) may be required. Once larger wounds have closed (in a few days or longer) and are already healing, tea tree oil, oregano oil or diluted onion or garlic juice can be applied to speed healing and help prevent scarring. When the wound has mostly healed, shark oil can be applied daily until completely healed. (Aloe vera can also be used, however the other remedies mentioned tend to be more beneficial.) See also #4, "Helpful Supplements and Dosages."

RECTAL OR VAGINAL BLEEDING   If bleeding rectally or bleeding excessively from the vagina, calm the person, use a menstrual pad for the bleeding, get the person to lie down in a vehicle while transporting to the hospital. See also "Helpful Supplements and Dosages."

NOSEBLEEDS   For nosebleeds, have the person lie comfortably on their back. Use a cotton swab to place a drop or two of tea tree oil or oregano oil (can be diluted) up the nostril. A drop or two of pressed onion or garlic juice diluted in water can also be put up the nose with an eyedropper. Plug the nostril that is bleeding with clean tissue or cloth or, if both nostrils are bleeding, plug both and have the person breathe through their mouth. Apply ice or an ice pack (frozen peas or corn in a bag are great covered in a tea towel) to the nose area to slow the flow of blood. If the bleeding does not stop in a short while, consult your doctor.

4. Helpful Supplements and Dosages
- For all wounds, while the person is bleeding, if time allows (if going to the hospital), serve them a cup of yarrow or comfrey tea or have them take these in capsule form with water followed by a cup of pleasure tea. If available, one of these can be administered quickly in

tincture form. Drinking unsweetened cranberry juice also helps coagulation of blood.

- For large wounds and/or excessive bleeding, when shock, trauma or severe upset occurs, take Rescue Remedy®, Traumeel®, or St. John's wort (one 300 mg capsule), immediately. Take brand name products according to package directions.
- Take water-soluble vitamin K for help with blood clotting as required. Ask a holistic doctor for the best dosage.
- Take 15–50 mg zinc daily to assist healing.
- Take 1,000–2,000 mg vitamin C one to four times daily, depending on the severity of bleeding or wound, until it is healed.
- Take 200–400 IU vitamin E once or twice daily, depending on the severity of bleeding or wound, until it is healed.

5. Cautions and Exceptions

If unsure how to proceed, or if complications arise, consult a doctor (or nurse if no doctor is available) immediately! If infection occurs and antibiotics are required, take acidophilus (or bifidus for children) daily as directed in the "Natural Remedies Glossary." To help prevent infection, if *not* taking antibiotics, (do not take *with* them, although after is okay) one of the anti-viral remedies can be used for a week or as long as a month, depending on the remedy used. See *Viruses* for more information.

6. Nutrition Aids and Recommended Foods

A wholesome, natural diet without excessive refined or fatty foods or junk foods is best for all kinds of healing. Eat lots of whole grains, legumes, vegetables, and fish.

7. Beverage and Herbal Tea Suggestions

Drink lots of pure spring water daily. Vegetable juices, 4–6 glasses weekly, especially with carrots, beets and a green food product are especially beneficial, help to speed healing. Helpful herbal teas include: red raspberry and black cohosh especially for female health problems that cause excessive bleeding. For other bleeding: alfalfa, white oak bark, yarrow or comfrey can be taken.

BLEEDING GUMS

See *Oral Hygiene Problems*

BLEMISHES

1. Condition and Cause

Major acne problems are not covered here. Blemishes—pimples, blackheads and whiteheads—are a common problem for most North Americans, especially teenagers and adults usually under age 40. These skin eruptions usually appear on the face, neck and back. Besides hormonal changes and imbalances, blemishes or skin problems can be caused or contributed to by: heredity, poor diet, fatty and greasy foods, stress, infrequent or improper washing and bathing, body toxin overload, dust and dirt, allergies, bowel problems, Candida yeast, parasites, drugs, environmental pollutants and other factors.

2. Ailment History, Signs and Early Treatments

Clay and oatmeal have been used, traditionally to draw out facial poisons and is still used today in cleansing masks. Clay powder (purchased at health stores) or ground oatmeal, is mixed with water, applied and left on the skin for 20 minutes or more before washing off. Oatmeal soaps are still popular, though not tremendously potent for pimples. A garlic clove sliced open has also been rubbed on blemishes, as the garlic juice is antibacterial and cleansing. This can still be used today and is beneficial for some individuals, although not very pleasant smelling. Sliced strawberries rubbed on the skin are also still considered to be good facial cleansers.

3. Modern Natural Treatments and Remedies

The skin is the largest organ of the body; it is a major organ for eliminating body toxins. Holistic health experts believe the outside of the body reflects the inner. Excessive skin problems are often linked to toxin overload in the body and sometimes to bowel problems. Cleansing is the best way to remove these poisons. See *Toxin Overload* for the basic cleansing methods. Some herbs and naturopathic remedies including: colloidal silver, oregano oil, olive leaf extract, colostrum, milk thistle and many others are also used to help cleanse the body.

Eat a good diet (See #6, "Nutrition Aids and Recommended Foods") and cleanse the outer skin several times a day. Regular saunas and steam baths can help remove body poisons and cleanse the skin. For mild skin blemishes (not acne), elderflower herb or Swiss Kriss® herbs can be good for adding to a pot of boiled water for a facial steam. Get tested for allergies (to food, environment and makeup), Candidiasis, parasites and also bowel problems if they are suspected, to rule out these contributing factors. If these tests are positive, alter the diet and do the required treatments. Blemishes should not be scratched, squeezed or picked at, as some skin specialists believe this may contribute to scarring. Avoid using base makeup on the face and use hypoallergenic, natural makeup if any is used. Wear natural (not synthetic) clothing near the face and other areas where blemishes are plentiful.

External treatments include applying 10 ppm or higher colloidal silver to blemishes. Also use 15 percent tea tree oil, diluted with about twice the volume of water, for external use, applied to blemishes with a cotton swab. Diluted oregano oil or propolis tincture may also be helpful for some individuals, applied topically to pimples. Fresh lemon juice applied with a cotton swab or aloe vera gel, special soaps and cleansers are also used for their astringent effects on blemishes. Fresh pineapple slices, containing bromelain, rubbed on pimples are another astringent skin cleaner. There are also many healing products, cleansers and soaps available at health stores for skin problems. Experiment and find the right external remedy for your skin type. If skin problems are severe, consult your doctor.

4. Helpful Supplements and Dosages

- Take 25,000 IU vitamin A and 25,000 extra beta-carotene daily for healing. (Reduce vitamin A to standard 10,000 IU after improvement.)
- Take two capsules acidophilus once or twice daily. See "Natural Remedies Glossary" for method.
- Take one B50 complex two to four times daily.
- Take 1,000 mg vitamin C one to four times daily, depending on severity.
- Take 15–30 mg zinc daily for healing.
- Optional: Take garlic capsules or better yet take one clove,

chopped not chewed, garlic according to directions in
Toxin Overload.
- Optional: Some digestive aids may be helpful for certain
individuals. See the "Natural Remedies Glossary" or
consult your holistic physician.

5. Cautions and Exceptions
Each person is unique and may respond differently to various treatments. For continued or severe skin problems see your holistic
doctor or a skin specialist.

6. Nutrition Aids and Recommended Foods
Proper diet is essential for individuals with skin problems. Eat plenty
of high-fiber foods: mainly vegetables, especially green and orange
ones and Jerusalem artichokes, fish, whole grains and legumes.
Include yogurt, miso, and/or sauerkraut in the diet. Add ground
flaxseed to cereals, yogurt or mixed with other foods, five or six
times a week. Do not eat fried, fatty and greasy foods, pork and
fatty meats and all processed cheeses. Avoid cream, milk, uncooked
cheeses (some cooked cheeses may be had once or twice a week),
margarine, pasta, junk foods, refined foods, spicy foods, sugar,
chocolate, artificial sugar substitutes, food additives and chemicals and sweet fruits. See my *For the Love of Food* and other books
for hundreds of delicious recipes you *can* eat! Eat high zinc foods
like pumpkin seeds, pecans, beans and oysters.

Beverage and Herbal Tea Suggestions
Drink six to eight glasses of spring water daily, between meals. Drink
five or six glasses of vegetable juice weekly with added green food
products especially. Soda pops are extremely bad for blemishes. Better
to drink a little diluted fruit juice, fresh grapefruit juice, vegetable
juice or water. Beneficial herbal teas include: elderflowers or leaves,
echinacea, dandelion herb (or coffee), lemon grass, peppermint and
spearmint teas. Vitex tea is good for PMS blemishes.

BLISTERS

See *Calluses, Corns, Bunions and Blisters*

BLOOD SUGAR PROBLEMS

See *Hypoglycemia* (Low Blood Sugar)

BOWEL PROBLEMS AND CONSTIPATION

The first signs of bowel problems are fatigue and weakness, then recurrent constipation, abdominal cramps or pain, blood or mucus in some stools, occasional diarrhea and sometimes other symptoms like undigested food in stools, rectal itching or flatulence.

A healthy individual who is eating *mainly* natural, whole foods has three to five bowel movements per day (less if not eating these foods). "Healthy," not "normal"; many Americans and Canadians think it is normal to have four to seven bowel movements per *week*, a clear sign of digestive troubles that lead to irritable bowel syndrome, colitis, diverticulitus, chronic fatigue syndrome, Candida yeast infections, other bowel problems, and immune deficiency diseases.

If a sink gets clogged, it backs up and eventually becomes totally closed unless cleaned out. This can happen with the digestive tract. Many people have doctors who recommend partial removal of the colon or a colostomy. According to *Healthy Healing* by Dr. Linda Rector-Page, V. E. Irons (a colon and cleansing expert who lived into his nineties) and countless other health specialists: "Ninety percent of all diseases generate from an unclean colon." Healthy bowel transit time should take about 12 hours rather than the 24 to 48 it takes most people in our society. The longer food takes to process and stays in the body, the more chance there is for putrefaction and disease to grow. (And the more calories are absorbed!) The colon can become a breeding ground for Candida and other yeasts, parasites, unfriendly bacteria and viruses.

A serving of white bread (or refined pasta) can make a paste in the intestines that is like glue and clogs the pipes. Not to worry. Many people drink a human variety of liquid Drano®, in the form of caffeinated colas and soft drinks. Eating lots of sweets and desserts is the equivalent of feeding a basement full of venomous snakes and then wondering why you cannot use your basement anymore. "Here, yeast, bacteria, and parasites. I have some nice sugar for you, so you can grow up big and strong."

It is no surprise when disease develops. It requires effort to become ill. One has to ignore all natural healing principles and ignore indigestion, gas, stomach upset, headache, discomfort, and pain—the body's warnings that you are on the wrong track and living poorly.

A diet of white bread, pasta, dry breakfast cereal, pastry, potato chips, corn chips, and white crackers has more to do with disease, in particular bowel disease, than occasional meat does. Meat is one of the hardest foods to digest, but it has more nutritional value than refined starches. A healthy individual can digest occasional meat and remain healthy. Eating excessive amounts or poor-quality meat is harmful, especially pork and other red meats. Eating meat can be especially toxic for individuals with clogged colons.

Refined foods are "dead foods" that give the body no vitality. We live in a "cold pasta" or "deli food" generation. Imagine this refined food sitting on a store shelf for months, even years, then sitting in your cupboard for months more; you expect to eat it and feel energized? The body cannot tell the difference between white flour and white sugar when digesting it. These items are among the biggest offenders when it comes to constipation: More than 75 percent of all constipation in North America could be healed instantly by eating four to six servings (1 cup raw or ½–¾ cup cooked per serving) of vegetables daily!

Some people with bowel problems cannot digest raw vegetables. Next to meat, raw vegetables, especially iceberg or head lettuce, are the hardest foods to digest! Raw vegetables can be agitating and damaging to colon problems and diseases. It is better to eat easy-to-digest vegetables in salads at lunchtime (rather than at supper) with yogurt, lemon or lime juice and non-oil dressings or to drink a glass of vegetable juice five or six days a week than to eat vegetables that cannot be properly digested. Easier-to-digest vegetables: spinach, exotic greens (minus endive, escarole and radicchio) grated or sliced zucchini, finely grated beets or carrots or Jerusalem artichokes or peeled kohlrabi, red or yellow or orange bell peppers (green ones are unripe and gassy) and occasionally—if tolerated—a little peeled and seeded tomato.

Raw nuts and seeds and popcorn are also damaging to the colon. It is better to use nut or seed butters like tahini, almond butter or sunflower butter in warm recipes like sauces, or to use ground nuts in casseroles than to eat a handful of these, especially with other foods if you have severe bowel problems. If you really must eat a handful of nuts, avoid the roasted ones like they are poison—they are similar to rocks in damaged intestines. Eat one small handful of raw nuts no more than once or twice a week and chew them to absolute water before swallowing. Remember, Gandhi said, "Drink your foods and chew your liquids."

A diet of well cooked complex carbohydrates, legumes and three to six servings of vegetables a day can nearly defeat constipation, unless there is physical damage. If the digestive tract has been severely damaged or is clogged with toxins, these must be flushed out before normal, natural digestion can take place. See a naturopathic doctor or natural health-care specialist about cleansing programs and read over the cleansing sections in this book in "Healing Aids" and under *Toxin Overload* in this section. Educate yourself on the pros and cons of enemas, colonics, laxative teas and other colon-cleansing processes. Some are easy, non-invasive and highly beneficial if done correctly. Health experts say, "Death begins in the colon" (as well as "Ninety percent of disease begins in the colon.") Health begins in the colon, too. It is possible to reverse even severe damage, sometimes, if caught before it is too late. Many individuals have experienced miraculous healings—with effort and some natural body wisdom.

Whenever cleansing (including during Candida or parasite treatment), you must have at least one bowel movement per day, every day. If you do not, poisonous toxins accumulate more quickly during the stresses of treatment and if your system gets clogged, especially at this sensitive time, more severe damage can be done to the colon than under normal circumstances! So eat vegetables—raw, juiced, and/or cooked—four to six times daily. If you cannot have a bowel movement, take flaxseed, acidophilus, laxative teas (like licorice, fennel or senna with flaxseed and sometimes cascara sagrada), or digestive aids. Do whatever it takes to bring on a bowel movement as soon as possible; keep them regular. Avoid drugs if possible. If constipation continues for several days and you cannot alleviate the problem, contact your doctor. Individuals who have had bowel surgery may not be able to have regular bowel movements or do regular cleansing and should consult their holistic doctor for safe cleansing methods or alternative options.

BRUISES

1. Condition and Cause
To injure the skin by a blow or by pressure, without laceration may form a bruise. Bumping into hard objects or falling can cause bruises or tissue damage and bleeding under the skin. The bruise starts out black and blue, and sometimes reddish. It turns yellowish as the healing process goes on. Bruises usually disappear within a few days to a week or longer depending on the severity of the injury.

2. Ailment History, Signs and Early Treatments
Herbalists have used compresses of comfrey, St. John's wort or lobelia herbs to cover bruises and help them heal. These herbs and compresses are still used today. Garlic and onions have also been used to rub on bruises.

3. Modern Natural Treatments and Remedies
Rub vigorously around (not on) the bruised area to help stimulate the circulation and allow energy to flow to the injured area and speed healing. Apply a cold pack to the bruised area next to get blood flowing to that area, here again, increasing circulation and enhancing healing. Tea tree oil is a potent healer for quick healing of bruises. Often within 24 hours, after applying tea tree oil a few times, the bruise disappears. Oregano oil can also be effective for bruises. Comfrey, witch hazel, horestail or calendula cream or compresses are a helpful healing aid and preventative. After initial treatments with tea tree oil, oregano oil and/or comfrey for two or three days, apply shark oil for added protection and healing of the skin and underlying tissues.

4. Helpful Supplements and Dosages
- Take 1,000–2,000 mg vitamin C one to three times daily, depending on the severity of the bruise(s).
- Take a bioflavonoid supplement daily to assist healing if not already included with the vitamin C supplement.
- Optional: Take 200–400 IU of vitamin E daily for healing.
- Optional: Take CoQ10, pycnogenol or grape seed extract daily for added oxygen and bioflavonoids for healing.

5. Cautions and Exceptions

Do not take aspirin or anti-inflammatory drugs. Bruising frequently and easily may be an early sign of cancer. Pale skin, tiredness, nosebleeds, pain and frequent infections are other signs of leukemia.

6. Nutrition Aids and Recommended Foods

A wholesome natural food diet is helpful. Eat lots of vegetables, especially, green ones. Take a high-chlorophyll green food product, especially, like alfalfa, barley green, spirulina, chlorella, or blue-green algae. Good foods include high vitamin C and K foods: citrus fruit, bell peppers, molasses, sprouts, dark green leafy vegetables, broccoli, Brussels sprouts and flaxseed.

7. Beverage and Herbal Tea Suggestions

Enjoy vegetable juices, especially those with carrots and green food products.

Healing herbal teas for bruises include: alfalfa, dandelion, horsetail, parsley, rose hips, raspberry leaf, yarrow and occasionally comfrey or St. John's wort.

BUNIONS

See *Calluses, Corns, Bunions and Blisters*

BURNS

See also *Sunburn*

1. Condition and Cause

First and second degree burns from heating elements, stoves, fires or other intense heat sources can be treated naturally at home. Severe second and all third and fourth degree burns should receive medical attention or emergency hospital treatment. Hot substances like wax or plastic can be removed from the skin with ice water before treating minor burns. For major burns, seek medical attention to remove hot substances if needed.

First degree burns are characterized by slight skin discoloration, sometimes redness, unbroken skin and slight burning or stinging sensation or sensitivity to touch. Second degree burns include broken skin, blistering, pain and redness. Third (and fourth) degree burns include damage to underlying skin tissues and sometimes muscle too and may appear white, yellow, red or blackened. There may be little or no pain due to nerve damage.

2. Ailment History, Signs and Early Treatments

Folklore claims the use of peeled potatoes, onion slices, mud, vinegar and raw chicken fat for soothing burned areas of skin. Butter is another old remedy still used today, although it is not recommend as it can seal in the heat, clog the pores and actually slow or deter healing.

3. Modern Natural Treatments and Remedies

Immerse all first and second degree burns in cool (not cold) water for a minute or two to sooth and reduce pain, then apply natural treatment. Two of the more commonly used treatments for burns are vitamin E oil and aloe vera gel from a live plant or bottled. However vitamin E oil, from a cream or squeezed out of a capsule that has been poked with a pin, can, like old fashioned butter treatments, clog the pores and sometimes slow healing or contribute to scarring. Aloe vera gel is temporarily cooling and soothing, however it does not speed healing, and scarring is still possible. Tea tree oil is usually the most potent, fast-acting burn remedy available. It actually reduces the swelling of blistered skin (in second degree burns) and saves the skin from breaking, preventing the need for new skin growth and scarring. Tea tree oil also increases healing action five to seven times more quickly than if the burns were left untreated or treated with other remedies.

After cool water immersion, apply 100 percent pure tea tree oil directly to wounds, generously. Use immediately, as soon after the burn occurs if you want to save the skin. Expect it to sting. The more damage, the more stinging, yet the stinging speeds healing. If possible, soak a bandage in tea tree oil and attach to wound for several hours or more. Re-soak with extra tea tree oil every few minutes or so during the first hour and for every hour as desired to speed healing and relief. Apply new oil every hour until stinging stops. Then apply new oil every four to six hours for the first day and two to four times daily for a few days after until healed. Most minor burns will "disappear" within four days. If tea tree oil is not available, use aloe vera as a second choice and vitamin E as a third choice using the same method as for tea tree oil except for between 4 and 14 days or until the scar is reduced as much as possible and blistering and redness have healed. (For large burn areas, a mister can be used with tea tree oil (15 percent) and distilled water (85 percent) spraying directly on or above the wounds.) Once third and fourth degree burns have closed and partially healed, tea tree oil can be applied to hasten healing and minimize scarring for several weeks or until no change appears in the skin.

4. Helpful Supplements and Dosages

- Take 2,000 mg vitamin C immediately after minor burns, and daily for several days after. For third and fourth degree burns, take 5,000–10,000 mg vitamin C directly after burns occur and 2,000–3,000 mg one to three times daily afterwards until healing occurs. Include bioflavonoids as well.
- Take one or two 15–30 mg capsules of zinc to speed healing after all burns. Then daily until healing occurs. Take 100 mg total if zinc lozenges are used.
- Take 100–200 mg vitamin B complex (two to four B50s) daily until healed.
- Take 10,000 IU vitamin A daily plus 25,000 IU beta-carotene (increase if doctor recommends) for severe second degree and all third and fourth degree burns.
- Take 200 IU vitamin E daily until minor wounds heal. For major wounds, take 200 IU the first three days, double to 400 IU for three more days, then continue with 600 IU and increase to 1,000 IU or more if doctor recommends. Decrease gradually before stopping.

5. Cautions and Exceptions

Unless allergic to the treatments, any of the above can be used as directed. For children, who might cry or object to the stinging action of tea tree oil as it heals, soothing words, kisses and a follow up of cool, soothing aloe vera gel can follow after the tea tree oil has done its main work. The tea tree oil can also be mildly diluted with pure water, to reduce stinging for children, if necessary.

6. Nutrition Aids and Recommended Foods

For minor burns, simply eat a more wholesome diet for several days following a burn. For severe burns, the Phase II or III diet in my *Complete Candida Yeast Guidebook* is a perfect healing diet until recovered. Avoid excessive amounts of dairy products (except yogurt) and include lots of green foods—vegetables and a healing green food product—daily in the diet. Avoid fatty foods, sugars, sweets and refined foods.

7. Beverage and Herbal Tea Suggestions

Daily vegetable juice of carrot, beet and green powder can assist healing. Daily teas can include chamomile for children or adults. For adults, daily teas include: a.m. gotu kola or for those over 40—ginseng, yarrow, organic green tea and (if doctor recommends) comfrey. Sleep aid teas include especially catnip for children and skullcap for adults.

C

CALLUSES, CORNS, BUNIONS AND BLISTERS

For these foot problems, do a foot bath several times weekly and coat these with one of the following two to three times daily: tea tree oil, aloe vera gel, colloidal silver (24 ppm or higher), oregano oil, propolis tincture or the juice from a fresh dandelion stem. Take green food products regularly and take echinacea while corns, calluses, bunions or blisters last. Make sure to wear comfortable shoes, and go without socks or stockings, barefoot at home especially and outside whenever possible. Let the feet breathe and avoid wearing dark socks too often and when you do, wear cotton. Use foot pads, bandages or protectors for these when wearing shoes. Elevate the feet and legs one or more times daily for five to ten minutes or so and do some feet stretches or massage several times a week.

CANDIDA

See also *Jock Itch* and *Yeast Infection, Vaginal*

1. Condition and Cause

Candida yeast is a type of fungus, a microorganism that is not beneficial for the body; therefore it is called "unfriendly" bacteria. Candida albicans exists everywhere in our environment—in the air and on everything we touch and most of what we consume. It only becomes a problem when it "overgrows" and then interferes with the balance of "friendly" bacteria in the body. Overabundance appears as dandruff, athlete's foot, white/flaky skin, coated tongue, jock itch, vaginal yeast infections, colic and thrush. It can also contribute to: digestive problems, gas, headaches, allergies, viral infections, skin problems, fatigue, depression, blood sugar problems, aches and pains, hyperactivity, earaches, acne, thinking difficulties, cravings, bloating, weight gain and dozens of other health problems and even diseases like cancer and AIDS. Excessive fruit, sugar, sweets, alcohol, antibiotics, birth control pills, other drugs, weakened immune system or disease, stress, lack of sleep and overworking can contribute to Candida overgrowth and resultant health problems.

2. Ailment History, Signs and Early Treatments

Although Candida has been around probably as long as humankind, it has not been widely recognized or understood, nor has it been a major problem, until the later part of the last century. The advent of increased sugar production and consumption and abundant antibiotic treatments can be considered major factors in the rapid advance of yeast problems. Garlic was used for some Candida symptoms in earlier years, as well as today as one helpful remedy, although garlic alone will not usually alleviate all symptoms of severe Candida overgrowth. Aspirin also helps control Candida and its increased use may very likely be due to Candida side effects like headaches and anxiety that are common in North American society.

3. Modern Natural Treatments and Remedies

Besides prescription drugs to kill the unwanted, troublesome yeast, there are possibly hundreds of effective natural treatments including: caprylic acid, aloe vera, oil of oregano, colloidal silver, citricidal, desensitization drops or injections, homeopathic remedies, ginger tea, oxygen therapies, taheebo (Pau d'Arco) tea, tea tree oil, vitamin C, garlic and many more. There are also combination products available in health stores for Candida treatment. Usually one or more remedies are taken for 30 days or more with a specific yeast control diet to "cure" Candida or minimize symptoms. See remedy bottle or package for how to take most treatments. One can try one or two drops (only!) tea tree oil with pure (spring or distilled) water once or twice daily or one to three cups taheebo tea daily (see recipe), or the garlic cleanse in this book for 30 or more days. See my *Complete Candida Yeast Guidebook* for more detailed treatments and tips. Proper diet and yeast killing remedies are both required for Candida to be effectively treated. See your holistic physician for specific treatments.

4. Helpful Supplements and Dosages

- It is essential for most people with Candida (unless they have high stomach acid, which is unusual) to take two high quality acidophilus capsules (may include bifidus) once or twice a day, one hour or more away from food with 4 to 6 ounces of pure water to replenish friendly bacteria and help digestion. Try to use a brand that includes added FOSs (fructooligosaccharides), which assist friendly bacteria growth. Take before and/or after breakfast and/or lunch, not after supper.
- Take digestive aids and/or laxative teas and flushing agents as needed.
- Vitamin C—especially Allergy C, Ester C or buffered C—can help reduce symptoms, energize and boost the immune system. Take 500–1,000 mg one to four times daily as needed, at least three or four hours before sleeping. Do not take chewable vitamin C. (For children, vitamin C powder can be mixed in some solid foods.)
- Take two to four vitamin B50 complex daily, spread during the day and/or bedtime.
- Take one 300–500 mcg biotin tablet with each starchy meal or snack. Up to three tablets or capsules daily taken with one B50 complex. (Maximum 1,500 mcg daily)
- Take energizing supplements if needed. See *Energy, Low.*

5. Cautions and Exceptions

Avoid any remedies, treatments or foods you are allergic to.

Temporary food intolerances (see *Allergies*), and some side effects like fatigue, indigestion or increased Candida symptoms sometimes appear initially while treating the yeast (or cleansing). Use the preceding supplements to help alleviate symptoms. Contact your holistic physician if severe symptoms persist. Remember that proper diet is essential to effective Candida treatment!

6. Nutrition Aids and Recommended Foods

A yeast-free diet without alcohol, smoking, sugar, artificial sweeteners, refined foods, junk foods, hard-to-digest foods, pork, processed meats, milk and cheeses, sweet and tropical fruits, natural sweeteners, desserts, potatoes, corn, oatmeal, breads, crackers and grain flour products is essential to treat Candida and be successful. Good foods to include are: whole grains, legumes (brown and black beans and lentils), abundant vegetables, limited sub-acid (tart) fruits, yogurt, butter, some seeds and nuts (like pumpkin, sunflower, sesame and flax seeds, home-roasted almonds or filberts), pure (spring or distilled) water and some other foods are required. See my *Complete Candida Yeast Guidebook* for complete diet details.

7. Beverage and Herbal Tea Suggestions

Helpful herbal teas include peppermint, spearmint, lemon grass, raspberry leaves, fennel or fenugreek seeds, alfalfa seeds, senna and flax and slippery elm. Stronger teas, which could be harmful for pregnant women or those who are sensitive should only be used with your holistic physician's advice are: burdock, comfrey, ginger, goldenseal, ginseng, eucalyptus, licorice and/or taheebo. Five or six glasses of vegetable juice weekly can be very helpful, especially with carrots, beets and green food (barley green, spinach, parsley, or others—some of these require a special juicer or blending in water before using). See *Juices*

CIRCULATION, POOR

1. Condition and Cause

Illness, disease (like heart problems), digestive problems, a weakened immune system, bad diet, smoking, alcohol, varicose veins and lack of exercise are the main causes of poor circulation. Poor circulation can contribute to tiredness, low energy, headaches, dizziness, shortness of breath, thinking difficulties, numbness, cold extremities, possible ringing in the ears and other health problems.

2. Ailment History, Signs and Early Treatments
Asian peoples have used ginseng for centuries to stimulate the circulation, retard aging and rejuvenate the body. See *Ginseng* under "Natural Remedies Glossary." Other Oriental herbs (like gotu kola), garlic, citrus fruits, bee products, massage, acupressure and acupuncture have also been used to help the circulation by ancient and modern peoples alike.

3. Modern Natural Treatments and Remedies
Chiropractic, massage, acupressure or acupuncture are excellent aids for improving the circulation. Vigorous as well as gentle stretching exercises, done daily, are also extremely beneficial and essential. Even bedridden individuals should do tensing and relaxing exercises and stretching techniques. Hot/cold showers, baths and packs are also extremely beneficial for stimulating the circulation. See "Healing Aids" for details on these and other options.

Dr. John Christopher, who was a world-renowned herbalist from the U.S., used and widely recommended the healing power of capsicum (found in cayenne pepper) for good circulation. (See his book entitled *Capsicum*.) Cayenne can be put in herbal tea (if you can handle the hot taste) or taken in capsules (not on an empty stomach!) to help stimulate digestion as well as improve the circulation. In winter, sprinkle cayenne on top of light cotton gloves and socks and cover with a thicker pair to keep fingers and toes warm while avoiding frostbite. Cayenne stimulates internally as well as externally. Do not place cayenne directly on the skin though as it may sting and burn temporarily. See *Cayenne* in "Remedies from Your Refrigerator and Cupboard."

Ginseng and gotu kola are two stimulating Asian herbs that can be used if over 40 or with a doctor's advice. For women, Dong quai is a better choice to avoid stimulating too many male hormones. Horseradish and ginger roots are also good for the circulation as a food or herbal tea.

4. Helpful Supplements and Dosages
- Take 2,000–5,000 mg vitamin C once or twice daily take the larger dose the more severe the problem is.

- Take 100–200 mg vitamin B complex (two to four B50s) daily.
- Take 300 mcg vitamin B12 daily (preferably with a B complex or two).
- Take 10,000 IU daily of vitamin A plus 25,000 IU beta-carotene (increase if doctor recommends).
- Take 200 IU vitamin E for the first three days, double to 400 IU for three more days, then continue with 600 IU and, increase to 1,000 IU or more if doctor recommends. Decrease gradually before stopping within 30 days or so.
- Take one 15–50 mg capsule of zinc daily for immune function.
- Take digestive aids, flushing agents and energizing supplements as needed.
- Optional: Do a 14–30 day garlic cleanse to assist circulation and healing. (See *Toxin Overload*.)

5. Cautions and Exceptions

Consult your physician for any serious circulation problems or extreme symptoms! Get authoritative advice before using Asian herbs and medicines.

6. Nutrition Aids and Recommended Foods

Eat smaller, nutritious meals including lots of cooked vegetables and vegetable juices, citrus fruits (except oranges), tender warm whole grains, tender warm legumes, fish, seaweeds, yogurt and kefir, and non-sweet/non-tropical fruits. Avoid red meats, shellfish, refined foods, sugars, junk foods, fatty foods, cheese and milk, corn products, pasta, potatoes and all nuts and hard-to-digest foods like lettuces, raw broccoli and other excessive raw foods. All foods must be chewed extremely well. Use digestive aids if needed. Take one or two teaspoons flax meal on your food (especially good on salads) four to six times weekly. See *Digestive Problems* if needed.

7. Beverage and Herbal Tea Suggestions

Ginkgo biloba, hawthorn, chickweed, (organic) green teas and mint teas are good herbal stimulants that just about everyone can take. For children, use peppermint, spearmint and rose hip teas. Vegetable juices and protein energy drinks can provide a stimulating boost.

Cleansing, Cleansing Reaction or Healing Reaction

See *Toxin Overload*, also *Cleansing* in the "Healing Aids" section

Cold Extremities

See *Circulation*

Colds

See also *Sore Throat, Coughs, Flu, Infections*

1. Condition and Cause
A cold is an upper respiratory infection that can be caused by dozens of different types of viruses. Side effects may include runny nose, sneezing, coughing, congestion, fatigue and sometimes body aches. Most colds last three to eight days.

2. Ailment History, Signs and Early Treatments
A traditional cure for colds is hot chicken soup, which has been scientifically proven to be effective and is still employed today to ease the symptoms of a cold. As far back as the 12th century, Moses Maimonides, a physician and philosopher, used chicken soup as a healing remedy, according to *Chicken Soup and other Folk Remedies,* by Joan and Lydia Wilen. Part of the reason it is beneficial is that it is hot and steaming, which when sipped or drunk, improves nasal clearance. Hot soup also helps the circulation, which when increased, speeds healing.

Other old-fashioned remedies have included hot rum with lemon and honey, apple cider vinegar mixed equally with honey, or garlic (chewed) taken alone or with cayenne, or long-simmered onions with added lemon juice and honey.

3. Modern Natural Treatments and Remedies
There is no real "cure" for a cold, only prevention, treatment or suppression.

COLD PREVENTION Preventing a cold is usually a first choice.
When you feel one coming on, rest, dress warmly, keep dry, avoid
junk foods, dairy products and sweet fruits/sugars, slow down your
life pace and employ one of the following:

1. Take the fresh juice of a small lemon or lime (about 3–5
    tablespoons), squeezed, and drunk straight or undiluted,
    (can be swished in the mouth to kill bacteria there before
    swallowing). Do this on an empty stomach and follow
    with a sip or two of water (which will taste sweet after
    the tart citrus). Fruit or food can be had 30 minutes
    after. The lemon or lime will kill much of the bacteria in
    the mouth and throat and if taken enough before the
    cold sets in, will often wipe it out. (Have the lemon
    treatment once or twice during the day sometime before
    supper for a day or two.)

2. Garlic capsules can be taken, but they are not nearly as
    effective as chewing an organic garlic clove which, like
    the lemon or lime juice, kills bacteria in the mouth and
    throat. Chew a clove of garlic daily, after a meal (right
    after or wait awhile) and spit out the pulp, to kill bacteria
    in the mouth and throat and soothe symptoms (and
    hopefully causes).

3. One can also boost the immune system with one to
    two grams vitamin C one to three times daily and
    1,000–2,000 mg echinacea daily plus an optional:
    500–1,000 mg royal jelly or a good dose of ginseng
    taken earlier in the day.

4. For antibacterial protection, take one of the following:
    300-600 mg propolis daily, goldenseal with echinacea,
    unsweetened elderberry or cayenne capsules. (Lemon
    and/or lime juice, as well as garlic, are also antibacterial.)

5. Cleansing when your body is low and you feel susceptible
    to a cold can also help clear body poisons that contribute
    to colds and help boost the immune system. Choose
    cleansing items that also help kill infection like *one* of the
    following: astragalus, cayenne, citricidal, colloidal silver,
    garlic (chopped/not chewed), olive leaf extract, OR
    oregano oil. Take a small or average dose because, if you

take too much, it will throw you into a full-scale cleanse or make you *more* susceptible to a cold. See *Cleansing* in the "Natural Remedies Glossary" for directions on how to take these. (See *Toxin Overload* for how to take garlic.)

Once the cold begins, these treatments will lessen the severity of it, but they will not halt a cold. Recent medical studies have reported that total *suppression* of colds, as with certain drugs, while alleviating colds, may increase risk of cancer and other serious diseases. Holistic doctors and health experts know that the common cold is actually a form of cleansing the body uses to clear toxins and poisons from the system.

COLD TREATMENT   Once a cold has begun, your best hope is to ride it through (rather than suppress it—see preceding), reduce the symptoms and shorten its length. Daily vitamin C and echinacea, small doses of an anti-viral remedy—an amount best suited for you (large doses will increase symptoms and cause major cleansing), and specific foods and beverages will lessen the length and severity of most colds. Health food stores also sell combination cold formulas if you prefer a pre-made remedy. (See "Cold Prevention.")

Helpful aids include:
1. foot baths.
2. keeping the air warm (not hot) but not too dry (use a vaporizer, boil water or put water or wet cloths on or near heat source) and airing out the house daily for fresh air.
3. using compresses and/or poultices with one or more of the following: grated ginger or ginger tincture, cloves, eucalyptus, yarrow or astragalus (add a sprinkling of cayenne, if desired).
4. drinking hot liquids many times a day.
5. bathing or showering daily and cleansing the skin to clean the pores and remove toxins.
6. resting and taking it easy, but not *too* easy, as lying around too much lessens circulation and stimulation for healing.
7. wash your hands frequently and dispose of facial tissues properly so they are not re-handled and spread the cold virus.

NASAL CONGESTION   At the end of a cold, the nose usually gets stuffed up for a while and it may be difficult to breathe through it; sometimes it is necessary to breathe through the mouth. Eucalyptus oil, peppermint or tea tree oil can be *sparingly* put on the chest, temples and around the nose. (Avoid nose area for children.) Aromatherapy oils, including those mentioned above and menthol as well, can be inhaled or placed in a disperser. Make sure your living space is well aired out at least once a day. Use a vaporizer to add moisture to dry air or boil water on the stove, place water or wet towels on or around heating vents or radiators. Eating horseradish, garlic and cayenne pepper can help clear the sinuses. The face, especially the cheeks, can also be massaged to help open sinus areas. Carrot and cucumber juices are especially good for clearing congestion. Also enjoy blueberries, as their nutrients are a helpful decongestant for stuffed up noses.

CHEST CONGESTION   Consult your doctor immediately if chest congestion occurs as lung infections can be dangerous!

4. Helpful Supplements and Dosages
- Take 500–1000 mg vitamin C one to four times daily or more, as required. A Vitamin C Flush can be a good preventative or treatment for colds (See *Vitamin C* in the alphabetized section of the "Natural Remedies Glossary")
- Take 1000–2000 mg echinacea once or twice a day or more, as required.
- Take 15–50 mg zinc daily, as a supplement or in lozenges.
- Take one or two B50 complex daily for healing and stress reduction.
- Take acidophilus (bifidus for children) or digestive aids *if needed* while cold lasts and up to a few days after.
- Optional: Take garlic capsules daily, or take one small clove garlic (chopped/not chewed) according to directions in *Toxin Overload*.
- Optional: Take a multivitamin and mineral supplement.

5. Cautions and Exceptions
Be careful not to begin a deep or rigorous cleanse (use one cleansing/infection herb or treatment at a time and do not take too much)

while trying to prevent or treat a cold, as this will weaken the immune system and may increase the length and severity of a cold. If a secondary bacterial infection develops, chest congestion, or if symptoms are severe, contact your doctor immediately!

6. Nutrition Aids and Recommended Foods
It is important to eat properly during a cold to keep your strength up and assist healing. Hot liquid soups are especially helpful. See the healing soups in "Remedies from Your Refrigerator and Cupboard." Avoid all junk foods, sweet fruits, sugars, excessive breads (which increase mucus), pasta, sushi, dairy products (these also increase mucus), very hard-to-digest foods, excessive meats, pork, cold meats, lettuces, cold beans, cold whole grains, and fatty foods, when sick, as these prolong colds. Enjoy mainly soups, stews, quality lamb and veal, blended and mashed warm beans, warm cooked whole grains, lots of cooked vegetables and fresh vegetable juices, and just a little butter or yogurt if desired.

7. Beverage and Herbal Tea Suggestions
Drink lots of water, six to eight glasses daily to flush the system. Hot herbal tea, drunk may times daily without milk/cream/dairy, and with lemon and/or honey (and an optional dash of cayenne to break up mucus) is the most beneficial. Enjoy one or more of the following: rose hips, raspberry leaf, yarrow, elderberry, lemon grass, slippery elm, ginger or mint teas. Also enjoy Vitamin C Magic, Cold Classic, Warm Cold Classic, vegetable juices, especially those with carrots, and other beverages from "Remedies from Your Refrigerator and Cupboard." Avoid drinking milk, cream and all dairy-based drinks and avoid using these in soups or other recipes as well because they increase mucus and prolong runny nose, sinus problems and sore throat. Drink orange juice for extra vitamin C unless you have Candida yeast problems too; then, drink grapefruit juice instead. Drink lemon or lime juice as directed under *Cold Prevention*. Organic green tea is better than coffee during colds.

Cold Sores

1. Condition and Cause
Cold sores or fever blisters, are caused by herpes simplex virus 1

(HSV-1), which is related to but different from the virus that causes genital herpes, says *Prescription For Nutritional Healing* by Phyllis and Dr. James Balch. After the first appearance of cold sores (which last a few days to a week if treated properly, or longer), the virus remains in the body in a dormant state and can be activated again when the immune system is low, during a cold, flu, fever or virus, during illness or disease, from stress, from nutritional deficiencies, hormone imbalances, or from extreme temperature and weather changes. They can appear on the lips, gums, tongue or inside cheeks. Cold sores usually begin with itchiness and redness, then a sore bump, next they become a hard crusted blister, and finally a swollen sore. Cold sores are contagious through skin contact, especially if touched when the sore is oozing.

2. Ailment History, Signs and Early Treatments

Applying red wine to sores was and still is considered helpful by some health sources. A paste of ground raw walnuts and cocoa butter is supposed to make cold sores disappear in three to six days, if applied daily.

3. Modern Natural Treatments and Remedies

To prevent or lessen the return of cold sores, it helps to first boost the immune system by getting more than adequate rest and sleep, eating a nutritious diet sans junk foods, getting enough exercise and keeping the bowels healthy and clean with regular cleansing. Keep the area of and around cold sores clean and make sure air circulates around them to assist healing.

External applications of tea tree oil, oregano oil, colloidal silver, propolis tincture, or rubbing with a sliced garlic clove can help reduce the length of a cold sore's appearance. Comfrey cream and aloe vera gel can also be helpful but are not as beneficial as the aforementioned. Regular use of peelu toothpaste, propolis or neem powder with baking soda as a tooth powder and/or the mouthwashes and gargles mentioned in *Oral Hygiene Problems* can help reduce and even help eliminate many cold sores in the mouth. Also L-lysine, vitamin C and zinc and B vitamins are especially beneficial in "Helpful Supplements." Lysine cream, calendula cream or St. John's wort salve can also be applied externally.

4. Helpful Supplements and Dosages
- Take 500 mg lysine once or twice a day. (If unavailable, be sure to take one of the "Optional but Helpful" items.)
- Take 1,000–2,000 mg vitamin C two or three times daily as needed, to boost immunity.
- Take 15 mg of zinc one to four times daily for healing.
- Take 10,000 IU vitamin A and 25,000 IU beta-carotene daily until cold sores disappear.
- Take one vitamin B50 complex two to four times daily for stress and healing.
- Take acidophilus once or twice daily (See the "Natural Remedies Glossary" for dosage).
- Optional but Helpful: Be sure to take one of the following if no lysine is available: a clove chopped/non-chewed garlic daily (See *Toxin Overload* for method), or 500 mg propolis once or twice daily, or two goldenseal/echinacea tablets or capsules once or twice daily to fight infection while cold sores last.
- Optional: Do an anti-viral cleanse (See *Viruses*) when no cold sores are present to boost the immune system and help prevent future outbreaks.

5. Cautions and Exceptions
Remember that cold sores are contagious by touch. If cold sores last for prolonged periods and occur frequently, consult your holistic doctor.

6. Nutrition Aids and Recommended Foods
A wholesome, natural diet without excessive refined or fatty foods or junk foods is best for all kind of healing. Eat lots of whole grains, legumes, leafy salads, cooked vegetables, fish, seafood, seaweeds, pumpkin seeds, flaxseed and other natural foods. Eat some yogurt, kefir, miso and/or sauerkraut daily. Avoid all agitating foods, especially refined foods, junk foods, fatty and greasy foods, excessive meats, artificial foods and additives, caffeine, pasta, sugars and sweet fruits. Organic green tea is better for cold sores than coffee.

7. Beverage and Herbal Tea Suggestions
Drink lots of spring water. Enjoy fresh vegetable juices five or six

days weekly. Beneficial herbal teas include: chamomile, raspberry leaf, elderberry of leaf, lemon grass, lemon balm, and occasionally as needed—white oak bark, licorice, comfrey, goldenseal and myrrh.

COLON PROBLEMS

See *Bowel Problems*

CONGESTION

See *Colds*

CORNS

See *Calluses, Corns, Bunions and Blisters*

CONSTIPATION

See *Bowel Problems*

COUGHS

See also *Colds*

1. Condition and Cause
Coughing is the body's protective mechanism that helps clear excessive mucus or foreign matter from the throat, lungs and bronchial tubes. A cough is often generated by a respiratory infection or irritation and can be nature's way of clearing and stimulating healing. Coughs can also sometimes be caused by Candida yeast infections or parasite problems. Like colds, coughs should not always be suppressed as they serve a purpose. Short-term coughs are often due to colds. Long-term coughs can be due to bronchitis.

Croup and whooping cough are contagious and require medical attention. Epstein-Barr in its contagious stage is accompanied by a cough that may spread the infection to others. Coughing can also be from smoking, asthma or other health problems. Poor diet, excessive dairy products or bread products, not drinking enough water and fluids, excessive sugars and sweets, toxin overload, dry air, and not dressing warmly enough can all contribute to coughs.

2. Ailment History, Signs and Early Treatments
Folk medicines for coughs include cough syrups made from honey and lemons, with olive oil or apple cider vinegar or (raw or simmered) onion juice or grated horseradish juice added, and given every two to three hours. Chewing on ginger root, whole cloves, ginseng root or drinking mulled wine was also employed.

3. Modern Natural Treatments and Remedies
Avoid some minor, occasional coughs by pressing your tongue firmly against the roof of your mouth and holding it there several seconds up to about 30 seconds or use your finger to press firmly below the nose, above the lips for the same amount of time.

You can also gently massage the shoulders, neck and face to relieve pressure build-up that aggravates coughs.

Besides taking traditional cold remedies (see *Colds,* preceding), licorice, slippery elm or wild cherry throat lozenges can be taken. Health stores have an array of cough syrups including Chinese cough syrups and excellent brands from Hyland's® and Olbas®. Use the mouthwash/gargles mentioned in *Oral Hygiene Problems* to kill throat bacteria, once or twice daily as required. Use a propolis throat spray or break open a propolis capsule in the throat (or chew a tablet) one to three times daily to help kill any infection and speed healing of any throat irritation, as well as helping other respiratory symptoms. Another option instead of propolis is to take cayenne capsules. Take two capsules once or twice a day during the middle of a regular meal (so it will not give you "hot" side effects) and sprinkle a little cayenne (one small shake) in herbal tea one to three times daily. A third option is chewing one clove of garlic daily after a meal (right after or wait awhile) and spitting out the pulp to kill bacteria in the mouth and throat and sooth cough symptoms (and hopefully causes).

4. Helpful Supplements and Dosages
- Take 500–1,000 mg vitamin C one to four times daily or more, as required.

- Take 1,000–2,000 mg echinacea once or twice a day or more, as required.
- Take 15–50 mg zinc daily as a supplement or in lozenges.
- Take one or two vitamin B50 complex daily for healing and stress reduction.
- Optional: Take garlic capsules daily, or take one small clove garlic (chopped/not chewed) according to directions in *Toxin Overload.*

5. Cautions and Exceptions

For persistent, hacking coughs or coughs that leave the throat raw, or if blood is coughed up, see your doctor immediately. Be sure to spit out any mucus coughed up in the throat instead of swallowing it, as it is loaded with bacteria and usually infection as well.

6. Nutrition Aids and Recommended Foods

Follow the same diet as for *Colds,* but be sure to include flaxseed in the diet.

7. Beverage and Herbal Tea Suggestions

Besides the beverages under *Colds,* add dill weed (works especially well), comfrey, myrrh and black cohosh to the list of herbal teas.

CRAVINGS

See also *Weight Problems*

1. Condition and Cause

Cravings can be caused by vitamin or mineral deficiencies (or overabundances) and protein deficiencies. When there is a drain on the body's nutrients as: during health problems or disease, when there are body or energy imbalances, under times of excessive stress or tiredness, during pregnancy, when dieting incorrectly or eating nutrient-depleted foods, cravings are likely to arise. Cravings are a signal from the body that your nutritional and/or physical needs are not being met. What you crave for however, is not necessarily what you need. People often crave what they are allergic to (foods like chocolate, sweets, milk, strawberries or seafood) or addicted to (coffee, alcohol, drugs or cigarettes). False cravings and cross-cravings (craving one thing but really needing another) can also arise when the body is exhausted or not in the best state of health.

Dieters who ignore needed fats in the diet often develop unnatural cravings for sweets and starches and often end up eating those excessively instead of needed fats in the diet. Avoiding all starches, is just as dangerous in different ways, the brain can become starved. Lack of water can also cause cravings. When *any* (one or more) nutrients (fats, proteins, starches, fiber, water, vitamins, minerals) are deprived, cravings are inevitable.

Starving and bingeing will cause cravings. Fasting, if done correctly, surprisingly will *not* cause cravings. Cleansing and Candida yeast treatment does cause cravings, often intense ones, however these need to be ignored as they are not "true" cravings, rather a sign of the body showing major purging. Sometimes in the case of Candida yeast or parasites infestation, when these critters are being killed off, they get very hungry, disruptive and *they* instigate some of the cravings!

2. Ailment History, Signs and Early Treatments
One long-standing joke says that pregnant women crave pickles and ice cream. Assuredly, there is no real nutritional need for pickles and ice cream, alone or together.

Gargling with a teaspoon of baking soda in a glass of warm water is supposed to stop cravings for sweets. Chewing gum, fennel or cardamom seeds, or whole cloves are claimed to abate many cravings.

3. Modern Natural Treatments and Remedies
The best cure is prevention. Keep healthy, eat a well-balanced diet, do not overeat any one food, or eat sweets on an empty stomach! Get enough rest, exercise, play and work. Take nutritional supplements and do not eat when nervous, excited, tired or not busy. Eat high-quality foods that are nutritious, not nutrient-depleted foods such as sweets, sugars, pasta, refined foods, fatty foods and junk foods. Add a green food product to your daily diet and increase your whole foods—whole grains, legumes and vegetables—intake. See *Weight Problems* for more information.

If cravings are prolonged and unnatural, and do not respond to eating properly for a month or two, see your holistic doctor for testing. Get allergy testing, hair analysis for mineral deficiencies or abundances, vega testing or blood and urine testing for vitamins and disease testing, parasite testing or Candida/Candidiasis testing and other diagnostic tests if needed to make sure health problems are not responsible for your cravings.

4. Helpful Supplements and Dosages
- Take a balanced multivitamin and mineral daily.
- Take 500–1,000 mg of vitamin C daily, or more if required.
- Take one or two vitamin B50 complex daily.
- Take 500 mg of calcium and magnesium daily, or more if required.
- Add one green food product to your daily diet, like blue-green algae, barley green, wheat grass, spirulina, chlorella or another. See *Toxin Overload* for more information on green foods.

5. Cautions and Exceptions
Sometimes you actually do crave something you need! If cravings are extreme and cause serious physical discomfort, contact your doctor immediately.

6. Nutrition Aids and Recommended Foods
Eat two or three wholesome, well-balanced meals daily and do not eat sweets on an empty stomach. See my books: *For the Love of Food* for relatively healthy peoples' complete eating plans and *Complete Candida Yeast Guidebook* for eating plans for those with health challenges including: cancer, allergies, chronic fatigue, digestive and bowel problems and many other health problems. Meat eaters should also get: *Jeanne Marie Martin's Light Cuisine* for wholesome seafood, poultry and egg recipes. For more information, see #3 "Modern Natural Treatments and Remedies" preceding.

7. Beverage and Herbal Tea Suggestions
Drink four to eight glasses of fresh spring water daily, more in hotter weather. Wholesome vegetable juices (four to six glasses weekly), supply many satisfying nutrients and can help alleviate some cravings. See drink recipes in "Remedies from Your Refrigerator and Cupboard."

Herbal pleasure teas such as peppermint, chamomile, lemon grass, rose hips, spearmint, alfalfa and others can be enjoyed often for flavor and nutrients.

CUTS AND WOUNDS

See also *Bleeding, Excessive*

1. Condition and Cause
Small, clean cuts can be treated simply at home. Large and/or deep wounds or cuts from rusty or unclean objects should be examined by a doctor and treated accordingly. Infected wounds may require antibiotics and possibly a tetanus shot. Large cuts may need stitches.

2. Ailment History, Signs and Early Treatments
Large cuts and wounds in past centuries were often treated by cauterizing—burning with fire, searing with a hot iron, or using caustics—to close and seal the wound. However, this usually did leave quite a scar, often a permanent one. Cauterizing is still used today, though relatively rarely. An electrical current, laser beam or a chemical is used to cauterize in special cases.

3. Modern Natural Treatments and Remedies
If the cut or wound is small and you are treating it at home, first run pure, cool water over the wound, and clean it. Use an antiseptic like tea tree oil, rubbing alcohol, colloidal silver or oregano oil and coat the wound. This may sting a bit (except the colloidal silver, which makes it great for children). Put a little of the antiseptic on the bandage on the spot that will cover the wound too. Use a bandage that is snug enough to apply pressure and stop the bleeding, but that will also allow airflow that will encourage wound healing. Change the bandage once or more daily and reapply a healing antiseptic (usually not rubbing alcohol after the initial wound is treated), until the wound fully closes and until the skin heals completely. Use a cotton swab to apply antiseptic, remember that excessive amounts of tea tree oil applied externally can have a cleansing effect. Internally, take: goldenseal, preferably with echinacea or take propolis or garlic (fresh or capsules) to assist healing. Use propolis or garlic capsules for children. (See "Natural Remedies

Glossary" for varied dosages.) Take for one or two weeks, or as required.

For larger wounds, bandage and pack in ice (a bag of frozen peas or corn works perfectly as it is not too freezing) to stop bleeding, and proceed to emergency room. If the wound is not too large or you question the need to go to the hospital, consult your doctor immediately to be sure!

To prevent bruising use witch hazel, comfrey, horsetail or calendula creams.

See also *Bleeding, Excessive,* if there is a problem closing the wound.

4. Helpful Supplements and Dosages

- Take 1,000–2,000 mg of vitamin C one to three times daily, depending on how big the wound is. If the wound gets infected, double these amounts.
- Take one to three vitamin B50 complex capsules or tablets daily for stress, calming and healing.
- Take a multivitamin supplement daily while healing.
- Take 15–50 mg of zinc daily to speed healing and for wound repair and preventing scarring.
- For major wounds, take: Rescue Remedy®, Traumeel®, or St. John's wort to calm and stabilize the patient.
- Optional: Take one or two of these: arnica, MSM or DMSO, and glucosamine sulfate for pain and to assist wound healing.

5. Cautions and Exceptions

A major cut may require stitches. If the cut (even a small one) is infected or suspected of being infected, a doctor's exam is necessary. Contact your doctor or the nearest hospital emergency room, if either of these is a possibility.

6. Nutrition Aids and Recommended Foods

No major diet changes are required for small cuts, however a wholesome diet is always important to healing. Make sure the digestion is good so the body can concentrate on healing without leaving a scar. As always, avoid too many fats and junk foods. A little flaxseed in the diet is helpful. Lots of green vegetables and some green food products are excellent for wound healing.

7. Beverage and Herbal Tea Suggestions
Vegetable juices, especially those with carrots are particularly beneficial. Helpful herbal teas include: peppermint, bilberry, chamomile, echinacea, fenugreek, alfalfa, senna (in combination with others), yarrow and sometimes comfrey, horsetail and/or myrrh are beneficial.

-D-

DANDRUFF

See also *Candida* and *Hair Problems*

Dandruff has many contributing causes, however, it is usually a sign of Candida yeast problems. The dry flaking scalp usually associated with seborrhea skin problems is actually too much oil clogging the sebaceous glands. Brush scalp for several minutes before shampooing. Be sure to wash your hair with a tea tree oil shampoo or a shampoo that contains selenium. Rinse very thoroughly, because poor washing and insufficient rinsing can contribute to the problem. Avoid using hair sprays and gels, especially if they contain alcohol.

Helpful Supplements include vitamins A, B complex and E; selenium; horsetail or silica; zinc; and either evening primrose, salmon or flaxseed oil. Make sure to eat a wholesome diet including fish, lecithin, natural flax and pumpkin oils, ground flaxseed and yogurt. It is best to follow the diet and treatments for Candida. Good herbal teas include: horsetail, lemon grass, peppermint, spearmint and yarrow.

DEPRESSION

Depression is considered a disease and can have many causes, including: heredity, hormone and chemical imbalances, improper absorption of foods, nutrient deficiencies or overabundances, toxin overload, excessive cleansing, heavy metal poisoning, parasites or Candida yeast, allergies, blood sugar problems, alcoholism, excessive sugar or junk foods in the diet, thyroid problems, drug abuse, addiction and excessive stress. Some forms of depression require medical attention and may require drug treatment. For lesser problems: See *Anxiety*, and see *Insomnia* for sleep aids.

DIARRHEA

See also *Bowel Problems*

Diarrhea is frequent soft or watery stools, sometimes accompanied by stomach pains, fever, tiredness or even vomiting. It can be caused by: indigestion, bowel problems, parasites, allergies, alcohol abuse, bacterial or viral infection, caffeine, drugs or laxatives.

Activated charcoal tablets like Eucarbon® can be helpful. Bulking agents such as psyllium seeds or Awareness Products's Experience® capsules can be beneficial, as can sea kelp tablets, whey liquid or acidophilus. Try one of the following anti-viral treatments: colloidal silver, oregano oil, olive leaf extract, garlic, citricidal or cayenne capsules.

Beneficial foods that help to naturally halt diarrhea include whole grains like brown rice and millet, cooked orange and white vegetables (including potatoes) and carob. Helpful teas include: elder, fenugreek, ginger, peppermint, raspberry leaf, slippery elm, yarrow and occasionally comfrey or St. John's wort. Avoid flower teas. Drink lots of spring water daily. Let mild diarrhea run its course for two to three days before trying drugs. Consult your doctor if symptoms continue or are severe.

DIGESTION AND DIGESTIVE PROBLEMS

You have to work with your body to develop eating habits that suit your personal needs and level of health, and that will benefit you and complement your lifestyle. Once you understand the principles of wholesome eating, you can devise your own diet plans for optimum health and enjoyment from eating. This section teaches important, basic principles for most healthful diets. Ask your health specialist, if necessary, to assist you in determining your needs.

Digestion and How It Works

The body breaks down foods in two basic ways. Carbohydrates (grains and starches) and some other foods such as vegetables, fruits and legumes need to be mixed with a good amount of saliva to break down properly when they get to the small intestine, where they are assimilated by the body. These foods pass through the stomach but are not primarily digested there. Proteins and some other foods (like acidic fruits) need to be in the mouth only long enough for you to chew them into small bits so that they are digested properly when they reach the stomach, where they mainly break down and are absorbed. These foods include meat, seafood, eggs, nuts and dairy products. Red meats including pork, lamb and beef take the longest to digest, taking up to six hours in the stomach. Acidic fruits like grapefruit, lemons, limes, tomatoes, cranberries and pineapples help break down meats and dairy products.

To assist digestion, follow principles of food combining: eat foods that are broken down like carbohydrates and those that are digested like proteins at separate meals. There are some exceptions. For instance, most vegetables are complementary to either carbohydrate-digested or protein-digested foods. Food-combining principles are based on the body's natural processes (see also "Food Combining" under *Weight Loss*).

Many doctors, even some holistic ones, do not believe in food combining. But the proof of its value comes when you use it: It works! It *does* help those with digestive problems and impaired health. There are many different schools of thought about what comprises proper food combining. The methods presented under *Weight Loss* are tested and have been found quite effective when properly utilized and adapted to the individual.

Without proper digestion, good health is not possible and healing is slowed or halted. A healthy person who is happy with their weight does not need to worry about how they combine their food. Poor food combining requires extra body energy for digestion and if one is healthy, one can get away with this. However, during cleansing or illness or when trying to lose weight, the body is under added stress. This may interfere with digestion, creating more toxins in your system and making digestion more difficult. The more energy that is taken up by digestion, the less goes to healing the body. Digestion requires a great deal of body energy for most individuals who do not use food combining. In the average healthy individual, it can take up to 40 to 60 percent of the body's physical energy each day. An unhealthy individual, with impaired or extremely poor digestion, may use up to 80 percent of the body's physical energy to digest food.

When you use the principles of good nutrition and digestion (see "Tips for Good Digestion" following), digestion time and the energy it takes can be reduced. Excellent digestion requires little more than 20 percent of physical body energy.

Good-Tasting Foods Help Digestion

Digestion begins in the mouth. If you like the flavor of a food, you salivate more, releasing larger amounts of digestive enzymes into your mouth. Chew food well, and mix with lots of saliva for better digestion, less constipation and less gas.

As children we have about 7,000 active taste buds in the mouth, and in our sixties as few as 700. Eating wholesome natural foods, avoiding artificial food additives and preservatives, and cleansing can revitalize our taste buds. No healthful diet or eating plan should be composed of bland and unappealing foods! It is an erroneous belief that you have to eat foods you dislike to be healthy. You are supposed to enjoy your food, even (and especially) while healing. Healthful foods should always be delicious if prepared properly.

Tips for Good Digestion

1. Prepare and eat meals in a positive frame of mind. Food is harder to digest when one is under stress. Do not eat when upset, angry or tense. Or, if you must eat while under stress, eat lightly and chew foods carefully.

2. Eat in a calm, peaceful atmosphere. Pleasant, low music can be a plus. Avoid watching TV or reading while eating; it takes concentration away from digesting food. Casual, low conversation is fine during eating. Looking at outdoor views can be relaxing.

3. Eat only when you are hungry and eat only enough to feel good. Never stuff yourself. It is better to let food spoil in the garbage than to let it spoil in your stomach. Spoiled food is perfect food for Candida yeast. Excessive food clogs the system, robs the body of energy and, of course, adds inches to your waistline.

4. Chew food well. Digestion begins in the mouth. If you eat more slowly, you generally eat less and absorb more nutrients.

5. Do not eat when you are overtired, or because you are restless, bored or have nothing else to do. Try cooking when you feel like nibbling; the process of cooking satisfies in a way that actually helps decrease food cravings.

6. Do not eat a big meal before sleeping or lying down. Digestion can take twice as long while the body rests. Let your stomach and intestines rest with you. If your body type, health or low blood sugar requires that you eat before bedtime, try cooked yams, winter squash, whole grain crackers, a little cooked whole grains or other cooked vegetables.

7. After eating, get some mild exercise to help stimulate digestion: walking, gentle bike riding, or washing the dishes. If digestion is sluggish, try digestive aids or teas, self-burping, self-massage or a few minutes of deep breathing, 30 minutes or more after eating. If before bedtime, try sleep-inducing deep breathing. These techniques are found in the "Healing Aids" section.

Severe Digestive Problems

People with severe digestive problems have such low energy that it takes them twice or even three times as long as the average person to digest a meal, and even then foods are not completely broken down and their nutrients utilized. Stools may contain chunks of food, and the constituents of the last meal may be clearly recognizable.

Some people with low energy (due to bad health and/or poor food combining) have so much trouble digesting because their bodies cannot adjust the temperatures of foods eaten to an acceptable temperature for digestion. Healthy individuals can drink a hot beverage and cool it in their system or eat ice cream and warm it in their system for proper assimilation. Have you ever eaten ice cream and had the momentary response I call "cold throat"—you are eating too fast and suddenly your whole mouth and throat react? You have to stop what you are doing; it is so cold you cannot stand it. Individuals with severe digestive troubles usually have food allergies and a sensitive reaction to foods that are too hot or too cold. A sip or two of ice water can throw the body temperature off so that these people feel cold for hours. Severe digestive problems like this require Rotation diets (rotating different foods so that the same ones are not eaten each day) and basic, wholesome foods cooked very simply and eaten not too hot or too cold.

High quality or, even better, organic whole grains, legumes and vegetables are essential, and should be prepared with seasonings that are not too fancy, complicated or spicy. Whole grains should be well cooked with extra water and eaten warm. Puree grains and add them to soups for easiest digestion. Brown, beige and black legumes are best (avoid the white ones), blended into soups or mashed and eaten warm. (These beans are higher in nutrients like proteins, calcium, phosphorus, potassium, iron and zinc and are less starchy.) It is best to eat grains and legumes singly rather than mix two or more whole grains or two or more legumes together at one meal.

Vegetables must be juiced raw or cooked very tender before eating, by steaming, baking or broiling. No raw salads, nuts, seeds, wheat, dairy or meats should be in this diet for severe digestive problems (you may also follow this diet while ill or cleansing). A few herbs and seasonings are okay; in fact, they are important because they make the food tasty and so aid digestion. As the body begins to heal, other foods can be reintroduced into the diet.

Exercise, self-massage, deep breathing and digestive aids and other healing aids are imperative for speedy and complete healing.

-E-

EARACHE AND EAR INFECTIONS

See also *Allergies* and *Candida*

1. Condition and Cause
Ear infections or recurrent infections of the middle ear, are common in infants and young children. Swimmer's ear, an infection of the outer ear, is more common in older children and adults. Allergies, especially food allergies, to dairy products and wheat,

are a common cause of ear infections. Candidiasis or yeast infection is another cause. Living with smokers can contribute to ear infections, especially for children. A cold or flu or other illnesses can contribute to earaches.

2. Ailment History, Signs and Early Treatments

A century ago and less, castor oil or bran and salt poultices were used on ear infections. Got a bug in your ear? Shine a light in it to guide the critter out, or pour warm water or warm olive oil in and tilt your head to pour it out. This old-fashioned treatment still works today.

3. Modern Natural Treatments and Remedies

One of the most common natural treatments is putting a few drops of freshly squeezed (preferably organic) garlic or onion juice into one teaspoon of pure spring or distilled water, and using a cotton swab to dab it just inside the ear. Or make an earplug out of cotton, wet the tip in the water/juice mixture and insert in the ear. A dropper can also be used to drop the mixture in the ear. Castor oil is also applied in the same way as garlic. A more pleasant smelling way (there is no smell to this) to ease ear infection and pain is to pour one half to one teaspoon of colloidal silver into the ear while lying on your side, and to then keep the infected ear up for about 10 minutes. An ear dropper can also be used to add the colloidal silver to the ear. Use 10 ppm colloidal silver—or, for greater potency, 24–30 ppm. This is one of the best methods.

Other treatments that may be applied by eardrops or cotton earplugs—and that *do* have a smell—are warm lobelia tincture or extract (without alcohol), St. John's wort tincture or extract (without alcohol) or one or two drops of oregano oil diluted in two or three teaspoons of water. Homeopathic remedies for earaches are also available from health stores.

Wax buildup and/or Candida in the ears can also cause irritation and contribute to infection. Your doctor can use a warm water flush or suction to remove them, or you may try ear coning or candling by a qualified ear candling specialist.

Doing a Candida treatment along with the Candida diet can also help to kill many infections. Also get tested for allergies and Candida and take energizing supplements to boost the immune system.

Note that treatment with antibiotics usually makes ear infections worse instead of better, since they increase Candida problems in adults and older children and thrush in young children.

4. Helpful Supplements and Dosages

- Take 1,000–2,000 mg vitamin C two or three times daily as required, to boost immunity and speed healing.
- Take 500–1,000 mg echinacea once or twice a day to boost immunity.
- Take 15–50 mg zinc daily, all at once or spread through the day, for healing. Zinc lozenges may be used.
- Take a vitamin B50 complex two or three times a day to relieve stress and promote healing.
- Optional but helpful: Take one of the following daily: a clove of garlic, chopped and not chewed, as described under *Toxin Overload*; 500 mg propolis; or citricidal or olive leaf extract (See the "Natural Remedies Glossary" for dosages of citricidal and olive leaf extract) or two capsules or tablets of goldenseal once or twice a day. For children, a small amount of colloidal silver taken internally is better. Children may alternatively take garlic capsules, citricidal tablets or a daily drop of oregano oil diluted in a tablespoon of pure water.

5. Cautions and Exceptions

Severe ear infections may cause a ruptured eardrum. Diving in water or air (as in skydiving or bungee jumping), sudden changes of air pressure, extremely loud noises, an injury or fall or a blow to the side of the head can also cause eardrums to rupture. Consult your doctor if earache does not subside in a day or so, if pain becomes severe or if dizziness, ringing, bleeding or hearing loss occurs in one or both ears.

6. Nutrition Aids and Recommended Foods

Avoid dairy products, breads and all other high mucus causing foods. Follow the recommendations for foods and nutrition aids for Candida.

7. Beverage and Herbal Tea Suggestions
Follow the beverage recommendations for Candida. These herbal teas are also beneficial: alfalfa, chamomile, echinacea, horsetail, lemon grass, peppermint, spearmint, yarrow and hops.

ENERGY, LOW

1. Condition and Cause
There are multiple causes for low energy, including exhaustion or overtiredness from overworking, overplaying, overexertion or not enough sleep. In addition, digestive problems, allergies, stress, disease, excessive cleansing, increased body toxins, depression, vitamin and mineral imbalances, Candida, parasites, weakened immune system, heavy metal poisoning, blood sugar problems, pregnancy, aging, substance abuse and bacterial or viral infections can all contribute to, or be a major cause of, decreased energy levels. Frequent energy lows are common symptoms of chronic fatigue syndrome, fibromyalgia and many other diseases.

2. Ailment History, Signs and Early Treatments
Until the early years of the 20th century, most people worked from sun up until sun down, six days a week as a normal routine. According to holistic health experts, overall energy levels have decreased in the North American population as a result of more sedentary lifestyles; increased consumption of sugar, sweets, refined starches and junk foods; and more frequent use of drugs for everything from headaches and indigestion to major diseases.

Early Egyptians and Greeks used garlic for strength and stamina. In the last century, supposedly rejuvenating liquid elixirs were sold from wagons and general stores for everything from backache to old age as "miracle cures" for "whatever ailed ya."

3. Modern Natural Treatments and Remedies
There are actually several modern-day energy-increasing elixirs sold in health food stores, including Bio Strath® liquid or tablets (take according to package directions), Essiac® or Floressence® liquids (take one to two tablespoons with boiled water according to bottle directions).

My favorite supplement is royal jelly, which is produced by bees.

Russian athletes use it for strength and endurance, and it also makes a great aphrodisiac. Take 300–500 mg of pure royal jelly once or twice daily, but not within a couple of hours of sleeping. The Montana brands are the highest quality North American varieties and surpass most Asian imports. Garlic also increases energy.

Other energizers include ginkgo biloba, an antioxidant that increases oxygen in the body and especially the brain. It is well known for its anti-aging properties and for improving the memory. Take 60 mg of the extract one to three times daily or as directed by your physician. Gotu kola, an Asian energizer and immune system stimulator, should be taken only under the supervision of a holistic physician. For energy for those over 40, see *Ginseng* in the "Natural Remedies Glossary." Adults as well as children can also use peppermint aromatherapy oil (a drop at a time on the wrists) for mild stimulation.

4. Recommended Supplements and Dosages

- Vitamin C—especially Allergy C, Ester C or Buffered C, can boost energy and bolster the immune system. Take 500–1,000 mg one to four times daily as needed, at least three or four hours before sleeping. Children can take chewable vitamin C or vitamin C powder mixed in some solid foods.
- Green food products can sometimes aid energy levels. See *Cleansing* in the "Healing Aids" section for directions on how to take them.

5. Cautions and Exceptions

Do not give ginkgo biloba, gotu kola, ginseng or the packaged energizers to children. Children may take royal jelly under the guidance of a holistic expert. Amino acids like L-glutamine, L-phenylalanine and L-tyrosine can be helpful for some individuals but can be dangerous for certain health conditions and are best taken on a holistic physician's recommendation.

Do not take energizing supplements before sleeping as they may keep you awake. Remember that energizers are not a replacement for rest and sleep. Do not use too many different energizers at one time. Do not use energizing supplements with drugs or alcohol. Take them preferably four hours or more away from prescription drugs.

6. Nutrition Aids and Recommended Foods

A high-nutrient diet of whole foods supports and enhances high energy levels. Sugar, sugar substitutes, excessive amounts of any sweets, refined foods and junk foods deplete energy and weaken the immune system. Eat lots of vegetables, whole grains, seeds and legumes, especially orange and green vegetables, brown rice, millet, pinto beans, adzuki beans, black beans, chickpeas, yogurt, miso and bee pollen. Avoid foods that require extra energy to digest, like cheeses, milk, red meats, corn products, fried foods, iceberg/head lettuce, raw broccoli or cauliflower and large quantities of raw salad.

7. Beverage and Herbal Tea Suggestions

Vegetable juices three to five times weekly and protein power drinks two to four times weekly are great pick-me-ups. Ginseng (for those over 40), mint and ginger teas are also stimulating.

Organic green tea provides a more beneficial form of caffeine than coffee as green tea contains tannins, which have astringent and antibacterial qualities.

EYE PROBLEMS

Many holistic health practitioners and doctors use *iridology* to assess a person's overall health, and health history. Iridology involves reading the health condition of the whole body by examining the lines and circles in the eyes.

Weak, swollen, bloodshot, itchy or watery eyes can be caused by tiredness or sleep deprivation, environmental or household poisons, dust or dirt particles in the eyes, allergies, poor diet or liver malfunction, among other things. Health stores carry eye drops and eyewashes with MSM and healing herbs. Or you can make your own eyewash with strained, room temperature chamomile, raspberry leaf or witch hazel tea.

Most dairy products are detrimental to eyesight. North American herbalists and Asian physicians remove or decrease dairy products from the diets of individuals who wear glasses or have eyesight problems as these high mucus foods contribute to decreased vision and blurred vision as well as digestive problems and decreased energy that can and does interfere with vision. Eating dairy products, especially cheeses and milk should be avoided indefinitely. A little occasional butter or yogurt is okay for most individuals unless eye problems are extreme. This is particularly important for individuals with cataracts. Vitamins A, B complex, C and E, along with zinc and some amino acids, may be helpful for many eyesight problems. Eat wholesome whole grains, legumes, tofu, fish, a little high-quality meat (no pork, processed, ground or luncheon meats), lots of green and orange vegetables, sprouts, green food products, orange fruits, blueberries and yogurt several times a week. Healing and soothing herbal teas include bayberry, bilberry, calendula, chamomile, eyebright, dandelion (or dandelion coffee), lemon grass, raspberry leaf and slippery elm, and occasionally white willow bark or goldenseal.

-F-

FAINTING

Fainting is caused by a diminished flow of blood and oxygen to the brain. It can be brought on by: shock, upsetting news, low blood sugar, improper eating or a fall or injury, among other things. If a person faints from a fall or injury, get them immediate medical help.

Give the person who has fainted some juice or fruit as soon as possible to raise their blood sugar. Give them a tea of ginger, peppermint, spearmint or lemon grass with possibly a dash of cayenne to revive them. If they need to sleep, give them chamomile, catnip or skullcap tea. They can be given Rescue Remedy®, Traumeel®, valerian capsules or St. John's wort if they have had a shock or upsetting news.

FEVER

See also *Colds, Flu* and *Infections*

1. Condition and Cause
A fever, or elevated body temperature, is a symptom of a disease or of a toxin-overloaded body. Slightly higher temperatures can actually help the body by "burning off" or destroying bacteria and

harmful microorganisms. It is sometimes best to let a fever run its course and clear out body poisons. Low-grade fever (lasting several days or more) may occur while parasites and/or viruses are active in the body. A moderately high fever (over 102°F or 39°C for adults, over 103°F or 39.5°C for children and over 100°F or 38°C for infants) of long duration (more than two full days) can be a possible health problem for young children, pregnant women (especially during the first three months) and people with heart problems. Contact your doctor immediately if this occurs, especially if there are other accompanying side effects such as vomiting or breathing difficulties.

2. Ailment History, Signs and Early Treatments

"Starve a fever, feed a cold," is an old-fashioned, famous quote that often gets turned around (to say "feed a fever…"). In fact, a liquid diet is best when one has a fever. Folk remedies for fever include wrapping onion and garlic slices to the bottoms of the feet, which was used to bring down the temperature. Grapes and grape juice were consumed during the day, or orange juice with honey and cayenne were taken together to break the fever. Another popular treatment was drinking the strained liquid from cooking barley (half a cup every two hours or less) to reduce a fever, and this remedy is still used today. Barley water was also used in an enema.

3. Modern Natural Treatments and Remedies

The best course of action for a mild or moderate fever is to ride it out, unless it lasts more than two days. Take two or three baths and/or showers a day to purge poisons and be sure to cleanse the skin as explained under *Skin Cleansing* in the "Healing Aids" section. Include one bath a day with Epsom salts or a few shakes of tea tree oil to purge body toxins, and/or (for all but young children) take a daily sauna or steam bath to increase circulation.

Stay with liquid foods, such as: clear or light blended soups, vegetable juices (especially those with carrots and a bit of beet) and herbal teas with honey and fresh lemon juice, if desired.

Take sponge baths with cool water as needed and rub yourself with a towel afterwards. If bedridden, sponge baths (some with warm water and soap) must be given several times daily in place of baths, showers and saunas. Use cool compresses for the head and, if required, use body poultices with peppermint, ginger, fenugreek or catnip teas (with a touch of cayenne added if desired).

Take lobelia tea made with an equal part of one of the following: peppermint, ginger or dandelion herbs, a few teaspoonfuls every 3–4 hours. (Reduce the dosage if it upsets your stomach.) Sometimes the juice of a small lemon or ½ large lemon helps sweat out the fever, taken either full strength or (for the more sensitive) diluted in an equal amount of hot or very warm water. Barley water can also be used as described above. Catnip tea enemas can be given if needed, to reduce high temperatures.

4. Helpful Supplements and Dosages

- Take 10,000 IU of vitamin A or 25,000 IU of beta-carotene twice a day to fight infection.
- Do a Vitamin C Flush. See *Vitamin C* in the "Natural Remedies Glossary." After the flush, take 1,000–2,000 mg vitamin C every four hours or so while awake.
- Take acidophilus for adults and bifidus for children once or twice a day as described in the "Natural Remedies Glossary."
- Take a clove of garlic a day (minced and not chewed). See directions in *Toxin Overload.* Or take echinacea (1,000 mg daily), citricidal (one to three times daily in small doses), propolis or royal jelly (300–500 mg daily for either).

5. Cautions and Exceptions

If temperature exceeds the highs or duration given earlier, or if there are uncomfortable side effects or complications (such as shortness of breath, spots in the throat, swollen glands or excessive chills) consult your doctor immediately! Do not take any mineral supplements, especially iron, during fevers, as they may nourish the infection and prolong the fever.

6. Nutrition Aids and Recommended Foods

Until the fever breaks, stick with clear or light blended soups, vegetable juices, herbal teas and freshly squeezed grapefruit juice or unsweetened cranberry juice. Avoid all dairy products, especially milk, as well as junk foods, fatty foods and sweet or sugary foods; raw vegetables except for juices; and fruits other than those mentioned here. If you must eat solid food, try a little soft, ripe avocado, well-cooked, mashed yam, carrots or winter squash, or well-cooked, very tender green vegetables like broccoli or asparagus.

7. Beverage and Herbal Tea Suggestions
Good fever teas include feverfew, fenugreek, catnip, chamomile, lemon grass, elderberry or elder flower, white willow bark, sassafras, peppermint, echinacea, ginger, dandelion, yarrow and sometimes licorice. Also see the suggestions in "Modern Natural Treatments and Remedies" above.

FLATULENCE

1. Condition and Cause
Flatulence is the presence of gas in the digestive tract that creates an unflattering sound as it exits the body, often accompanied by a foul smell. Flatulence is caused by improper digestion of food, which may be due to eating while tired, digestive problems, health problems, bad food combining, eating too fast, eating improperly cooked or prepared food, eating spoiled food, not chewing foods enough, eating while stressed, drinking too much liquid with foods or lying down after eating.

2. Ailment History, Signs and Early Treatments
There have been jokes about flatulence through the ages, and attitudes toward gas have run the gamut from embarrassment to pride. Folk cures include eating an onion sandwich, drinking liqueurs and placing hot compresses on the stomach area.

3. Modern Natural Treatments and Remedies
Prevention is the best help for gas. If you are doing any of the things listed in "Condition and Cause" above, stop! Digestive aids, herbal teas and good food combining can also help correct the problem (see *Indigestion* for digestive aids). Rather than sitting or lying down after eating, take a walk, do mild exercise or do the dishes after

eating. A little light self-massage on the digestive organs and stomach area can help stimulate digestion one half hour or so after eating.

4. Helpful Supplements and Dosages

- To replenish friendly bacteria and help digestion, take two high-quality acidophilus capsules with four to six ounces of pure water once or twice a day, an hour or more away from food. (Don't take acidophilus if you have high stomach acid.) Try to use a brand that includes added FOSs (fructooligosaccharides), which aid the growth of friendly bacteria. Take before and/or after breakfast and/or lunch, not after supper.
- Take digestive aids and/or laxative teas and flushing agents as needed. See the "Natural Remedies Glossary" for different digestive aids and see the "Healing Aids" section as well for self-massage and other aids.

5. Cautions and Exceptions

Avoid eating improperly cooked beans (see my other books for proper cooking methods), eating beans and meat in the same meal (as in chili dishes), eating overly spicy foods and eating improper food combinations.

6. Nutrition Aids and Recommended Foods

Follow the major food combining rules. See my books for complete rules. The two main rules are:

1. Do not eat heavy proteins and heavy starches (like poultry and rice) at the same meal, as this slows digestion and causes you to absorb more calories while interfering with the proper breakdown and absorption of foods. For protein-digested meals, include meat, vegetable salad and/or vegetable soup and/or vegetable side dishes and optional nuts, eggs or dairy products. For carbohydrate-digested meals, include whole grains and/or legumes (or tofu), vegetable salad and/or vegetable soup and/or vegetable side dishes.

2. Do not eat raw fruits with other foods. Eat them alone or as a first course, never after a meal. Fruit digests very

quickly when eaten alone, but when eaten with other foods, it can spoil in the system, creating toxins or contributing to gas and indigestion.

(Other food-combining rules and exceptions should also be considered. See *Weight Problems* for more details on Food Combining.)

7. Beverage and Herbal Tea Suggestions
Peppermint, spearmint, fennel, fenugreek, ginger or chamomile tea, drunk 30 minutes or more before or after a meal, can help stimulate digestion. Avoid drinking liquids *with* meals, as they dilute digestive enzymes and interfere with digestion. If you must drink during meals limit yourself to three to five ounces of water, club soda or wine (if wine is suitable for your body type and you are not allergic). With protein meals it is okay to drink a little tomato or fresh grapefruit juice or vegetable juice (three to five ounces). With carbohydrate meals you may drink a little vegetable juice (three to five ounces). See the digest aid drinks in "Remedies from Your Refrigerator and Cupboard."

FLU

See also *Colds, Coughs, Fever, Infections* and *Sore Throats*

1. Condition and Cause
Influenza, commonly known as the flu, is caused by contagious viruses that infect the respiratory tract. You can get infected, if your resistance is low, from a touch, a kiss, or from airborne viruses from a sneeze or cough either directly encountered, or left behind in an elevator, car or room, during the early stages of the disease. Flu symptoms may include fever, muscle aches, headaches, fatigue, chills, sore throat, cough and runny or stuffy nose. In some cases, mental confusion, ear infections, nausea and vomiting occur. The most dangerous complication is pneumonia.

2. Ailment History, Signs and Early Treatments
Influenza is the fifth-highest cause of death in North America, and more than 20,000 people a year die as a result of flu in the

United States alone. Many more people are hospitalized and millions of North Americans get the flu each year.

3. Modern Natural Treatments and Remedies

During the first three or four days, eat a light vegetarian diet; mainly steamed vegetables (no raw vegetables), hot soups, vegetable juices with a green food product and herbal teas. A little fish may be eaten if desired. Avoid all dairy products, breads, pasta, cereals, refined foods, fried or fatty foods, sweet fruits, sweets, sugar and junk foods. After the first four days, you may eat some heavier foods if you feel like it, but do not eat a lot of meat. Still none of the "avoid foods" preceding should be eaten.

Use the antibacterial mouthwashes and gargles listed under *Oral Hygiene Problems*. Rest, keep warm and out of drafts and take baths and saunas as recommended under *Colds* and *Fever*, and also see these sections for more information.

Take one of the following remedies daily:

1. Drink the freshly squeezed juice of ½ large or one small lemon or lime once or twice a day (swish the juice around the mouth to kill bacteria before swallowing). Drink it straight or, for more sensitive individuals, dilute the juice in equal parts of hot or very warm, spring or distilled water. Take the remedy on an empty stomach and follow with a sip or two of water (which will taste sweet after the tart citrus), if desired. You can eat non-sweet fruit or other food half an hour later.

2. Once a day, halfway through a meal, eat a clove of garlic, minced finely (not pressed) and not chewed but washed down with water. (You can also chew a clove of garlic a day, right after a meal or a little later. Spit out the pulp. Chewing garlic kills bacteria in the mouth and throat and sooths coughs and sore throats.) Taking garlic that is not chewed or pressed during a meal kills bacteria, parasites and viruses in the intestines.

4. Helpful Supplements and Dosages

- Take 10,000 IU of vitamin A or 25,000 IU of beta-carotene twice a day to fight infection.

- Do a Vitamin C Flush. See *Vitamin C* in the "Natural Remedies Glossary." After the flush, take 1,000–2,000 mg vitamin C every four hours or so while awake.
- Take acidophilus for adults and bifidus for children once or twice a day, as described in the "Natural Remedies Glossary."
- Use *one* of the following daily—in small doses—after the first four days: cayenne, astragalus, goldenseal (can be with echinacea), propolis, oregano oil, olive leaf extract or colloidal silver. (If garlic is taken as mentioned above, this remedy may not be necessary.)
- Zinc lozenges, 15–50 mg total daily, can be used after the first four days if there is no fever.

5. Cautions and Exceptions

Flu, like fever, can be especially detrimental to pregnant women, young children, those with a weakened immune system or other health problems and the elderly. These people should take preventative measures to avoid the flu. Cold prevention methods, listed under *Colds*, can also help prevent flu. If you are in one of these risk categories and contract the flu, consult your doctor. If complications arise or if you show signs of pneumonia—shaking, chills, high temperature, rapid or difficult breathing, chest or stomach pain—consult your doctor immediately!

6. Nutrition Aids and Recommended Foods

See #3 in the treatments section, above.

7. Beverage and Herbal Tea Suggestions

Do not drink any soda pop, alcohol or sweet fruit juices (like peach, pear or tropical juices), especially those with added sugar or other sweeteners. Drink six to eight glasses of water a day to flush the system. Lots of hot herbal tea is very beneficial. Drink it without milk or cream, and with lemon and/or honey (and an optional dash of cayenne to break up mucus). Enjoy one or more of the following: echinacea, raspberry leaf, yarrow, elderberry, lemon grass, slippery elm, ginger, mint or skullcap. Skullcap tea is particularly good for flu, as it helps induce sleep and relieve anxiety.

Also enjoy vegetable juices, especially those with carrots and a green food product, and other beverages listed in the refrigerator remedies section. Avoid drinking milk, cream and all dairy-based drinks, and avoid using dairy products in soups and other recipes as well because they increase mucus and prolong runny nose, sinus problems and sore throat. Drink grapefruit juice rather than orange juice (especially if you also have Candida yeast problems), for its better antibacterial properties. Take lemon or lime juice as described in the treatments section above. Organic green tea is better than coffee during flu.

FOOD COMBINING

See *Digestion Problems* and *Weight Problems*

FOOD POISONING

For serious problems call your doctor. For minor discomfort see *Stomachache* or *Nausea.*

FUNGAL INFECTIONS

See *Candida, Jock Itch* and *Yeast Infections*

-G-

GAS

See *Digestion Problems* and *Flatulence*

-H-

HAIR PROBLEMS

See also *Dandruff and Nail Problems*

For dull, unhealthy hair that breaks easily, be sure to add enough natural oils to your diet: flaxseed oil, pumpkin seed oil, olive oil and sesame oil in particular. The best way to use these is in salad dressings. Salads and vegetables are particular beneficial. Good digestion and bowel health is imperative to healthy hair as well. Oregano oil, even just one drop taken internally, daily for 30–90 days, will transform your hair (as well as your nails) and make it strong, shiny, full and thick, and healthy. By the third day or so of taking oregano oil you will probably notice how exceptionally soft your hair is.

You may also try a Chinese remedy called Shen Min® from BioTech Corporation, which is made from a 10-12-year-old Asian root. The product, which contains anthraquinones and resveratrol, is a hair nutrient that causes hair to grow in thicker, and is especially good for growing new hair, for men and women. Olive oil with an optional drop or two of oregano oil can be massaged into the hair and left on for 15–20 minutes, once a week or so (be sure to wash it out thoroughly after) also. Gelatin capsules (filled with unflavored gelatin) are another long-established treatment for stronger, healthier hair (and nails). See the "Natural Remedies Glossary" for how to take gelatin. Nutrients for nails are also beneficial.

Be sure to use quality natural shampoo. Avoid the cheap stuff or two-in-one shampoo and conditioner combinations, and get split ends cut off regularly to help keep your hair healthy. Brushing and massaging the hair and scalp regularly will make your hair shiny and healthy. Brushing helps to distribute the natural oils in your hair evenly as well.

DRY HAIR CLEANER If you can't wash your hair because you are sick, or if you just do not want to get your hair wet, beat two or three egg whites until stiff peaks form, massage into the hair, let sit for 15 minutes or so and then brush out over a bathtub. Oiliness will be gone and your hair will look good for two to four days. My mother actually taught me this old folk remedy. I have used it many times.

Good medicinal teas for preventing hair loss are horsetail, nettle, rosemary, sage, yarrow and burdock. Ginger or cayenne tea or tincture can be massaged into the scalp and left in for 20 minutes or so to stimulate hair growth. Pleasure teas include chamomile, ginger and lemon grass.

HALITOSIS

See *Bad Breath*

HANGOVER

See *Alcohol Problems* and, in the refrigerator remedies section, the recipes for Hangover Helpers.

HAY FEVER

Hay fever season usually begins in the spring—around March, April or May depending on the area of the country. Hay fever is an allergic reaction to pollen and can cause runny nose, itchy and watery eyes, sneezing, fatigue and jitters. Many people find relief by taking the Hay Fever Helper drink in the refrigerator remedies section for three months *before* hay fever season begins. It usually alleviates future problems with pollen. Most people can desensitize themselves to pollen by taking *local* honey and/or bee pollen long enough in advance of hay fever season.

If hay fever season is already in progress, try garlic or another antiviral treatment. Cleansing can also help relieve some or even all the symptoms of allergies to pollen. An annual or twice-yearly cleanse can boost the immune system and assist healing. It is best to cleanse *before*—not during—hay fever season as the side effects could be quite severe if cleansing is done during that time. Take energy supplements like vitamin C, ginseng or dong quai, and drink energizing teas such as ginger, peppermint, spearmint, eucalyptus, lemon grass and ginseng. Avoid drinking flower-based herbal teas such as chamomile, calendula and elderflower.

HEAD LICE

Head lice are contagious and are frequently passed among young school children. Treat with tea tree oil shampoos and head-lice kits, which can be purchased at your health food store.

HEADACHE

1. Condition and Cause
Headaches include tension headaches, with symptoms of pain, throbbing and/or aching, and sinus headaches, with symptoms of congestion and inflammation. Headaches are caused by stress, upset, allergies, indigestion, hunger, eye strain, muscle tension, pinched nerves, improper or extreme fasting or cleansing, constipation and bowel problems, circulation problems, too much sugar or salt, caffeine, lack of water or fluids, artificial food additives, blood sugar problems, PMS, alcohol, illness and diseases.

2. Ailment History, Signs and Early Treatments
Head, neck and forehead compresses of apple cider vinegar, chopped onion or garlic, or horseradish were used traditionally for some headache treatments. Folk remedies also include standing in the bathtub in ice-cold water until you are so cold you forget the headache! This remedy would actually relieve some headaches by boosting the body's circulation.

3. Modern Natural Treatments and Remedies
First see if you can figure out the cause of your headache. Think about it. If you have not eaten all day, an ocean of aspirin or natural painkillers will not help. If you have eaten poorly, quickly make and slowly drink one of the power protein drinks from the refrigerator remedies section. If you have not had enough sleep, get it. Take a sleep aid if needed (see *Insomnia*). If you are not digesting well, take digestive aids with your next meals and right away take three capsules of acidophilus with half a glass of water at least an hour before eating again. Then take two capsules acidophilus once or twice a day. If your headache is caused by an allergic reaction, immediately take 2,000–4,000 mg vitamin C or 1,500 mg Allergy C.

White willow bark and feverfew are two natural headache remedies usually found in packages at your health food store; take one of them as directed. (Never take both together.) Do not take aspirin together with these natural remedies, because they antagonize one another. Vitamin C (especially Allergy C) can help relieve headaches, as can other energizing supplements; experience has shown that

750–1,500 mg of Allergy C, like Twin Labs Allergy C®, is really effective for wiping out many types of headaches, and not just those caused by allergies. Vitamin B complex and calcium with magnesium may also help relieve stress and some headaches, though they may not eliminate all the pain. Clinical studies show 5-HTP to be effective for headaches and migraines. Peppermint oil can be put on the wrists and temples to stimulate and to boost energy, which may help alleviate headaches as well.

4. Helpful Supplements and Dosages
- Take 750–2,000 mg vitamin C as required.
- Take two vitamin B50 complex when headache appears, to relieve stress and for calming.
- Take 1,000 mg calcium with magnesium.

5. Cautions and Exceptions
Migraines may require a doctor's attention. For excessive pain, recurrent headaches or headaches that will not go away, contact your doctor as soon as possible.

6. Nutrition Aids and Recommended Foods
A wholesome diet and two or three balanced meals a day are the best protection against headaches. Meals like pasta and/or shellfish, I call "headache foods" or "headache makers." Make sure you are eating *real* meals. Dry breakfast cereal or rice cakes are not a meal and neither is processed cheese spread on celery or crackers. Eat whole grains, legumes, tofu and lots of vegetables. Include flaxseed, lecithin and yogurt in your diet.

7. Beverage and Herbal Tea Suggestions
Drink five to eight glasses of spring water every day—the more the better. Enjoy four to six glasses of fresh vegetable juice a week, especially those that include carrots and green food products. Beneficial herbal teas include elderberry or elder flower, ginger, lemon grass, raspberry leaf, peppermint, spearmint, rosemary, ginseng and ginkgo. Chamomile is good for those without allergies.

HEARTBURN

See also *Digestion Problems.*

Heartburn is a burning sensation and pain in the stomach or chest that comes with gas, bloating, nausea and acidic aftertaste. Drink a glass of water or, better yet, have one of these teas: chamomile, fennel, ginger, peppermint, spearmint or ginseng. If you are willing to brave the fiery taste, add a dash or two of cayenne. Have yogurt with some meals. Daily acidophilus is helpful, as are mealtime digestive aids, especially bromelain, papain and plant enzymes. Eat a wholesome diet, avoiding aggravating foods, such as junk foods, refined foods, heavy meats and caffeine. A good cleanse (and, especially, a regular cleansing regime) will really help! Avoid high calorie and low fat diets as these have recently been discovered to contribute to heartburn. If heartburn is frequent and these treatments do not help, see your doctor to make sure it is not a sign of more serious problems.

HEAVY METAL OVERDOSE

Toxic metal overdose is becoming more common as pollutants in water, air, clothing, paint, hair dyes, canned foods and drinks and workplace and household items are becoming more common. The most problematic metals include: lead, aluminum, mercury, copper, arsenic and cadmium. Symptoms may include stomach and digestive problems, hyperactivity, skin rashes, depression, irritability, anger or lethargy, thinking difficulties, cold extremities and sometimes hair falling out or breaking.

One of the most accurate forms of testing for metal overload, or other mineral overabundances or deficiencies, is hair analysis. Often a local laboratory will do this testing. Check with your holistic doctor for other sources. Other tests include urine and blood tests and, from a holistic doctor, vega testing.

Heavy metals can be removed with chelation therapy treatments administered by a holistic doctor or with chelating substances (usually in tablet or capsule form or a liquid) that bind with the offensive metal and draw it out of the body. Zinc supplements are antagonistic to many heavy metals, including lead, mercury and copper, and will usually help expel them. Chelating enzymes, like Chelazyme®, can be purchased at some health stores and holistic pharmacies or from some holistic physicians—but they often take all major metals *and* minerals from the body and can deplete precious calcium, magnesium and other needed minerals as well. High doses of vitamin C also expel heavy metals, as does a lemon juice cleanse (such as the one described in this book) or garlic cleanse. Lemon juice has an astringent effect that draws out metals. Often a metallic taste will be noticeable on the tongue within the first seven days of cleansing to remove heavy metals. Be sure to brush the tongue thoroughly during this cleanse (as with others), and clean the skin carefully too because many of the heavy metals will be expelled through the pores of the skin. Garlic is a great chelator and detoxifier, and a 30-day or longer garlic cleanse is another alternative. Another method is to use colloidal silver for about 30 days. Vitamin C can be taken any time, but it is best not to mix lemon juice, garlic and colloidal silver—use them one at a time. Lemon juice and colloidal silver are antagonistic and do not work well together as citrus expels silver as well as unwanted minerals.

Other tips:

1. Pour pop out of cans immediately after opening, rather than drinking out of them—or, better yet, buy glass (or plastic) bottles.
2. Never leave leftovers in a can in the fridge.
3. Avoid using aluminum cookware.
4. Do not buy or use cheap china for hot foods, because they may have a high lead content.
5. Do not buy cheap, toxic, chemical-smelling, pressboard bookcases, cupboards or drawers.
6. Avoid cheap, poor-quality hair dyes.
7. Never drink water from the hot water tap, because lead and copper (and sometimes cadmium) from pipes are more prevalent in hot water.
8. If living in a house, run tap water for two minutes before drinking or, better yet, drink tested spring water for good health.
9. Replace mercury dental fillings with porcelain or other non-toxic substances over a safe period of time.

10. Get a shower filter for your bathroom (or a water filter for the whole house from water companies), because many toxic metals enter the body through the skin while bathing.

Eat a wholesome diet, and avoid hard-to-digest or aggravating foods, especially shellfish, caffeine, sugars, junk foods, canned foods and foods cooked in aluminum cookware. Eat lots of vegetables, especially organic ones, and green food products in particular. Beneficial teas include lemon grass, ginger, peppermint, spearmint, dandelion (or dandelion "coffee") and burdock.

HEMORRHOIDS

See also *Digestion Problems* and *Bowel Problems* (good digestion and bowel health are essential for dealing with hemorrhoids)

Hemorrhoids, or "piles," are swollen veins and capillaries around the anus that may protrude from the anus and in the rectum. They may be itchy, bleeding, inflamed and painful. Herbal suppositories using: goldenseal, slippery elm, white oak bark or garlic can be used. Alternatively, you can rub garlic on the affected area or apply: oregano oil, colloidal silver or tea tree oil. A paste of water and goldenseal or comfrey can also be applied. As healing progresses, apply shark oil. Aloe vera can also be used, though it is not a first choice.

Sitz baths can be soothing and beneficial. Vitamins E, C and B complex can be beneficial, and digestive aids and/or laxatives may help or may be required. Regular cleansing will help eliminate hemorrhoids. As usual, avoid foods like refined and junk foods that aggravate the condition and eat a high-fiber, whole foods diet, including whole grains, legumes, lots of vegetables, flaxseed, lecithin and yogurt. Drink about six glasses of water a day between meals. Good teas include fennel, ginger, parsley, raspberry leaf, white oak bark, burdock, yarrow and myrrh.

HERPES, COLD SORES

See *Cold Sores*

HERPES, GENITAL

1. Condition and Cause

Herpes simplex II (HSV-2), or genital herpes, is a sexually transmitted disease characterized by itchy, irritating, burning blisters filled with a clear fluid that spreads the contagious disease. The small, multiple clusters of herpes blisters can cover the genital and anal area. The blisters or sores open and become more irritating, and eventually become crusty before disappearing. Tingling, burning or pain urinating can be the first signs of infection, or it may be barely noticeable, depending on the individual and the strength of the immune system. Symptoms may include headache, fever and flu-like side effects.

Herpes is the most common STD in Canada and the U.S. The initial outbreak happens within a month of exposure and may last between one and three weeks. Anyone can contract herpes; it only takes one sexual encounter. Herpes is not life threatening. Repeat outbreaks may occur only once a year or less, or may be present monthly for several weeks at a time. It depends on the individual's state of health and how strong their immune system is.

2. Ailment History, Signs and Early Treatments

Hot sitz baths were traditionally used to soothe the itchiness and discomfort of herpes outbreaks, and are still used today. Onion and garlic slices were placed on the blisters to soothe the infection. This treatment may still be used today, though it is smelly and not a first choice for comfort or convenience.

3. Modern Natural Treatments and Remedies

HERPES PREVENTION   It is imperative to avoid sexual contact when the sores are present (which is harder to detect in women because they may be inside the vagina), as this will spread the disease to whomever comes into physical contact with it. In less than 10 percent of cases, an individual may "shed the infection" without ever experiencing any symptoms. Condoms can help a little, but they protect only a small area of the genital region. It is a game of Russian roulette to have sex during a herpes outbreak. If unsure after a sexual encounter if herpes may have been contracted, chew a clove of garlic as soon as possible, and repeat daily for a few days after (or gargle with tea tree oil—see *Oral Hygiene Problems*). Also, after possibly infectious sex, take a shower and apply full strength or diluted tea tree oil all over the genital and anal areas and, for women, put some tea tree oil on the fingers and insert as high up in the vagina as possible. The full strength tea tree oil will tingle a bit for 10 or 20 minutes but it may wipe out infection. Freshly squeezed garlic or onion juice works internally in the same way, but many find the smell unpleasant.

PREVENTING REPEAT OUTBREAKS   Once herpes has been contracted, keeping the immune system boosted and healthy is the most important prevention against future outbreaks. Take multivitamin supplements and at least one daily energizing supplement (see *Energy, Low* for energizers), keep the genital area clean and dry, wear comfortable, light-colored, cotton underwear and be cautious with each new sexual partner. Take oral garlic supplements, chew a clove of garlic or take garlic as a cleansing and boosting agent (see *Toxin Overload*).

HERPES TREATMENT   If you feel the familiar beginnings of tingling or itching, take some energy-boosting supplements and start right away with oral garlic supplements, as described above. Take the supplements recommended below while the blisters are present and for several days after they disappear. Two to six times a day, dab the blisters with a cotton swab soaked in 100 percent tea tree oil (or diluted if desired) or freshly squeezed garlic (or onion) juice. Some individuals may find colloidal silver (preferably 24–30 ppm or more) which has no scent, or oregano oil to be effective. Vitamin E, vitamin A, aloe vera, comfrey, zinc and especially in lysine ointments or creams can also be applied to the blisters (rotate or use one or two of them) between use of the infection-inhibiting treatments described above. Some individuals may use health food store–quality DMSO, though it is not the best choice. SOD is also used for herpes. Do not use either of these if pregnant. There are also individual natural remedies and combinations, and homeopathic products, available in health stores and holistic pharmacies for both oral and topical treatment of herpes.

Keep the infected area clean and dry. Change cotton underwear several times a day and try to dry it in the sun—or put it in the sun for an hour or two after washing—to be sure to kill infectious bacteria. Do not sleep without underwear and pajama bottoms or nightgown. Change sheets twice weekly during infections or more if desired.

4. Helpful Supplements and Dosages

- Take 500 mg lysine two or three times daily as treatment. Take with vitamin C and vitamin B complex.
- Take 1 vitamin B50 complex three or four times a day for stress, prevention and healing.
- Take 2,000–3,000 mg vitamin C two or three times daily as treatment. (Take half this amount once or twice a day as prevention.)
- Take 30 mg bioflavonoids once or twice a day as treatment.
- Take 10,000 IU vitamin A plus 25,000 beta-carotene daily as treatment.
- Take 15–50 mg zinc once or twice a day as treatment for healing.
- Take two capsules acidophilus twice a day as treatment (see the "Natural Remedies Glossary" for method).
- Optional but helpful: Take one of the following to boost immunity and help heal infection: 500 mg propolis once daily, two capsules or tablets goldenseal (without echinacea) once daily, 300–500 mg royal jelly once or twice daily, astragalus tea or tincture two or three times daily or as directed, or a clove of garlic internally (chopped and not chewed) once daily.

5. Cautions and Exceptions

If pregnant, there is a possibility of giving herpes to the baby if an outbreak is present during childbirth. A cesarean section may be required.

6. Nutrition Aids and Recommended Foods

Eat a diet high in lysine-rich foods, such as: fish, seafood, poultry, soybeans, legumes, sprouts, green beans and potatoes. Avoid aggravating foods that are high in arginine, such as meats, dairy products, almonds, cashews, chocolate, gluten (oats, barley, wheat and rye), corn, buckwheat, sunflower and sesame seeds, peanuts and coconut.

Eat a balanced, natural diet, avoiding aggravating foods including: pork and fatty meats, and all processed cheeses, uncooked cheeses (some cooked cheeses may be eaten once or twice a week), cream, milk, margarine (a bit of butter is okay), pasta, junk foods, refined foods, spicy foods, fried foods, fatty and greasy foods, sugar, chocolate, artificial sugar substitutes, food additives and chemicals and sweet fruits.

Proper diet is essential for healing. Eat plenty of high-fiber foods: mainly vegetables, especially green and orange ones, Jerusalem artichokes, cooked leafy greens, green salads, sprouts, fish, brown rice, millet, natural oils and legumes. Include yogurt, kefir, miso and/or sauerkraut in the diet. Add ground flaxseed to yogurt or mix with other foods five or six days a week. Add lecithin granules or liquid to blender drinks or mix with foods four to six days a week until outbreak is passed.

7. Beverage and Herbal Tea Suggestions
Drink six to eight glasses of spring water daily. Drink five or six glasses of vegetable juice a week, especially those that include green food products. Alcohol and soda pops are extremely bad during herpes outbreaks. Better to drink a little diluted, non-tropical fruit juice (such as apple, peach or pear), fresh grapefruit juice, vegetable juice or water. Beneficial herbal teas include: alfalfa, astragalus, dandelion herb (or "coffee"), lemon grass, eucalyptus, peppermint, and spearmint. Sometimes take black cohosh (for women) or saw palmetto (for men). Organic green tea is better than coffee.

HICCUPS

1. Condition and Cause
Occasional hiccups are usually not a problem however frequent hiccups can be troublesome. They are a spasmodic contraction of the breathing muscle—the diaphragm. A fast rush of air and sudden closure of the throat creates the familiar "hic" sound associated with hiccups. Hiccups can occur while stressed, scared, nervous, speaking with your mouth full, eating too fast, eating foods that are too cold or too hot, eating foods to which you are allergic, eating gassy foods or hiccups can happen when the stomach is upset. Conditions

like lung disorders, alcoholism and pregnancy can cause more frequent hiccups. The actual cause of the hiccups is not always known.

2. Ailment History, Signs and Early Treatments
Old-fashioned remedies for hiccups include putting a brown paper bag over your head, breathing into a brown paper bag, getting a shock or scare, holding your breath, making yourself burp by pounding your chest with the flat of your hand or your fist, drinking water from the opposite side of a glass, drinking little sips of water while holding your breath, drinking cream of tartar in warm water, sucking on an ice cube and various other methods of self-torture that may actually work on occasion.

3. Modern Natural Treatments and Remedies
Chewing on a little piece of ginger root or ginseng root can be a helpful, stimulating healing aid. If ginger or ginseng is not handy or desirable, take one or more energizing supplements (see *Energy, Low*) to boost the immune system and provide the energy you need to relax and overcome the effects. If the hiccups are still there, follow this five or ten minutes later with a cup of stimulating or alternatively a calming herbal tea (see the beverage suggestions below). Rescue Remedy® or Traumeel® can work quickly for some hiccups that will not go away.

4. Helpful Supplements and Dosages
- Take an energizing supplement such as vitamin C, royal jelly, ginseng, gotu kola, Bio Strath®, Essiac® or Flor Essence®, or apply peppermint oil externally to wrists and possibly the temples (of an adult).
- Alternatively, take calming and soothing supplements or teas like catnip, chamomile, skullcap, hops, valerian or St. John's wort.

5. Cautions and Exceptions
For recurrent, troublesome hiccups, see your doctor.

6. Nutrition Aids and Recommended Foods
Eat slowly and chew your food well. Eat a wholesome diet.

7. Beverage and Herbal Tea Suggestions
Drink slow sips of water. Drink one (or a combination of two) of these anti-spasmodic and stimulating teas, with a dash of cayenne, which is also anti-spasmodic, if desired: fennel, ginger, ginseng, peppermint or spearmint. Teas for soothing, as well as anti-spasmodic properties are: catnip, chamomile, celery seed, black cohosh, buchu, skullcap, valerian and St. John's wort. Lobelia tea also has the same effects, but you should drink only one or two teaspoons every 5 minutes for the first 15 minutes, then every half hour if hiccups continue.

HYPOGLYCEMIA (Low Blood Sugar)

1. Condition and Cause
Hypoglycemia can be hereditary or caused by poor diet, stress or other health problems. The body's cells are nourished by glucose or blood sugar. Blood sugar levels are regulated by the amount of insulin released by the pancreas. If the pancreas is impaired for the above reasons, it may become overactive or "trigger happy"(as it does with hypoglycemia), and send out too much insulin. For a person with hypoglycemia, eating even a little sweet or refined food can cause the pancreas to overreact. This diminishes the amount of glucose sent to the cells—the condition we call low blood sugar—with the result that they are not properly fed. Low blood sugar may have some or all of these symptoms: decreased energy, tiredness, light-headedness or "spaciness," faintness, dizziness, irritability, restlessness, anxiety, headaches, over-emotionalism, depression, mental confusion, nervous habits, aggression, cravings and insomnia.

2. Ailment History, Signs and Early Treatments
Hypoglycemia is definitely a major 20th-century disease. In past ages, it was rare and would most likely have resulted in the sufferer being considered mentally unbalanced. The advent of eating primarily processed and refined foods has taken low blood sugar problems to startlingly dangerous heights in the last one hundred years. The average Canadian and American consumes about 160 pounds of sugar annually, much of which is hidden in canned and frozen foods, processed foods and snack foods. According to Dr. Joseph Mercola's "Healthy News You Can Use" newsletter, February 7,

2001: "about 90 percent of the money that Americans now spend on food goes to buy processed food."

Just a little over two decades or more ago, hypoglycemia was treated with spoonfuls of sugar, the reasoning being that since the cells were suffering from diminished glucose, eating sugar would help. The error in this thinking was that in a person with hypoglycemia, any amount of ingested sugar triggers the pancreas to release overabundant amounts of insulin that deplete the glucose going to the cells even further. All up-to-date medical doctors have abandoned this inadequate treatment.

3. Modern Natural Treatments and Remedies

No drugs or even natural remedies are required for hypoglycemia, though some supplements can be helpful. In the near future, however, I expect to see the discovery of healing remedies and treatments that will help to heal the pancreas completely.

The primary way of treating low blood sugar today is with proper diet, along with exercise, fresh air and the usual human needs for adequate rest, sunshine and other health aids. In a proper hypoglycemic diet (see the nutrition aids section, following), all foods that trigger overreaction of the pancreas are eliminated or limited. The present allopathic nutritional approach (or traditional medical treatment) merely limits the amounts of white bread, fruits and sugars that can be eaten. The more effective holistic approach eliminates all (or most) foods that overstimulate the pancreas and concentrates on foods that help the body to heal (foods that nourish the whole body and do not overwork the pancreas). The holistic approach aims to help the person with hypoglycemia to function as healthily as people without low blood sugar problems.

Modern testing methods for low blood sugar are inadequate—a person may have hypoglycemia even after testing negative for the condition. If there are evident blood sugar problems, it is important to undergo proper medical tests to rule out other health concerns with similar side effects, such as: Candida, parasites, digestive problems, allergies, or vitamin or mineral imbalances. Pregnant women and those with major health problems or diseases may experience temporary problems with the regulation of their blood sugar and will be helped by using the low blood sugar diet that follows.

4. Helpful Supplements and Dosages

- Take one to four vitamin B50 complex daily as needed, to help the body to handle carbohydrate foods that can upset blood sugar levels. B vitamins also have a calming effect on those with low blood sugar.
- Take 300 to 600 mcg chromium picolinate a day to aid glucose absorption.
- Take 500 to 1,000 mg calcium/magnesium daily.
- Take 15 to 30 mg zinc picolinate (or, if it is unavailable, zinc gluconate) daily or several times a week.
- A multivitamin, a green food product, amino acids, digestive aids, biotin, energizing supplements and/or sleep aids may be helpful, taken as needed. You may take L-glutamine if your doctor approves.

5. Cautions and Exceptions

Never eat sugar, sugar substitutes, sweet foods or refined foods on an empty stomach! Always eat sweet or starchy foods partway into a meal. If you eat natural (or sweetened) desserts an hour to 90 minutes after a full meal, blood sugar levels will be affected very little or not at all. Alcohol, artificial sweeteners, smoking and unnecessary drugs are especially harmful for those with low blood sugar. If you indulge in these things (except for smoking), at least do not do it on an empty stomach. Some individuals who maintain an excellent diet can tolerate occasional sugar desserts (one to three times a week) after a full meal.

6. Nutrition Aids and Recommended Foods

To keep their blood sugar levels stable, people with hypoglycemia require two or three full meals a day plus two to four snacks, or five or six small meals spread throughout the day. Beans and peas (cooked from dried, rather than canned), especially soybeans, chickpeas and black, pinto, kidney and adzuki beans, are high in protein, calcium, phosphorus, potassium, iron and zinc. Beans, according to *The Wellness Encyclopedia of Food and Nutrition*, by Sheldon Margen, are extremely beneficial for hypoglycemia, because they balance blood sugar levels like no other food. So eat lots of nutritious beans, and make sure they are cooked correctly (soft enough that you can mash them with the tongue against the roof of the mouth) so they can be digested. Take digestive aids if needed, but do eat beans!

A natural whole-foods diet is absolutely essential for everyone with low blood sugar. Diet is the main treatment for hypoglycemia. Eat a diet that consists mainly of the following: properly cooked, warm whole grains (7–14 servings a week), especially chromium-rich millet; beans and peas (6–12 servings a week); vegetables (3–6 servings a day); limited meats—preferably lamb or veal (1–2 servings a week) with some poultry (1–2 servings a week) and fish (2–4 servings a week); seaweeds; warm nut and seed butters and well-chewed raw nuts and seeds (2–4 times a week); flaxseeds and flaxseed oil; popcorn (with only butter and/or salt); cooked warm tofu; eggs; cooked cheese; occasional butter; carob; blood sugar–balancing Jerusalem artichokes and garlic; and non-sweet fruits like citrus (except for oranges), apples, pears, watermelon and berries. Vegetarians may exclude meat and those with allergies can exclude dairy if desired, using substitutions. For low blood sugar diet particulars, see pages 151 and 488 of my *Complete Candida Yeast Guidebook* particularly and follow—for life— the Phase II or Phase III diet I describe in that book, with only a few exceptions, to maintain balanced blood sugar levels, normal energy and optimum health. Some whole grain–/whole food–based natural desserts can be had three to five times a week, an hour to 90 minutes after a full meal—never on an empty stomach. Chew foods very well to assist digestion. Take digestive aids if needed.

Foods that aggravate low blood sugar problems include: pork, excessive amounts of red meats, processed meats, shellfish of all kinds, fatty foods, refined foods, junk foods, processed foods or foods with additives and preservatives, white and multigrain (hard to digest) breads and crackers, all pasta, all dry breakfast cereals, all potato chips, pretzels (unless 100 percent whole wheat), rice wraps, rice cakes, oatmeal, processed cheeses, cheeses not cooked into a recipe, milk, roasted nuts and seeds, refined oils, chocolate, candy, ice cream, cakes, pies and tropical and sweet fruits (especially bananas, mangos, coconut, lychee nuts, kiwi, cantaloupe and honeydew melons, grapes, oranges and dried fruits).

7. Beverage and Herbal Tea Suggestions

Drink mainly tested spring water. Vegetable juices, especially those that include carrot, beet and green vegetables or a green food product, are particularly helpful. Power protein drinks that are not too sweet are good energizers. For parties, or for snack beverages, try club soda with a wedge of lemon or lime, fresh grapefruit juice or veggie juices. Blender drinks with yogurt and fruit can also be occasional treats. Blueberry leaf tea reduces high blood sugar. Other helpful herbal teas include peppermint, spearmint, alfalfa, lemon grass, chicory, fennel, fenugreek, raspberry leaf and dandelion root. Dandelion "coffee" is also excellent for low blood sugar.

-I-

INDIGESTION

See *Digestion Problems*

INFECTIONS

See *Earache and Ear Infections, Candida* and *Yeast Infections, Vaginal* (for Candida yeast infections), *Viruses* (for viral infections) and *Skin Problems* (for skin infections)

INSECT BITES OR STINGS

See *Bee Stings, (Other Insect Stings)* and *Insect Stings and Bites*

INSOMNIA

1. Condition and Cause
In *Healthy Healing*, Linda Rector Page, N.D., states, "Americans consume over one and a half million pounds of tranquilizers annually!" Fifteen percent or more of the North American population suffers from sleep problems at any given time—the inability either to fall asleep or to stay asleep. Anxiety, emotions and busy thoughts are more to blame than physical problems when it comes to sleep deprivation. Sometimes, however, overeating—or not eating enough nutritious meals—can be the cause. It depends on a person's body type.

2. Ailment History, Signs and Early Treatments

Remember the fairy story of "The Princess and the Pea"? One little pea under her twenty mattresses kept her tossing and turning all night. Traditionally, and still today, warm milk at bedtime is used to induce sleep, mainly because it contains the natural amino acid tryptophan, which helps encourage sleep. See the recommended foods below for more high-tryptophan foods.

Abraham Lincoln liked long walks before bedtime. People who do physical labor during the day usually have little trouble going to sleep. A hundred years ago, North America was full of farmers and day laborers, and most people could sleep soundly almost anywhere—even without special mattresses, padding, pillows, perfect temperatures and just the right food and quiet. Folk cures for good sleep include drinking boiled onion water, sniffing a peeled raw onion before sleeping and rubbing the soles of the feet with garlic at bedtime.

3. Modern Natural Treatments and Remedies

Exercising during the day can help you sleep better at night. Being sedentary during the day and exercising at night can actually keep you awake most of the night. You will usually sleep better if you go to bed at about the same time at night and wake up around the same time every morning rather than going to bed at a different time each night and sometimes sleeping in. Too much fresh air—or too little—in your sleep environment may also keep you awake. Too much daytime napping can also interfere with night sleep.

Be sure not to take energizing supplements like vitamin C (especially in its chewable form), echinacea, royal jelly, ginseng, dong quai, gotu kola or gingko before bedtime. Also avoid taking acidophilus or too many digestive aids near bedtime, or eating the wrong foods (see following). There is an abundance of remedies, herbs, foods and natural teas that help to induce sleep or to keep you asleep, though none of these work if you are thinking way too hard or are really upset about something. Avoid working late at night, or having emotional discussions late at night, or thinking about what you have to do tomorrow and other distracting, wakeful thoughts. Try listening to calming music, reading a few pages of a soothing book, doing relaxing breathing exercises or thinking about all the things you are happy about or thankful for. Nighttime meditation helps some people sleep better, but energizes others. Wind down your day, but try not to lie around too much on the couch or to doze before actually going to bed.

For gentle sleep aids, try kava kava herb or capsules, passion flower herb or capsules, sleep teas (below), or Hyland's Calms® (usually take two or three with food and/or water). Stronger sleep inducers include valerian root capsules or tablets (300–600 mg taken with food and/or water before bedtime) or melatonin. Also try some of the suggested herbal teas in the beverage section, following.

Melatonin is actually a synthetic hormone that is used for anti--aging and rejuvenation. Take 1–3 mg with only a little water— not with food, or it will actually *keep* you awake. Sublingual tablets (those dissolved under the tongue) work faster and are more effective. Otherwise, take melatonin with a digestive aid like a non-coated acidophilus tablet, or just take the melatonin an hour or more before bedtime so it has time to break down and do its work. (Non-sublingual capsules work better than tablets usually.) Get your doctor's okay to take melatonin during pregnancy.

The strongest sleep aid—which can also help calm you down if you are upset or really stressed or depressed—is St. John's wort. I recommend using it as a last resort, only if all else fails to get you the desired sleep. St. John's wort is powerful and does not work well with some prescription drugs and for certain health concerns and sometimes not during pregnancy. Check with your holistic medical doctor or naturopath (not traditional doctors or pharmacists, who may be biased), to get the most accurate assessment of your need for St. John's wort and your ability to handle it. It can make you groggy and a bit disoriented the next day, especially if too much is taken. Try one 300 mg capsule (containing 0.9 mg hypericin). Take up to 900 mg (3 capsules) daily if needed. Do not exceed this amount!

4. Helpful Supplements and Dosages

- Take two to four vitamin B50 complex daily, including some before bedtime for a more restful sleep. Take a 300-500 mcg of B12 with one just before bedtime for addition help to enhance drowsiness. (Some very hardy individuals are energized by B50 complex while most average or sensitive people find it calming and relaxing.)

- Take 500–1,000 mg calcium/magnesium daily, or before bedtime for undisturbed sleep.

5. Cautions and Exceptions

Check with your holistic physician before taking melatonin or St. John's wort, especially if you have health problems, are taking drugs or are pregnant. It helps to rotate different sleep aids rather than rely on one all the time for better sleep. Do not take more than two different sleep aids for one night. Take melatonin at least three to four hours away from other sleep aids. Do not use natural sleep aids with drugs that induce sleep. Take all natural or holistic doctor–approved sleep aids at least four hours apart from any drugs. For serious sleep disorders like sleep apnea (temporary cessation of breathing while sleeping), restless or jumpy limbs or severe depression, see your physician.

6. Nutrition Aids and Recommended Foods

High-tryptophan foods help encourage sleep when eaten in the evening, usually a couple of hours or more before bed. Tryptophan is found in turkey, tuna, dark leafy greens like collard and turnip greens, kelp, spirulina, milk, yogurt, pumpkin, whole grains and seeds and seed butters like pumpkin and sunflower.

Average, healthy individuals should not eat too much too late at night, though those with blood sugar problems, some allergies and other health concerns require a small meal later in the evening to sleep soundly throughout the night. It is important for most individuals to eat two or three solid meals a day, or the body's hunger for nutrients may wake you after four or five hours of sleep. Taking too many digestive aids can have the same effect. Improperly balanced, incomplete meals—such as those containing pasta or seafood, instant foods, frozen foods, and other refined and junk foods—are so nutrient-deficient and unsatisfying to the body that it may be hard to fall asleep, or to stay asleep for more than a few hours. Eating too heavily late at night can also disturb sleep and cause nightmares.

Hard-to-digest foods eaten late at night can disturb the digestion and agitate the body, causing you to lie awake or causing nightmares. Such foods include: nuts and seeds—especially roasted ones—soy nuts, corn nuts, corn chips, fatty foods, potato chips and dips, multi-grain breads, cheeses, milk, and especially raw vegetables. Sweet and tropical fruits like bananas, mangoes, oranges and other citrus fruits, lychee nuts, coconut, dried fruit, plums, peaches, cherries, berries—and other fruit with seeds—can also disturb sleep. It is best to avoid eating *all* fruits and raw vegetables at night. Sugars—refined or natural—and artificial sweeteners should also be avoided at night. Sweets and fruit sugars can give you a quick, unstable surge of energy and keep you awake at night, especially if you have blood sugar problems, allergies, Candida, parasites or other major health concerns.

Eating fatty foods can cause internal throbbing and/or insomnia for some people, especially those with impaired livers or gall bladders or those with no gall bladders. Taking a bile salt tablet with the last meal of the day can eliminate this problem for most of these individuals.

7. Beverage and Herbal Tea Suggestions

Herbal sleep teas include: chamomile, hops, skullcap, valerian, passion flower, kava kava and special melatonin tea blends. These teas may be used singly or in a double combination, instead of other sleep aids. For children, use chamomile or natural catnip teas. Catnip also helps prevent nightmares. Avoid caffeinated coffee, tea, chocolate or cola, too late in the day. While alcohol may feel initially like a good relaxant, later in the night it may have stimulating effects to some organs, such as the liver.

INSECT STINGS AND BITES

See *Bee Stings and Insect Bites*

-J-

JITTERS OR JUMPINESS

A cup of celery seed tea, with one teaspoon of seeds per cup of water, is a potent way to calm the jitters. See "Herbal Teas, Tinctures and Treatments" for the method. Also see *Anxiety* for more detailed information.

Jock Itch

See also *Candida* and *Yeast Infection, Vaginal*. Also see *Digestion Problems*, as these conditions can be related.

Candida yeast is generally the culprit here. Jock itch can be a form of sexually transmitted Candida and may keep reoccurring if both you and your partner are not treated for Candida. Take internal Candida treatments and external applications of oregano oil, colloidal silver, tea tree oil, aloe vera gel or cream, or MSM lotion. Daily acidophilus, in conjunction with a Candida diet, will help. Be sure to wear loose-fitting, comfortable, light-colored, cotton underwear.

Helpful supplements include: vitamins A, C and B complex, digestive aids, multivitamins and lecithin (in capsule form or, better yet, as a food supplement in granular or liquid form). Vegetable juices are good, as are the energy and power drinks described in "Beneficial Beverages." Helpful teas include chamomile, echinacea, peppermint, spearmint, ginger, ginseng, fennel, fenugreek and horsetail. See your doctor if the problem persists, to ensure that more severe health problems, such as cancer, are not underlying.

Joint Aches and Pain

Eat a wholesome, high-fiber diet including whole grains, legumes, lots of vegetables and some vegetable juices, green food products (especially alfalfa), fish, and include flaxseed, lecithin and yogurt in the diet. Take daily multivitamins, calcium and magnesium, extra vitamin B complex as well as vitamin C. To bring down inflammation, try Anti-Flam®, Flammaforce® or Infla-Zyme Forte®. Pain remedies include arnica and MSM. Glucosamine sulfate and SOD can help repair cells, tissue and cartilage. For external application to soothe aches and pains, use: aloe vera, tea tree oil, MSM or arnica lotion, and, as healing progresses, shark oil. Hot castor oil packs and/or witch hazel poultices can also sometimes be helpful during treatment. See *Anti-Inflammatories* under "Stocking Your Natural Medicine Chest."

Beneficial teas include: alfalfa, catnip, fenugreek, slippery elm, horsetail and parsley. A dash or two of cayenne may be added to teas, or it may be taken in separate capsules with meals. Walking, yoga and other similar exercises are helpful—and necessary. If you suffer from arthritis, see the health books listed in the bibliography. Epsom salts or other therapeutic baths can also be helpful, as can saunas or steam baths. Doing a cleanse will also help. Get tested to make sure that an overabundance of heavy metals is not an underlying cause of your symptoms.

-L-

LAXATIVES

See "Herbal Teas, Tinctures and Treatments" and "Fast Finger Remedies"; also see *Digestive Aids* in the "Natural Remedies Glossary"

LIPS, CHAPPED

See also *Cold Sores*

1. Condition and Cause
Extremely hot or cold weather can cause chapped, cracked, peeling, blistered or even bleeding lips.

2. Ailment History, Signs and Early Treatments
Beeswax was traditionally used to protect lips from chapping, and is still used today in many lip glosses and lip protectors.

3. Modern Natural Treatments and Remedies
Use one of the many lip balms or chapped lip-protectors that are available in health food stores in a variety of natural flavors. Extracts of echinacea, calendula and vitamin E are often added for their healing properties. Vitamin E oil or cream can also be used separately. Add a drop or two of oregano oil to a teaspoon of olive oil and apply to the lips. Use shark oil alone on the lips as often as required.

4. Helpful Supplements and Dosages
- Take 100–200 IU vitamin E once or twice a day for protection and healing.

- Use ground flaxseed, flaxseed oil and/or pumpkin-seed oil in the diet with salads several times a week.

5. Cautions and Exceptions

Do not lend your lip balm, lip gloss or lipstick to anyone else, as bacteria and infection can be spread easily this way. In particular, do not lend them to people with cold sores or chapped, bleeding lips. Do not lick the lips without wiping them afterwards, as it invites chapping. Avoid touching your lips with dirty hands to prevent spreading bacteria to the lips and mouth.

6. Nutrition Aids and Recommended Foods

Eat a wholesome, varied diet with lots of vegetables and fiber. Avoid excessive amounts of citrus fruit, tomatoes or acidic foods.

7. Beverage and Herbal Tea Suggestions

Drink lots of water every day. Wipe your mouth after drinking beverages. Avoid drinking too much milk or acidic beverages.

-M-

MEMORY PROBLEMS

1. Condition and Cause

Loss of memory or forgetfulness occurs at one time or another for everyone. However consistent memory loss problems often occur with aging, although age itself is not the main cause of memory problems. Memory problems can occur due to: stress, fever, malnutrition, vitamin and mineral deficiencies or overabundances, alcohol or drug abuse, depression, sleep deprivation, thyroid problems, blood sugar problems, hyperactivity, menopause, anemia, allergies, Candida yeast, parasites, toxin overload, exposure to free radicals, severe health problems and diseases such as: stroke, senile dementia and Alzheimer's disease.

2. Ailment History, Signs and Early Treatments

Jokes and stories about memory loss have been around for centuries.

The lore includes tying a string around your finger to help you remember something; having a memory like an elephant; and getting a bump on the head and forgetting who you are and the ones you love. Eating a few prunes every day is an old remedy for memory loss, maybe because prunes have a laxative effect and we tend to think better when not constipated! Ginger and/or cloves, which have a stimulating effect, are supposed to improve memory as well.

3. Modern Natural Treatments and Remedies
Include lecithin spread, granules or liquid in the diet (see the power and energy drinks in "Beneficial Beverages"). Make sure there is plenty of fiber and natural foods in the diet. Avoid chemical additives and preservatives. Eat foods high in bioflavonoids like the inner skins of citrus fruits, berries, spinach, exotic greens and dark leafy greens. Take green food products—such as blue-green algae, barley green, chlorella and spirulina—regularly in rotation. Garlic helps improve mental clarity marvelously, as well as assisting the memory. Take a clove (chopped and not chewed, following the method described in *Toxin Overload*) either daily or every other day, and notice the difference. (There may be an initial "cleansing reaction" if the body is very toxic, but once that passes, your thinking will be clearer and sharper.) Also include energizing foods, supplements (see *Energy, Low*), teas and other drinks.

Do yoga, tai chi, qi gong or martial arts; swim, dance, go walking or bicycling; or do other stretching exercise several times per week. See the "Healing Aids" section for other ways (including acupressure, acupuncture and more) to stimulate better memory. See *Circulation, Poor* for aids to improving memory by increasing the circulation.

4. Helpful Supplements and Dosages
- Take two to four vitamin B50 complex a day, with extra choline and inositol.
- Take 1,000–2,000 mg vitamin C three or four times a day for its antioxidant effects.
- Take one 500 mg calcium and magnesium supplement two or three times a day.
- Take a balanced, natural multivitamin mineral supplement every day.

- Take 15–60 mg of zinc every day.
- Take 60 mg of ginkgo biloba, or take ginseng or dong quai supplements, every day.
- Optional: Consult with your holistic physician to help you decide which of the following supplements to take regularly or on a rotational basis for anti-aging and as memory aids: melatonin, royal jelly, bee pollen, CoQ10, SOD, garlic, amino acids, vitamins E and A, manganese, evening primrose oil, horsetail or silica, selenium, other antioxidants, Bio-Strath® (energizer and nutrients), DHEA, HGH (human growth hormone—for improved brain function), gotu kola, 5-HTP, and/or others. (Do not take too many of these supplements at once!)

5. Cautions and Exceptions

For major health problems and diseases, beyond occasional memory loss, see your doctor. If sudden memory loss is accompanied by slurred speech, vision changes, dizziness or severe pain, seek medical assistance immediately.

6. Nutrition Aids and Recommended Foods

Eat a well-balanced, wholesome diet of mainly green and yellow vegetables (4–6 servings daily), both cooked and with natural, raw flaxseed and/or pumpkin-seed oils in raw salads, as well as in juices. Also eat plenty of whole grains, legumes, yogurt, fish, seaweeds, flaxseed, pumpkin seeds, sesame seeds, tahini, sunflower seeds and green herbs. Avoid aggravating and energy-stealing foods like too much red meats or pork, shellfish, fatty or greasy foods, fried foods, caffeine, alcohol, dairy products, wheat, refined foods, junk foods, sweets, sweet fruit, sugars, artificial sweeteners and additives, and pasta.

7. Beverage and Herbal Tea Suggestions

Drink at least five or six glasses of spring water a day. Drink vegetable juices with green food products. Avoid soda pops, soft drinks and alcohol. Organic green tea is better than coffee for those with memory problems. Enjoy these beneficial herbal teas: lemon grass, peppermint, spearmint, raspberry leaf, rose hips, ginkgo, echinacea, ginseng, licorice and eyebright.

MENSTRUAL PROBLEMS

Menstrual problems may include: PMS (bloating, mood swings, irritability, depression, fatigue, weakness, headaches), cramps, aches, irregular cycles, very light or heavy flow, large clotting or spotting between periods. These and other problems can make the monthly menstrual cycle uncomfortable and even debilitating for some women.

My own experience and the experiences of my clients have been that most menstrual problems can be lessened and sometimes even eliminated with proper cleansing (unless you have a specific medical problem that requires medication or a doctor's attention). The first month after a 12–30 day cleanse, the period is usually heavier and *more* troublesome—but the periods that follow are usually much easier, unless the cleansing was ineffective (too short or done improperly). The time to start a new cleanse is the day after the menstrual cycle ends. *Never* start a cleanse just before or during a period.

Once menstrual problems are in progress, take energizers to boost your energy. See *Headache* for headache remedies, *Insomnia* for sleep aids and *Digestion Problems* if you have any problems with food. If your flow is very heavy or you experience spotting between periods, consult your doctor, as they can be signs of miscarriage, venereal disease or another STD, hormone imbalance or other health problems.

Health stores have many products to help women during the menstrual cycle, including natural aids for cramps and herb combinations to ease symptoms. Supplements that may help include vitamins C and B complex and, for some women, dong quai or evening primrose oil. Experiment with a trial period taking one of the latter supplements (at a time) or check with your holistic physician to see if these might be helpful for you.

A wholesome balanced diet with two or three proper meals is essential. Do not eat "headache foods" (see *Headache*). Vegetable juices with a green food product can be especially beneficial this time of the month. This is a good time to enjoy salmon, legumes, tofu, brown rice and/or millet and lots of green and orange vegetables. Include flaxseed, miso and yogurt in the diet and avoid too much fat, sugars and all junk foods. Try some of the power drinks described in "Beneficial Beverages." Helpful teas include alfalfa, parsley, peppermint, chamomile, raspberry leaf, black cohosh, chaste berry (vitex) and organic green tea.

For major problems or excessive flow, contact your doctor.

METAL OVERDOSE, TOXIC OR HEAVY

See *Heavy Metal Overdose*

MIGRAINES

See *Headache*

MORNING SICKNESS

See *Nausea*

MOTION SICKNESS

See *Nausea*

MUSCLE ACHES AND PAINS

See *Joint Aches and Pain*

-N-

NAIL PROBLEMS

See also *Hair Problems*

Most of the foods, herbal teas and supplements for hair problems—especially oregano oil, gelatin and horsetail—work well for nail problems too. The most important supplements include calcium, magnesium, iron, zinc, silica, vitamin A, vitamin C, vitamin B complex, acidophilus and flaxseed. A high-protein diet is important. Avoid using nail polish remover and do not leave the hands in hot detergents.

Your nails can indicate your overall state of health and indicate diseases. *Prescription For Nutritional Healing* by Phyllis and James Balch is a great guide to disorders that show up in the nails.

NAUSEA

Nausea may be caused by: motion sickness (from car rides, boating, air travel or other motion), food poisoning, overeating, alcohol problems, stomach upset, anxiety, flu, illness, allergies, intensive cleansing, morning sickness or other reasons. It may or may not be followed by vomiting. See *Alcohol Problems* for nausea related to drinking.

FOR NAUSEA FROM DIGESTIVE PROBLEMS   Digestive aids can help if the problem is food-related, and food combining may help to make foods easier to digest. Drinking tomato or grapefruit juice with protein meals, or peppermint tea (preferably one half hour) before any meal, can help digestion. Avoid most other liquids during mealtime. If nausea is common, take daily acidophilus. See *Digestion Problems.*

FOR NAUSEA FROM FOOD POISONING   If serious (continued or extreme), go to a hospital emergency room. If not, take three acidophilus capsules with half a glass of water and repeat two or three times a day until improved. Also take one of the following: garlic, propolis, lemon juice or citricidal for several days.

FOR NAUSEA FROM MOTION SICKNESS   Be sure to eat a good meal at least two hours before traveling, so the stomach is settled. (Take digestive aids if needed, especially if the meal is a heavy one.) Take two ginger capsules an hour or so before departing (or chew on a piece of fresh ginger if capsules are unavailable), preferably along with a B complex and an extra B6 supplement. If you are prone to motion sickness and know you are traveling the next day, eat balanced meals and take two ginger capsules once or twice the day before. Drink peppermint or fennel tea just before you depart and sip during travel—or drink club soda, preferably with some added fresh ginger juice or slices (see the Motion Sickness Miracle in "Beneficial Beverages"). If you are still nauseous after travel, have more tea or club soda. Eat a hot or warm starchy meal or snack after with brown rice, millet, orange yams, winter squash or potatoes. Miso soup is also a great stomach settler.

FOR NAUSEA FROM MORNING SICKNESS   Drink raspberry leaf tea daily, take digestive aids with meals if needed, and take a B50 complex three or four times a day, with an extra B6 supplement once or twice a day (twice if more nauseous). Take ginger tea or capsules when you get up, if you are nauseous or expect to be. Whole-grain crackers can help settle the stomach, but a breakfast of baked winter squash or steamed orange yam is better than dry toast, rice cakes or cereal. Daily acidophilus can also be very helpful.

FOR ALL NAUSEA   Relieve body pressure with an Epsom salt or other therapeutic bath with added fresh ginger juice or peppermint tea or tincture. Vitamin C and other energizers like royal jelly can help to boost energy levels and help alleviate nausea. Helpful teas include catnip, chamomile, dandelion (or dandelion "coffee"), ginger, fennel, peppermint, spearmint and lemon grass. Deep breathing can be a great help in calming and alleviating nausea.

NERVOUSNESS

See *Jitters or Jumpiness* and *Anxiety*

NOSE BLEED

See *Bleeding, Excessive*

-O-

OPERATION PREPARATION AND HEALING

For a speedy recovery from an operation, take acidophilus for at least a week prior to surgery and while you are healing. Acidophilus helps to replace friendly intestinal bacteria that are usually killed by antibiotic drugs, and will assist digestion and healing. Before surgery and during recovery, also take 1,000–2,000 mg of vitamin C two to four times a day (more around the time of your operation), at least 25 mg a day of bioflavonoids (especially pycnogenol or grape seed extract), 200–400 IU of vitamin E a day, 15–50 mg of zinc a day and one of the following daily if possible: a garlic clove (minced and not chewed) or 500 mg of propolis or take goldenseal with echinacea. (Do not take goldenseal for more than 10 days or so.) Eat a good diet with lots of veggies, lecithin, flaxseed, green food products and yogurt. Healing teas include alfalfa, dandelion (or dandelion "coffee"), echinacea, lemon grass, fenugreek, parsley and yarrow. Organic green tea is more beneficial than coffee. Do not take remedies that clash with prescription drugs.

ORAL HYGIENE PROBLEMS

See also *Toothaches* and *Bad Breath*

1. Condition and Cause
Oral hygiene problems include bleeding gums, gingivitis, tooth decay, loose teeth, plaque and tartar, infections, bad breath and jaw misalignment. Causes may range from genetic weaknesses in the teeth and gums to improper diet or poor dental hygiene habits. Remember, there are over 200 types of bacteria found in the mouth.

2. Ailment History, Signs and Early Treatments
Few ancient civilizations brushed their teeth—but none of them consumed 160 pounds of sugar a year like Canadians and Americans do either, not to mention the junk foods, refined foods, sticky sweets and other dental atrocities we consume daily.

East Indians still use a stick from the neem tree, also known as the "miracle tree," to clean their teeth. Gandhi used this marvelous antibacterial cleaning tool. In the past, people have cleaned their teeth by chewing on fennel seeds, cardamom, cloves and hard vegetables and fruits like carrots and apples, and have rubbed their teeth with strawberries and lemons. (Unfortunately, lemon juice residues strip away tooth enamel, with frequent use.) Before tooth-paste came into regular use, tooth powders of baking soda and/or salt, also papain powder or cream of tartar were common.

3. Modern Natural Treatments and Remedies
Prevention is the most important way to ensure good oral hygiene. Brush your teeth at least twice a day, morning and night, and floss or

use a water cleaning device daily. Do not brush too hard or too soft, do not use a hard bristle brush and try to brush for at least two minutes. Chewing on hard fruits and vegetables daily is still beneficial for your teeth. Stay away from overly sweetened toothpastes, citricidal toothpastes (which may strip off enamel and help make the teeth hypersensitive) and fluoride toothpastes (which holistic doctors do not recommend, because studies have shown that fluoride may not really be beneficial for tooth decay and may even be detrimental). Brush with baking soda (with optional sea salt) and warm water or with natural toothpastes that contain peppermint, peelu, tea tree oil, neem or other natural herbs. You can augment baking-soda tooth powder with added peelu, tea tree oil, neem, or propolis powder for more effectiveness.

Brush the tongue at least once a day with toothpaste, tooth powder or mouthwash. Morning is the best time, as toxins, bacteria and Candida yeast usually coat the tongue in the morning and can lead to bad breath, teeth and gum infections. Vigorously brush the middle and front of the tongue and make sure you remove any white coating. (There is no need to brush the edges of the tongue.)

Do not use commercial supermarket mouthwash brands. Use natural mouthwashes from health food stores or create your own. Here is a selection of **natural mouthwash** recipes:

1. sea salt in 6–8 ounces of warm water
2. a shake or two (several drops) of tea tree oil in 6–8 ounces of water
3. 10–20 drops of aerobic oxygen in 8 ounces of water (or follow package directions)
4. 1–2 teaspoons of peelu extract in 3–4 ounces of water
5. ¼ cup of aloe vera gel in 6–8 ounces of water
6. homemade goldenseal and myrrh tincture—see "Herbal Teas, Tinctures and Treatments" for information on how to make tinctures—(not to be used daily and not for pregnant women or those with severe illness, unless doctor recommends)
7. 1 tablespoon of 3 percent food-grade hydrogen peroxide in 6–8 ounces of water
8. a drop of clove oil in 8 ounces of water
9. one or two capsules (about 500 mg each) of neem powder in 6–8 ounces water

10. 1–2 tablespoons of 5–24 ppm colloidal silver in 6–8
     ounces water

It is best to use a variety of mouthwashes. Rotate so you use between
two and four different methods a week, to increase antibacterial potency
and to avoid the possibility of overusing any one natural remedy or
contributing to future allergies. Use mouthwash and gargle, one to three
times daily. Do not swallow. If using a mouthwash at bedtime, be
sure not to use a type that is too stimulating for you. See also *Bad Breath*.
     Most of the suggested mouthwashes can also be used to soak a
toothbrush for several hours, to kill bacteria build-up. Regular use
of the toothpastes and mouthwashes described above will also help
to avoid and heal bleeding gums. Treatments for Candida and/or
parasites may also help to heal bleeding gums.

4. Helpful Supplements and Dosages
It is best to have your holistic medical doctor or naturopathic physician recommend supplements for oral hygiene. They may include: bee
propolis, garlic, peelu, neem, tea tree oil, colloidal silver, vitamin C,
calcium, magnesium, phosphorus, aloe vera, and goldenseal with myrrh.
There are also throat sprays that may be employed (see *Sore Throat*).

5. Cautions and Exceptions
Note the cautions and exceptions given throughout this section.

6. Nutrition Aids and Recommended Foods
Do not leave sugars, sticky foods, dried fruit, citricidal, citrus fruit
or juice, club soda, tomatoes, chewable vitamin C (which is very
acidic), cheese or other sweet or acid foods on the teeth for long
periods, especially at night. Such foods are damaging and may help
corrode tooth enamel and contribute greatly to tooth decay. Eat
raw, hard fruits and vegetables every day. A wholesome natural foods
diet, preferably organic, is a natural defense against tooth decay and
other oral hygiene problems.

7. Beverage and Herbal Tea Suggestions
Drink lots of pure, tested spring water. Peppermint, spearmint, alfalfa,
lemon grass, raspberry leaf, organic green tea and other pleasure herbal

teas are beneficial. Parsley tea is especially strengthening for teeth. Vegetable juices, blender drinks and protein drinks are nutritious beverages that contain nutrients beneficial to healthy teeth and gums. Avoid alcohol, pop and soft drinks of all kinds, especially those with artificial sweeteners or lots of sugar. They corrode the teeth and are nutrient-deficient.

-P-

PAINS

See *Joint Aches and Pain, Toothache, Backache, Headache* or *Earache and Ear Infections*

Also try acupuncture for body pains—consult your doctor.

PANIC ATTACK

See *Anxiety*

PARASITES

Few books are available concerning parasites. The best are *Guess What Came to Dinner*, by Ann Louise Gittleman, and *Parasites: The Enemy Within*, by Hannah Kroeger. My *Complete Candida Yeast Guidebook* also contains some information on parasites. It is estimated that 90 percent or more of North Americans are host to one or more types of parasite. The most common is the microscopic Candida yeast. See *Candida; Yeast Infections, Vaginal; Jock Itch* and *Dandruff* for more information on Candidiasis and its symptoms, causes and cures.

Hundreds of other internal parasites range from the microscopic (protozoa such as giardia) to small or large worms (pinworms, round-worms, hookworms—or tapeworms up to 12 feet long), flukes (liver, lung and blood flukes) and many more. They are picked up chiefly from water, food (from restaurants or from some canned goods orig-inating in some Asian countries), soil and tropical travel. Parasites can sometimes be transmitted by pets and via toilets, sexual contact and other means. Side effects include everything from stomachaches and digestive problems, headaches, hyperactivity, fatigue, weakness, nutrient deficiencies, allergies, skin rashes, diarrhea, insomnia, bleeding gums, difficulty in thinking, irritability, depression, PMS, slow healing of wounds to toxin overload.

Treatment requires parasite cleansing. Cleansing products include Clear® and Experience® from Awareness Products; Parasave® and Bioxy® from Bioquest Imports; Paraway®, Paragone®, and the homeopathic Detoxosode D•P® by Hobon (a homeopathic product). Parasite experts Hannah Kroeger and Ann Louise Gittleman have developed their own products too, and many other anti-parasitic products are available from your health store, holistic pharmacy, holistic medical doctor, chiropractor, herbalist or other holistic health expert. You may also try taking minced garlic (not chewed—see *Toxin Overload* for method), colloidal silver, lemon juice, citricidal, black walnut or cloves. See *Toxin Overload,* the discussion of cleansing in "Healing Aids" and, for specific remedies, the "Natural Remedies Glossary." See package labels for how to take packaged products. Not every parasite product kills every type of parasite.

PMS

See *Menstrual Problems*

POISON IVY, POISON OAK AND SUMAC

1. Condition and Cause

These plants, vines, bushes and trees are found throughout most of North America and contain an irritating sap that is immediately toxic to humans, especially those of fairer skin. Keep children away from the plants and their tempting, but dangerous, white or grayish berries. Avoid all contact, as one light touch of the hand—or contact even via clothing or pets—can transmit the poison to anyone who subsequently comes in contact with it. The entire body can become affected, including the face and genitals. Symptoms may begin immediately or several days after exposure. They start with itching and burning, and are usually followed by an itchy red rash, swelling, bumps and oozing blisters. Severe cases include fever and inflammation. Most symptoms disappear in a week or two.

2. Ailment History, Signs and Early Treatments

These poisonous plants have been on the planet a long time. Common folk remedies to alleviate the itchiness and discomfort include packing mud, or powdered chalk mixed with water, on the sores to draw out the poison and cool the itchy skin; rubbing the sores with the inside of a pineapple skin or banana peel; and rubbing the sores with slices of lemon, onion or garlic. Folk herbal remedies are still used today.

3. Modern Natural Treatments and Remedies

Besides the ever-popular calamine lotion (which contains phenol and zinc oxide), many topical remedies based on herbal and household ingredients may be used to soothe and heal blisters. They include applying oatmeal and water packs, baking soda and water paste, cornstarch and water paste, goldenseal (with optional myrrh) and water paste, clay and salt water paste, rubbing alcohol or tea tree oil (full strength or diluted one part to nine parts of apricot kernel oil, almond oil or corn oil); rubbing with plantain leaves; soaking in apple cider vinegar or aloe vera gel, and last but not least–applying a cloth soaked in a strong tea of white oak bark mixed with equal parts lime juice. The last treatment is especially good for applying to sore genitals. Vitamin E oil or cream, calendula cream and comfrey cream may also be applied externally for cooling relief.

As well, you may soak in a soothing bath augmented by a cup or two of baking soda, cornstarch, oatmeal or Epsom salts.

Remarkably, the fastest-working, most potent, quickest-drying and healing remedy is to apply non–food grade hydrogen peroxide topically many times a day (use cotton swabs to apply) for instant relief of itching. It foams up on contact with sore, red skin and dries up poisons before they can ooze out of the sores and blisters and spread. All other remedies take a back seat to this potent treatment.

4. Helpful Supplements and Dosages

- Take 1,000–3,000 mg vitamin C once or twice a day, or more if the rash is severe.
- Take 1,000–2,000 mg echinacea daily until rash and sores disappear.

- Take 10,000 IU daily of vitamin A plus 25,000 IU beta-carotene daily.
- Take one 15–50 mg capsule of zinc daily, for skin repair.

5. Cautions and Exceptions

If children (or adults) should eat any berries or plant, contact your local poison control center or emergency hospital.

In general, do not try to use too many different remedies at once. Do not pick or scratch at sores, or let sores ooze on clothing or other people, as the rash can easily spread to other people this way. Change and wash clothing frequently along with bed sheets. Cover cloth furniture with plastic first and then sheets, to keep from spreading the rash. Use bandages, socks, thin cotton gloves from the drug store, long cotton pants and long-sleeved shirts to protect and cover infected areas.

6. Nutrition Aids and Recommended Foods

Eat a wholesome natural diet avoiding the usual agitating foods: fatty foods, sugars of all kinds, junk foods, refined foods, pasta, seafood, red meats, cheeses, nuts, alcohol and milk. Eat lots of vegetables, whole grains, legumes, seeds, yogurt, and non-sweet fruits. Taking a green food product like spirulina can help and may speed healing.

7. Beverage and Herbal Tea Suggestions

Jewelweed often grows near poison ivy and may be used as an antidote, either externally as a tincture or internally as an herbal tea. Other helpful teas include white oak bark, mint, raspberry leaf and fennel.

-R-

RASHES

See also *Allergies; Skin Problems; Poison Ivy, Poison Oak and Sumac* or *Insect Stings and Bites*

Rashes may be caused by digestive and bowel problems—either a reaction or a blockage—or by allergic reactions, tight or itchy clothing, toxic substances, poisonous plants, insect bites or stings, a healing reaction or side effect of excessive cleansing, or diseases or other problems. Some rashes are contagious and can be contracted from another infected person, clothing, pets or from various substances like food. It is best to consult your doctor to find the cause of the rash, if it is unknown. Proceed with appropriate treatment.

-S-

SEXUAL ENERGY, LOW

A good sex life depends in part on getting sufficient rest and proper food. Junk food diets do not provide enough energy, in the long run, for prolonged sexual enjoyment. Some of the couples with the best sexual health rely on vegetarian diets. Meat eaters can, of course, also be quite healthy provided they include some whole grains, legumes and lots of vegetables in their diets. Many sex drive–killing "headaches," as well as sore backs, yeast infections and jock itch, disappear when you eat a good diet. When it comes to good sexual health, all the vitamins and Viagra® in the world cannot make up for a poor diet. Prescription drug aphrodisiacs also have been proven to have many dangerous side effects. Health food stores sell some safer, healthier versions of sexual enhancers. Also see the aphrodisiac and power drinks in "Beneficial Beverages" for some great bedroom energy boosters. Take them preferably an hour or more before sex. Vegetable juices with green food products are very helpful, especially if you drink them regularly (three to six times a week).

APHRODISIAC SUPPLEMENTS   Royal jelly is an excellent aphrodisiac. After all, it's the food that makes the queen bee lay up to 500 eggs a day and makes her the biggest bee in the hive! Take 300–500 mg of royal jelly once a day for two to three months at a time, and then take a break, so it is more effective. Or, on "special days," when you want increased stamina for sexual performance, take extra royal jelly one to three hours before sex (not exceeding 1,000 mg a day). Vitamin C is also a helpful energy booster. 1,000–2,000 mg can be taken several times a day, as desired, any time. Take part of this amount one to three hours before sex as well. Vitamin B complex is also invaluable for sexual enhancement; take one or two capsules daily. Ginseng (for men) and dong quai (for women) are Asian secrets for peak sexual performance, and anti-aging too. Take as directed, since quality varies widely. Ginseng tea an hour or more before sex can also provide a boost. Gotu kola, bee pollen, oat extract products, saw palmetto, ginger, choline, vitamins E and A, zinc (especially for men), L-arginine and other amino acids are other aids known to boost sexual energy.

According to aromatherapy principles, various aromas enhance sexuality. Try ginger, jasmine and patchouli to stimulate sexual desire; ylang ylang and sandalwood to increase sexual potency; rose, and iris and amber enhance love.

Garlic and onions are sexual enhancers that are said to "excite the lower passions." Other aphrodisiac foods include: fresh globe artichokes (served hot), avocados, ginger, oysters, shellfish, caviar, truffles, exotic fruit, bananas, strawberries, peaches, grapes, pumpkin seeds, black beans, whipped cream and chocolate.

A recent poll found that 50 percent of American women preferred chocolate to sex—some nutritious foods and supplements could help change that! Remember, no matter how many supplements you take, they are valueless without a regular wholesome diet! See my other books for more information on good foods and healthful diets.

Energizing teas include echinacea, ginger, ginkgo, ginseng, lemon grass, peppermint (as well as peppermint oil on the wrists or temples) and spearmint, any of which can be supplemented with a dash of added cayenne, if desired. Teas of specific help to women include: black cohosh, raspberry leaf, false unicorn and chase berry (vitex). For men: sarsaparilla, saw palmetto and, for impotence, damiana.

Finally, sexual energy and function can be greatly enhanced by deep breathing exercises, yoga, tai chi, qi gong and martial arts.

SEXUAL PROBLEMS

Sexual function may be impaired by lack of energy (see the previous entry) or by poor nutrition, sexually transmitted diseases, major health problems (such as prostate problems, impotence or cancer), hormone imbalances, alcohol or drugs. These many and varied problems are not covered in this book. It is best to see your holistic doctor for help with sexual problems. Acupuncture can help some sexual problems.

SKIN PROBLEMS

See also *Rashes* and *Sunburn*

The skin is the largest organ in the body. Aging, allergies, rashes, infections, diseases, Candida yeast, sunburn, injury, poor diet, lack of water, lack of essential oils, and many other factors can affect skin health. Make sure you know what is wrong with your skin before you begin to treat skin rashes or problem skin.

Tea tree oil is very good for most skin problems including yeast infections and sunburn. However, it does not help—and actually enhances or aggravates—staphylococcus (staph) skin infections and some other skin irritations. For some individuals, goldenseal paste (made from the ground root and water), fresh garlic juice, colloidal silver or oregano oil can be helpful for staph and some other infections. Shark oil (squalane) is excellent for aging (wrinkled), sunburned, damaged and healing skin. Other skin aids include comfrey or witch hazel creams; vitamin E ointment or cream; MSM lotion or cream (for aging, injured or damaged skin); and clay packs, poultices or baths. Check with your health food store or skin care specialist for others.

Remember that the skin is an outer reflection of your internal health. Major skin eruptions and rashes may be the result of digestive and bowel problems. Cleansing is almost always beneficial for assisting the healing of most skin problems. Drink lots of water. Herbal tea recommendations vary depending on the skin condition. See your doctor if skin problems are severe.

SLEEP AIDS

See *Insomnia*

SORE THROATS

See also *Colds, Coughs, Flu* and *Infections*

1. Condition and Cause

Sore throats, like common colds, are often caused by a virus, and frequently accompany a cold. They may also be caused by an irritation of the membranes at the back of the throat. In rare instances a sore throat may be a forerunner of tonsillitis, mononucleosis, Epstein-Barr virus, chronic fatigue, cancer or another serious disease. Yelling, loud singing (if unprofessional), excessive talking, lack of fluids in dry temperatures, smoke, fumes, hot food that burns the mouth and throat, getting a chill (especially when wet), a weakened immune system, allergies, Candida yeast or mouth infections can all contribute to or cause some sore throats. Hoarseness is usually due to inflamed vocal cords. Laryngitis (temporary loss of the voice) may come with a cold. With strep throat (streptococcus infection), the throat is extremely sore, the glands are swollen and there may be accompanying fever and body aches.

2. Ailment History, Signs and Early Treatments

Folk remedies include gargling with various mixtures, such as triple-strength black tea, apple cider vinegar in warm water, horseradish juice and cayenne or onion juice and honey. Eating a slice of fresh pineapple and chewing on cloves or garlic are other old-fashioned remedies.

3. Modern Natural Treatments and Remedies

Some of the treatments prescribed earlier for colds and coughs work well for sore throats too. They include propolis, citricidal, garlic, cayenne, astragalus, and low-dose natural antibiotics like colloidal silver, oregano oil and olive leaf extract.

Try one of the following for a sore throat:

1. On an empty stomach, drink the freshly squeezed juice of half a large or a whole small lemon or lime, straight or undiluted. The juice can be swished around the mouth to kill bacteria there before swallowing. Follow with a sip or two of water (which will taste sweet after the tart citrus). Half an hour later, you can eat fruit or other food. The lemon or lime will kill much of the bacteria in the mouth and throat, helping to prevent or heal a sore throat. Take this remedy once or twice a day before suppertime for one to three days.

2. Chew an organic garlic clove daily, after a meal (either directly afterwards or some time later), and spit out the pulp. Like lemon or lime juice, garlic kills bacteria in the mouth and throat, soothes symptoms and hopefully tackles the causes. Garlic capsules may be taken instead, but they are not nearly as effective.

3. Use a propolis throat spray, break open a propolis capsule in the throat or chew a propolis tablet one to three times a day. It will help kill any infection and speed the healing of throat irritation, as well as helping other respiratory symptoms and bad breath.

4. Take two cayenne capsules, once or twice a day, during the middle of a regular meal (so it will not give you "hot" side effects), and sprinkle a little cayenne (one small shake) in herbal tea one to three times a day.

5. Take citricidal, colloidal silver, oregano oil, olive leaf extract or astragalus in small doses (smaller than you would usually take for cleansing, so as not to throw the body into an intense cleansing state) daily while the sore throat lasts, and for two or three days afterwards, following the directions in the "Natural Remedies Glossary." (If taking astragalus capsules or tinctures, take according to package directions or a little less than the package directs.)

Licorice, slippery elm or wild cherry throat lozenges can also be taken as well as traditional cold remedies. Health stores sell an array of cough drops. Use the mouthwashes and gargles listed in *Oral Hygiene* to kill throat bacteria, one to three times a day, as required.

4. Helpful Supplements and Dosages

- Take 500–1,000 mg vitamin C one to four times a day or more, as required. (Vitamin C capsules, especially Ester C or Allergy C, are sometimes a better choice. Avoid powdered or chewable vitamin C.)
- Take 1,000–2,000 mg echinacea once or twice a day or more, as required.
- Take 15–50 mg zinc daily, as a supplement or in lozenges.

- Take one or two B50 complex daily for healing and stress reduction.
- Optional: Take garlic capsules daily, or take one, small clove of garlic (chopped and not chewed) following the directions in *Toxin Overload.*

5. Cautions and Exceptions

For severe or persistent sore throats that do not go away, see your doctor. Be aware that aspirin can aggravate sore throats.

6. Nutrition Aids and Recommended Foods

It is important to eat properly while suffering from a sore throat (especially if you have a cold or other ailment as well), to keep your strength up and assist healing. Very warm (but not too hot) liquid soups are especially helpful. See the healing soups in "Remedies from Your Refrigerator and Cupboard." When sick, avoid all junk foods, sweet fruits, sugars, excessive amounts of bread (which increase mucus), pasta, sushi, dairy products (which also increase mucus), very hard-to-digest foods, pork, cold meats, any meats in excess, lettuce, cold beans, cold whole grains and fatty foods. Enjoy mainly soups, stews, quality lamb and veal, blended and mashed warm beans, warm cooked whole grains, lots of cooked vegetables and vegetable juices, and just a little butter or yogurt if desired.

7. Beverage and Herbal Tea Suggestions

Drink six to eight glasses of water a day to flush the system. Drink lots of herbal tea. Very warm (but not too hot) herbal teas, drunk may times daily, without added dairy products, and with lemon and/or honey (and an optional dash of cayenne to kill mouth and throat bacteria) are the most beneficial. Enjoy one or more of the following often: rose hips, raspberry leaf, echinacea, lemon grass, slippery elm, chamomile, ginger or mint teas. Also elderberry, myrrh, goldenseal, fenugreek, licorice, eucalyptus or yarrow teas may be had occasionally. Skullcap and valerian teas are good for relaxing the throat and body. Also enjoy Vitamin C Magic, Cold Classic, Warm Cold Classic, vegetable juices (especially those that include carrots) and other beverages from the refrigerator remedies section.

Avoid drinking milk, cream and all dairy-based drinks or using them in soups or other recipes, because they aggravate the throat. Grapefruit juice is better than orange juice for sore throats and for extra vitamin C, especially if you have Candida yeast problems too. Drink lemon or lime juice as directed above. Organic green tea is better than coffee for sore throats.

SPRAINS AND STRAINS

A doctor should examine all major sprains and strains.

Do not apply heat until swelling subsides for at least 1–2 days. Apply intermittent cold (no more than 20 minutes at a time). A bag of frozen corn or peas wrapped in a thin dish towel is better than a block of ice. Begin immediately after receiving the injury and repeat every few hours or so, until the swelling is gone. Heat can be applied after swelling subsides for no more than 20 minutes at a time.

For most sprains and strains, apply tea tree oil many times the first day and two or three times a day after that to reduce the swelling very quickly and heal bruises. Tea tree oil applied too much externally can have a cleansing effect on sensitive people. Other external applications may include: oregano oil, aloe vera, comfrey or witch hazel creams or compresses, MSM lotion, colloidal silver, clay poultices, onion slices, garlic slices or goldenseal paste (made with the ground root and water). For any tissue or cartilage damage take glucosamine sulfate. Take arnica or MSM if pain arises.

Take energizing supplements and anti-inflammatories, if needed. Taking calming teas or sleep aids at bedtime if pain interferes with sleep, and also to help relax muscles. Speed healing with extra vitamin C, echinacea, zinc, vitamin A and beta-carotene, bromelain, amino acids, multivitamins and possibly CoQ10. A nutrient-rich, wholesome diet with extra vegetables and green food products is most important. Vegetable juices and the power drinks described in "Beneficial Beverages" are helpful. Include flaxseed and yogurt in the diet several times a week. Herbal teas to take for sprains and strains include alfalfa, chamomile, fenugreek, feverfew, ginger, ginseng, organic green tea, horsetail, lemon grass and occasionally licorice.

STOMACHACHE

Stomachache can be caused by overeating, poor food combination, gas, food poisoning, parasites, viruses and many other factors. See *Digestion Problems, Heartburn, Nausea* and *Stomach Flu.*

STOMACH FLU

Stomach flu is not really a flu, but a stomach inflammation that may be due to a variety of causes, including viral infection, food poisoning, drug intake or allergies. It may include stomach pains or cramps, diarrhea and/or vomiting. Stomach flu usually lasts for between one and three days and can be treated like a virus. An antiviral remedy may be helpful; see *Viruses.* Fasting or light eating, as with flu, is recommended. See *Nausea* for ways to settle the stomach. Eat foods and drink teas recommended under *Flu* or *Viruses.*

SUNBURN

1. Condition and Cause
Too much exposure to sun can cause skin to get red and then burn. Continued exposure to too much sun can cause skin damage, and may contribute to or cause skin cancer. Choose a natural brand of sun block if possible. Commercial brands of sun tanning and blocking lotions are now claimed by holistic sources to have ingredients that actually contribute to skin damage and skin cancer.

2. Ailment History, Signs and Early Treatments
In ages past, people had more tolerance for the sun and were able to adapt to different amounts of sun and degrees of heat. But in recent decades, the incidence of sunburn, skin damage and skin cancer has risen, because more people are living away from their original climates, because we are spending more time indoors and because of the depletion of the ozone layer. More people are now oversensitive to the effects of the sun. A century ago, "refined" Europeans and North Americans shielded themselves from the sun to avoid freckling and because a tan was considered unattractive, lower-class and not healthy. North American Indians, who lived a

predominantly outdoor life, tanned a rich reddish brown, but also wrinkled at an early age.

People have used oils on their skin to protect it from the sun in past centuries. Sunburn was cooled with a soothing milk and ice mixture that was soaked on the skin, sometimes with the addition of salt. Yogurt, cream and green tea were also used to soothe redness from too much sun.

3. Modern Natural Treatments and Remedies

Today people regulate the amount of sun they get, to avoid skin damage and wrinkles. Certain skin types can tolerate more sun than others. It is healthiest to never let the skin get so much sun that it burns. Methods of prevention include covering easy-to-burn areas of the body with aloe vera gel, either from a bottle or from a fresh plant. Some potent aloe vera creams also offer good protection when used in advance. Vitamin E creams and oils are also used, however, they can sometimes clog the pores and interfere with tanning. If using vitamin E as protection, test a small area of the body first with it to make sure it is effective as some vitamin E lotions are not beneficial. Aloe vera and vitamin E creams, lotions, oils and gel are also used after burning to soothe the skin and help healing. Colloidal silver is also sometimes applied to the skin for sunburn.

One of the most potent skin protectors is cool, soothing, and non-greasy shark oil or (squalane). It can be used under other suntan lotions or all by itself. It can be used after a burn to speed healing and repair the skin as well. Shark oil has been used quite successfully to help heal some cases of skin cancer along with special diets. Apply it generously at least twice daily for burns.

Tea tree oil is a great burn remedy for healing and if applied soon enough after the burn will also prevent blistering and peeling. One drawback is that it stings a little while it heals. The worse the damage, the more likely it is to sting until healing begins to take effect. However tea tree oil speeds healing more effectively than either aloe vera or vitamin E. One approach is to use aloe vera first to cool a burn, and then wipe off the excess and apply tea tree oil for fast healing and reduced skin damage. Apply treatments many times in the first few hours after burning, and then twice daily or more often, as desired, until healed.

4. Helpful Supplements and Dosages

- Take 1,000–5,000 mg vitamin C with bioflavonoids once or twice a day. The more severe the burn, the more vitamin C should be taken.
- Take 100–200 mg vitamin B complex daily until the sunburn is healed.
- Take 10,000 IU vitamin A plus 25,000 IU beta-carotene a day (increase if doctor recommends) for severe sunburn.
- Take 200 IU vitamin E a day until minor sunburn heals or, for major sunburn, take 200 IU a day for the first three days, double to 400 IU for three more days, and then continue with 600 IU—and increase to 1,000 IU or more if doctor recommends. Decrease gradually before stopping.
- Optional: For severe sunburn take one to two 15–30 mg capsules of zinc to speed healing after receiving a sunburn. Repeat daily until the burn is healed. Take 50–100 mg total daily if zinc lozenges are used.
- Optional: Take 50 mg B6 daily for severe sunburn.
- Optional: Take 25 mg PABA (para-aminobenzoic acid) daily, preventatively or after burning.

5. Cautions and Exceptions

Never put butter, lard or creams on new sunburn. They seal in the heat, clog the pores and may hinder healing! Severe sunburn may require a doctor's attention. Use natural treatments on sunburn as soon as possible. If some measure of relief is not obtained within the first hour or so of treatment, seek a physician's advice or go to your hospital emergency room. Severe sunburn may be accompanied by fever, chills and nausea.

6. Nutrition Aids and Recommended Foods

Eat a more wholesome diet for several days after receiving a sunburn. Avoid consuming too many dairy products (except for yogurt) and include lots of green foods—vegetables and a healing green food product—in the diet every day. Avoid fatty foods, sugars, sweets and refined foods.

7. Beverage and Herbal Tea Suggestions

A daily vegetable juice of carrot, beet and green powder can help heal severe sunburn. Daily teas that can aid healing include chamomile for children or adults. For adults, daily herbal teas may include mint teas, chamomile, yarrow, organic green tea and (if your doctor recommends) comfrey. Sleep-aid teas include catnip for children and skullcap and/or hops for adults. See *Insomnia* for more sleep aids.

SWELLING

See *Sprains and Strains*

-T-

TONSILS, SORE

See *Sore Throat*. Consult your doctor.

TOOTHACHE

1. Condition and Cause

Over 200 different types of bacteria are found in the human mouth. Bacteria can lead to infection and contribute to tooth decay and toothache. Toothache can be caused by an infection of the gums or of a root canal, a cracked tooth, a dental cavity or a reaction to a dental treatment. Toothache can be constant, throbbing or intermittent.

In some rare instances, previous work on teeth or on a root canal can become painful because of problems elsewhere in the body. According to holistic health principles, all parts of the body are connected by energy medians—numerous lines of energy, each connecting many parts of the body, that run from the top of the head to extremities of the feet and hands. So a dysfunction of, for example, part of the colon, could result in stress or pain to teeth if they are located on the same median, especially if those teeth are weak or have sustained damage, as through root canal work. New developments in holistic dentistry present alternatives to root canals, and natural remedies can sometimes be effective instead of pain-killing drugs and antibiotics.

After extensive research and personal experience, I have found that some very healthy individuals have root canals and never have another ache or problem, while some more sensitive individuals have endless problems with recurrent pain and infections. Every time their body energy is quite low, previous dental work may become painful. These more sensitive individuals are best to look into alternatives to root canals.

2. Ailment History, Signs and Early Treatments

The art of dentistry was quite advanced for some early civilizations, such as that of the ancient Egyptians. But more primitive methods were employed in the Western world a mere century ago. Teeth were yanked out with nothing to dull the pain, except possibly a "stiff drink." Alcohol, as a beverage or applied to the tooth, was a common painkiller for toothaches. Its help was temporary. Home remedies for toothaches have included wrapping the tooth in a ripe fig, roasted onion or part of a brown paper bag soaked in vinegar and black pepper for 30 to 60 minutes.

3. Modern Natural Treatments and Remedies

There are numerous natural treatments for toothaches, each of which works to a greater or lesser degree. Different people swear by and are helped by different remedies. The quickest home remedies from the kitchen are a garlic clove, grated horseradish, a whole spice clove or lemon (or lime) juice. Try one of these at the first sign of pain, and then call your dentist immediately! Chew on a medium clove of garlic (one small part of a whole bulb of garlic) on the side of the mouth where the ache is. Chew well to release the anti-bacterial juice into the affected area, and then spit out the pulp. Use grated horseradish in the same way. Or place a spice clove between the affected tooth (or teeth) and the teeth above or below and chew slowly. Spit out the remains when done. Or swish the juice of half a lemon (or lime) around the mouth (and then swallow it). Do not eat starchy foods within half an hour of taking the citrus juice. Each of these foods has natural antibiotic qualities, and will often help relieve the pain of toothache.

Use one of the following natural remedies to relieve pain and to heal infection after dental work. Colloidal silver can be taken before, during a series of dental visits and after dental work. See the "Natural Remedies Glossary" section for how much to take internally. It can also be used as a healing mouthwash and gargle. Oil of cloves can be dabbed very sparingly on the offending tooth or gums with a cotton swab. It is quite concentrated and potent so use only a little. Add a drop or two of clove oil to olive oil if you want to dilute it a bit. Peelu extract is a potent natural antibiotic, and is especially beneficial for the gums. Clean the mouth, then swish a teaspoon or two of the extract around the mouth for several minutes and spit it out. Do not eat anything for a half hour or more after using these natural treatments.

Mild aids for toothaches include gargling with warm sea-salt water, aloe vera gel, a few drops of tea tree oil in four ounces of water or low potency (5–24 ppm) colloidal silver. Also see *Oral Hygiene Problems* for everyday care of teeth and gums.

4. Helpful Supplements and Dosages

- Take 2,000–3,000 mg vitamin C one to three times a day during toothaches. Do not take chewable vitamin C—it is acidic and can actually increase toothache pain and eat away at tooth enamel.
- Take 500–1,000 mg calcium/magnesium supplements daily.
- Take about 500 mg propolis powder, tablets or capsules daily.
- Take energizing supplements or sleep aids as needed. See *Energy, Low* and *Insomnia.*
- Optional: For healing after dental work, take 15–30 mg zinc daily.

5. Cautions and Exceptions

The treatments given here for toothache can be quite effective much of the time for easing pain, but they *cannot* be used as a replacement for dental care! Be sure to get treatment from your dentist and use these remedies only after making dental appointments and use them to assist healing and preventing infection after needed work is done. Antibiotics and drug-based painkillers may still be required. Find a holistic dentist who is willing to include natural remedies in your program, if possible. Take acidophilus daily while taking any antibiotic drugs, and for two weeks afterwards. (See the "Natural Remedies Glossary" for how to take.) Preventative dental care includes at least two dental checkups a year.

6. Nutrition Aids and Recommended Foods
Eat a wholesome diet including fresh, raw foods, lots of vegetables, yogurt, whole grains, legumes, fish, and limited amounts of poultry and red meats (about three to five times weekly total for both). Reduce fats and sweets in the diet, especially sugars, sugar substitutes, natural sweeteners, tropical and sweet fruits. Dried fruits contribute more to cavities than other sweet foods, because they stick to the teeth for much longer and therefore help erode the enamel. Lemon juice, while occasionally helpful for toothaches, should also not be left on the teeth, because it is very acidic and it too eats away at tooth enamel. Avoid dried fruit and lemon juice at night, unless you make sure to brush the teeth soon after.

Although cheddar cheese is rumored to be beneficial for preventing dental cavities, it can actually contribute to infections and tooth decay if it is left on the teeth for long periods of time, especially at night. The mold content in the cheese can contribute to Candida yeast infections in the mouth and increase bacteria.

7. Beverage and Herbal Tea Suggestions
If you are suffering from toothache or other dental problems, avoid drinking all kinds of carbonated pop or soft drinks, which are acidic and damage tooth enamel. This includes everything from club soda to orange pop and root beer, and especially all cola drinks. Avoid drinking very cold or hot beverages. Drink cool or warm drinks instead to avoid added tooth pain. Vegetable juices (except for tomato) served at room temperature, three to six times a week, can help healing.

Goldenseal and myrrh herbal tea can be made like a strong tincture and swished around the mouth several times a day for minor relief. It can also be applied to teething babies' gums to ease pain. Adults can also drink a few ounces, once or twice a day. Babies can be given a teaspoon or two up to a few times a day.

Chamomile, peppermint and yarrow herbal teas have a natural anti-inflammatory effect. Cayenne can be added to tea for healing effects if you can handle it. It stings at first, but then soothes pain.

TEETH CLEANING

See *Oral Hygiene Problems*

TOXIC METAL OVERDOSE

See *Heavy Metal Overdose*

TOXIN OVERLOAD

1. Condition and Cause
The average American and Canadian consumes 14 pounds of food additives and chemicals each year, not to mention the hundreds of pounds of toxic substances that are inhaled, the amount depending on what urban or rural area of North America you reside in. Toxic substances build up in the body, weaken the immune system and cause or contribute to disease. Cleansing is a natural way to rid the body of toxic buildup.

Cleansing involves using special herbs, natural remedies and internal cleaning agents, along with a whole-foods diet, to remove stored poisons and toxins from the body, aid the digestion and elimination organs, slow down the aging process, increase energy and circulation and complement healing processes. Cleansing is rather like performing surgery on yourself, and must be done very cautiously with expert advice from a holistic doctor or qualified cleansing expert.

Cleanses include food cleanses (the easiest and safest); herbal and supplement cleanses; liver (using milk thistle, dandelion, artichoke extract and other herbs), colon, other organ and full body cleanses (often purchased in kits from health food stores); anti-viral and parasite cleanses (see *Viruses* and *Parasites*); toxic or heavy metal cleanses; and anti-aging cleanses. Cleansing is not the same as fasting. It does not require abstention from food, but a special healing diet is required while cleansing. It is safest to use only one kind of cleansing herb or product at a time, and not to exceed two to four cleanses (or 90 days of cleansing) within a year. (See the "Healing Aids" section for more information on cleansing.)

If you have regular symptoms of bad health that might be caused by toxic overload, consider cleansing but *always* consult a holistic doctor or qualified cleansing expert first! Such health problems include severe allergy problems, indigestion, chronic fatigue, poor circulation, extreme illness or disease, skin rashes, constipation or diarrhea or frequent headaches.

2. Ailment History, Signs and Early Treatments

Although fasting has been around for many thousands of years, cleansing is a fairly new development of the last century that only became necessary because of our toxic atmosphere, increased additives and poisons in our water and food and increasingly unhealthy living habits.

3. Modern Natural Treatments and Remedies

Two to four cleanses per year are recommended by many health experts today, including myself. Ann Louise Gittleman, M.S., author of numerous health books, including *Super Nutrition for Women/Men* and *Your Body Knows Best* recommends two parasite cleanses a year for North Americans. However, one parasite cleanse is usually sufficient unless you do a lot of international travel. Cleanses can last from 24 hours to, more commonly, 12 to 30 days, depending on the results you wish to achieve. The primary food cleanse—and everybody's first cleanse—should be an improved diet! Simply changing the diet for the better will help expel some stored body poisons and gradually improve overall health. This process takes anything from one month to many months, as you choose. Complete guidelines for improving the diet step-by-step are provided in my book *For the Love of Food.*

Other food cleanses that may be utilized *after* changing the overall diet include the daily use of garlic, lemons or limes, green foods or products based on them (barley green, wheat grass, green kamut, spirulina, chlorella, blue green algae, aloe vera or others), seaweeds, cayenne pepper, as well as a variety of other less well-known food cleanses. The primary cleanses listed here are outlined for individual use, preferably under an expert's supervision, once the overall diet has been changed. For other cleanses see the alternatives listed above, the "Natural Remedies Glossary" and your holistic doctor or qualified cleansing expert.

GARLIC   Garlic is one of the most powerful everyday foods. It is easily available and most people tolerate it well. When it is used in cooking, the beneficial effect is minimal, but when eaten raw, it provides positive healing reactions. During colds, flu or Candida problems, chewing raw garlic kills bacteria and fungi in the mouth and throat. It's easy to add raw garlic to a salad or salad dressing. Or chew garlic by itself and spit out the pulp—though one does have to deal with garlic breath after chewing raw garlic. Chewing raw parsley shortly after a meal that includes raw garlic can help reduce the smell (and taste).

Another way to ingest garlic is in supplements. However, even the most potent capsules are limited in their capacities because the garlic must be processed, which destroys certain qualities of the garlic (exactly which qualities is yet to be fully determined). Certain other qualities may be enhanced by processing.

One potent method of taking garlic is to eat it raw *without* chewing it, but you will need to take precautions to avoid stomach upset with this method. Take one medium clove of garlic and chop or mince it very finely; do not press or crush it. This releases the juice, which contains healing allicin. (Allicin is the essential element in garlic oil, responsible for its antibacterial and anti-inflammatory qualities.) Garlic also helps to normalize blood sugar levels.

Never take raw garlic this way on an empty stomach! Halfway through a regular meal, take chopped garlic on a spoon and put it on the back of your tongue. Wash it down with water, without chewing, so the precious juice remains in the garlic until it reaches the small intestines, where it can do the most good, killing Candida and other parasites and purging toxins from the body. (Carbohydrate-digested foods like garlic break down mainly in the small intestines.) Avoid putting garlic on the front part of the tongue if you want to avoid the strong flavor and garlic breath. You may take one to three cloves of garlic a day for weeks or a month or more at a time with no garlic breath. After ingesting the garlic, continue with your meal.

Garlic works best when taken daily for periods of one or two months (usually 30 to 45 days is enough). Do not exceed this time period, because overextended use of garlic (and other natural remedies) can contribute to sensitivities or allergies and anemia.

One may experience healing reactions or apparent side effects while taking garlic this way during the entire time period. These reactions usually indicate that the garlic is doing its work and bacteria and parasites are reacting to it. As a test for parasites I suggest taking a medium clove of garlic (about three-quarters to one teaspoon minced) daily for 10 to 14 days. If you experience no reactions, you probably do not have a yeast or parasite problem.

Often, within 3 to 10 days of eating garlic, an individual with Candida yeast or parasite problems may become nervous, irritable, hyperactive, easily angered, emotional and/or queasy in the stomach. This may indicate a yeast problem, and their doctor will usually confirm this suspicion. Slight reactions may simply indicate that the garlic is helping the body cleanse itself of toxins. For the sensitive, choose a smaller clove of garlic (about half a teaspoon minced), or take the garlic every other day to reduce cleansing side effects.

Use only the regular type of garlic (not elephant garlic) and be sure it is organic. Organic garlic often, but not always, has a purplish color in the outer skin. Non-organic garlic may have been treated with formaldehyde and other unnatural additives and pesticides.

LEMON JUICE OR LIME JUICE CLEANSE   Lemon juice is a potent antibacterial, cleansing and healing food. It can kill bacteria and fungi, especially in the mouth and throat, and also in the stomach. Unfortunately, it loses its full potency before it reaches the intestines. Many people mix lemon juice with hot water, which reduces its value even more. To be fully effective, lemon juice (or lime juice, which is equally effective) must be ingested full strength. (However, people who are very sensitive may need to dilute the juice if they have too strong a reaction while cleansing.)

Squeeze one small lemon or one-half of a large lemon (three or four tablespoons) and drink the juice straight down on an empty stomach (do not use bottled or canned juice!). It can be drunk first thing in the morning (after nothing but water), at midmorning or midafternoon—but never at night. Do not leave juice in the mouth any longer than necessary (about half an hour), as it can strip enamel from the teeth if it is regularly left in contact with them for long periods. If you like, you can drink the juice with a straw, but it is best if you gulp it quickly all at once. After drinking the juice, take two or three sips of water and notice how sweet it tastes in your mouth.

This treatment is often effective for avoiding minor throat irritations that can lead to coughs and colds. It is most effective if it is taken for 7 to 21 days in a row. You may notice a metallic taste on the tongue after several days of this treatment, as lemon juice is a potent expeller of heavy metals from the body. If this occurs, gargle with sea-salt water, aerobic oxygen in water, or antibacterial mouthwash or other cleansing gargle to remove traces of metals being brought up in the mouth for the body to eliminate. For the sensitive, the juice can be reduced to two tablespoons, and/or the juice can be taken every other day. As noted above, the extremely sensitive may dilute the juice with an equal amount of spring or distilled water, though this is not nearly as good at killing mouth and throat bacteria.

After drinking the lemon juice, followed by a few sips of water, do not eat for at least 15 minutes! Even then, eat only tart or subacid fruits (like apples, pears or berries), or wait 30 minutes before eating any other foods.

If slight dizziness occasionally occurs after taking the lemon juice, it is a natural sign that the juice is doing its work. The wave of dizziness is generally quick and temporary. If dizziness persists, eat subacid fruits promptly or yogurt if needed or desired. Whenever possible, purchase organic lemons, but only if they are high-quality, fully ripe and fresh, otherwise it is better to buy non-organic.

ALOE VERA GEL, BARLEY GREEN JUICE, WHEAT GRASS JUICE AND OTHER GREEN FOODS   These green foods are listed together because they serve similar purposes in healing—but it is best to use only one of these treatments at a time. Many people have strong healing reactions to these foods, much more so than to garlic or lemon juice, and I do not advocate mixing several green food products together—except for very hardy individuals.

Aloe vera is generally more potent in gel form. Care must be taken to select a product that is full strength, not watered down or processed so heavily that it has lost its medicinal properties. Ask your health-care specialist for recommended brands. Aloe vera is a wonderful stomach soother and is claimed to heal ulcers and internal and external wounds. Like other controversial foods, aloe vera and some other green foods are not right for everyone. Since aloe vera has an astringent effect, it is not always beneficial for those with dry skin, those on fat-reduced diets or some body types. Get checked and tested by your holistic health-care specialist to see if it is right for your body type and health concern.

Barley green juice and wheat grass juice work similarly. Barley is generally preferred, as wheat is a common allergen. These juices have been used for cancer treatment, cleansing and healing diets. They contain high amounts of chlorophyll, protein and beta-carotene, with some vitamin C, vitamin B12 and other trace nutrients. Barley green juice is particularly high in potassium and calcium, while wheat grass has more iron. It is best to take these healing "green drinks" (the aloe may be clear, but it comes from a green plant like the others) 30 to 60 minutes after meals to lessen reactions. Start with half an ounce (1 tablespoon) at a time; increase to 1 ounce or more, if tolerated and approved by your doctor or health-care specialist. Take the initial smaller dose for two weeks or more before increasing amounts. Stay with the new amount for at least two weeks before increasing again. For green food powders, start with one-quarter of a teaspoon or less, and increase after two weeks only if you are very comfortable with this amount. Adjust amounts to a comfortable level or leave at a small dose. To stop taking green drinks, slowly reduce the treatment by cutting it in half every three to seven days, until amounts are one-half to one tablespoon of liquid or one-eighth to one-quarter of a teaspoon of powder, as preferred.

Other green foods that may be used include spirulina, chlorella, blue-green algae, green kamut and astragalus. The first three are micro-algae and are high in protein, iron, other minerals and vitamin B12, as well as healing chlorophyll. They protect the immune system, balance blood sugar and help lower cholesterol.

ALL GREEN FOOD PRODUCTS   Using one type of green food at a time is more beneficial than taking a "green mixture" that may contain anything from a dozen to 60 ingredients, including various green foods and additives (not all of them natural). Many of these mixtures also contain large amounts of sweeteners, again not always natural. These products do not agree with many people, especially those with food sensitivities, allergies, or other health problems. (Some people get a "buzz" or feel "high" from taking green products for the first few months or longer; this often passes once the body gets enough of the green nutrients that it has been deficient in. Most North Americans do not usually include enough green vegetables or herbs in their diet.) It is best to use one green product at a time, for 30 to 60 days, skip a couple of weeks, and then switch to another type of green. Rotating between different greens allows you to enjoy the benefits unique to each green product. As noted above, remember to build up green food dosages slowly, and decrease gradually before stopping.

KELP, DULSE AND OTHER SEAWEEDS   These foods are used widely in East Asian countries like China and Japan, and are natural anti-fungals and heavy metal–expellers. Kelp, also called sea kelp, is used to help with weight loss and thyroid healing, and to regulate the metabolism.

Kelp contains iodine and high amounts of magnesium, calcium, phosphorus and potassium, as well as sodium and trace B vitamins. Other seaweeds have the same nutrients, in lesser amounts than kelp, but with no recognizable magnesium and higher iron content. Dulse has the least value, with only calcium and iron as special nutrients. Seaweeds have been used as healing foods for centuries. They are most helpful when eaten two to five days a week for a month or longer.

Note: Seaweeds are not recommended with certain types of thyroid medications! Consult your doctor if taking prescription thyroid drugs.

CAYENNE PEPPER   Cayenne is a stimulant, and is beneficial to the circulation and the heart. It helps to keep the arteries clear so the blood flows smoothly. It is also good for ulcers. Dr. John Christopher, one of the world's most renowned herbalists, devoted a book entitled *Capsicum* to the wonderful benefits of cayenne. Capsicum is the name of the potent healing agent in cayenne.

Cayenne aggravates and kills the Candida yeast and some parasites; they do not like spicy foods. Spices have been used for centuries to preserve foods, long before refrigerators came to be, especially in hot countries. Note the traditional spicy foods of the Middle East, India, Thailand, Mexico, and Caribbean countries in particular. Cayenne, along with spices such as cloves, curries, ginger, garlic and horseradish, fight yeast and some other parasites as well. (Consult your holistic doctor before taking ginger or clove supplements or teas on a regular basis.)

Cayenne can be used almost daily in meals. Use it frequently in recipes, and sprinkle it in herb teas occasionally to break up mucus in the throat. Or take it in capsules, on a full stomach. If you take cayenne capsules on an empty stomach, it may feel like you have swallowed a bomb: Your eyes may water and it can bring on a downpour of tears as well as temporary stomach pains. As with garlic, take cayenne capsules halfway through a meal or cayenne (not garlic) can be taken immediately afterwards.

4. Helpful Supplements and Dosages
Additional remedies are not usually needed while food cleansing. However, the following may be helpful if needed:
- Take digestive aids and/or laxative teas and flushing agents as needed.
- Vitamin C—especially Allergy C, Ester C or buffered C can help reduce symptoms, energize and boost the immune system. Take 500–1,000 mg one to four times a day as needed, at least three or four hours before sleeping. Do not take chewable vitamin C. For children, vitamin C powder can be mixed into solid food.
- Take energizing supplements if needed. See *Energy, Low*.

5. Cautions and Exceptions
Do not take any of these foods if you are allergic to them. Only use one special food (or other) cleanse at a time, and only after establishing and while still following an overall improved diet! Do not exceed the amount of time suggested for each food (or other) cleanse. Negative health symptoms may actually increase slightly during the first three to eight days, but they should improve after that. If severe negative reactions occur, consult your holistic health practitioner immediately and, slowly or immediately, as advised,

end the specific food cleanse—but continue the improved diet! For packaged cleansing herbs and remedies, follow the directions given with the product in regards to altering and ending these cleanses or consult the "Natural Remedies Glossary."

A "cleansing or healing reaction" is a set of side effects that occur while using cleansing herbs or products. These reactions are generally harmless signs that the body is purging poisons and healing. They may include slight nausea, headaches, indigestion, light-headedness, fatigue, irritability, minor aches and anxiety. However, cleansing too much, too often or too fast can be very dangerous. It is best to start with easy food cleanses or small doses of herbs or remedies (as suggested above), adjusting the amounts if needed.

Similarly, a "green reaction" may occur as a cleansing side effect of taking green food products. If *major* side effects occur, consult a holistic doctor immediately!

6. Nutrition Aids and Recommended Foods
For the most effective cleansing, follow the Phase II or Phase III diet in my *Complete Candida Yeast Guidebook*. Enjoy a mainly whole-foods diet, avoiding too many sweets, junk foods and other agitating foods.

7. Beverage and Herbal Tea Suggestions
Drink all the usual pleasure herbal teas like mint, raspberry or strawberry leaf, lemon grass, rose hips, chamomile, fennel, fenugreek and other mild teas (except, of course, any you are allergic to). Organic green tea is better than coffee during food cleanses. It is best to avoid coffee and alcohol, or at least to have them four or more hours away from any cleansing foods. While on any other cleanses than food cleanses, do not drink *any* coffee or alcohol. You should never smoke while on *any* cleanse.

-U-

URINARY INFECTION

See *Bladder Infection*

-V-

VARICOSE VEINS

See also *Circulation*

Varicose veins are helped by extra vitamin C, bioflavonoids, vitamins A and E and zinc. Eat a wholesome, well-balanced diet, including especially: green and orange vegetables, salads, sprouts, green food products, whole grains, legumes, fish, lecithin, flaxseed and yogurt. Apply topically, one of the following (or alternate between two) on swollen veins one to three times a day: tea tree oil, aloe vera gel, oregano oil or colloidal silver. Add a dash or two of cayenne for added stimulation. Enjoy ginger, bilberry, hawthorn, peppermint, spearmint, lemon grass, raspberry leaf or fennel tea.

Aid circulation by practicing the shoulder stand from yoga, or raise the legs above the head against a wall for several minutes, one to three times a day. Try learning and practicing yoga, tai chi, qi gong or other similar stretching movements. Take walks and wear supportive shoes. Go barefoot at home. Hot/cold: packs, baths and showers help, as can massage, chiropractic, acupressure or acupuncture.

VIRUSES

1. Condition and Cause

According to *Alternative Medicine*, by the Burton Goldberg Group, "a virus is the smallest of parasites..." A virus is a living microorganism, which in its simplest form is a strand of DNA or RNA surrounded by protein and often fats. It invades and rapidly reproduces in body cells; usually it eventually explodes body cells, then reproduces in surrounding cells. Viral symptoms include fever (usually low grade), general aches, tiredness, chills and sometimes headaches and mental fatigue. Viruses are spread mainly through the air or by saliva, blood and sexual contact. The common cold, chicken pox, diarrhea, ear infections, herpes, AIDS, measles, mumps, mononucleosis, pneumonia, tonsillitis and some kinds of warts are all examples of viral diseases.

2. Ailment History, Signs and Early Treatments
In the recent past, viruses have been unsuccessfully treated with antibiotics. Most traditional allopathic medical doctors will tell you there is no exact drug or cure for a virus. Doctors recommend rest, sometimes good diet and waiting it out. Ancient and medieval treatments included garlic and herbs.

3. Modern Natural Treatments and Remedies
Holistic treatments for viruses include dozens of naturopathic, homeopathic, herbal and food treatments, many of which have proven quite successful in reducing viral symptoms and promoting more rapid recovery. Some natural anti-virals include: garlic, lemons, limes, cayenne, green food products, citricidal, goldenseal, myrrh, oil of oregano, colloidal silver, olive leaf extract, colostrum, vitamin C, tea tree oil and aloe vera. Usually 14 to 30 days of treatment with one or two of these will do the trick if accompanied by a proper healing diet and possibly some digestive aids, acidophilus, extra vitamin C and energizing supplements. See the listing for each item in the "Natural Remedies Glossary" for how to take these natural anti-virals. Also, because most of these anti-virals are also cleansing products, see *Toxin Overload* for how to cleanse properly and safely.

4. Helpful Supplements and Dosages
- Take 2,000–10,000 mg vitamin C a day, depending on the severity of the virus.
- One or more cloves of fresh, raw garlic a day, chopped and not chewed, taken as directed in the "Natural Remedies Glossary" will help any other natural anti-viral treatment to be more effective. (Use lemons or limes if allergic to garlic.) You may also take high-quality garlic capsules (two to six daily), though they are typically not as beneficial as fresh garlic.
- Take two capsules of high-quality acidophilus, if possible with bifidus, with four or five ounces of water, once or twice a day, an hour or more away from meals and before supper.
- Optional but helpful: Take 15–30 mg zinc daily to assist healing.

- Optional: Use laxative or digestive aids and energizing supplements if needed.

5. Cautions and Exceptions

Avoid all treatments you are allergic to. Pregnant women and individuals with heart problems or on special medications must avoid using goldenseal as well as many other anti-viral treatments. (See "Natural Remedies Glossary" for safe use and recommendations for each anti-viral.) If you have any major health concerns whatsoever, consult your holistic physician before taking any treatment (except vitamin C, which is safe for everyone). Do not take anti-viral remedies along with conflicting drugs. Consult your holistic doctor to avoid possible complications from herb/drug interactions.

Echinacea may be helpful for some minor viruses, but it is detrimental to others. Use only if recommended by your doctor. Lemon or lime juice, grapefruit or citricidal should not be taken during the same period as colloidal silver, because citrus expels and counteracts silver and some other metals.

6. Nutrition Aids and Recommended Foods

Healing from viral infections requires a nutrient-rich diet of all-natural foods for the best results and healing. No fried foods, junk foods, refined foods, sugar or sugar substitutes, dairy products except yogurt, raw foods except in moderation, red meats, corn products, pasta, potatoes or other non-healing foods. Make 40 to 60 percent of your diet vegetables, plus additional whole grains and legumes. For mild viruses, use the Phase III diet from my *Complete Candida Yeast Guidebook*, and for major viruses use the Phase II diet.

7. Beverage and Herbal Tea Suggestions

Herbal tea suggestions include: fennel, fenugreek, peppermint, spearmint, ginger or raspberry leaf for general consumption, and licorice (if allowed), or senna leaves with flax for laxative effect. To aid sleep, skullcap or valerian tea is best. Vegetable juices three to six times a week are highly beneficial. Fresh grapefruit juice or club soda with a slice of ginger, lemon or lime can be a helpful digestive aid if taken with protein meals or between meals.

-W-

WARTS

1. Condition and Cause

Warts are usually, though not always, caused by a type of virus. One of 50 different viruses may be the culprit. A few types of warts are linked to possible cancer. Most warts are bumps or growths that may be light or dark in color, flat or slightly raised, and may appear singly or in clusters. Warts vary in size from a pin head up to about one-third of an inch in diameter. Body warts usually appear on the hands, arms, legs, feet or elsewhere on the body. Genital warts are the most contagious of sexually transmitted diseases. They are often pink or reddish in color, and may be raised and puffy like small cauliflower florets. Most warts are contagious, especially if they break open and their fluid contacts other parts of the body or another person. Plantar warts are only contagious to the feet and usually cannot be spread to other parts of the body. Babies may be infected with warts by their mothers during the birthing process.

2. Ailment History, Signs and Early Treatments

Washing your hands at midnight by the light of a full moon was one folk cure for ridding yourself of warts. This would probably be helpful if you managed to get a wart from handling a toad! Other folk cures involved covering the wart with crushed figs for 20 to 30 minutes a day until the wart disappeared or, for a similar amount of time, soaking it in spit or dandelion stem juice, covering it with garlic or onion slices, rubbing it with raw potatoes or pineapple chunks, covering or rubbing it with the inside of a banana or papaya skin. Some of these treatments are still used today as home remedies and natural treatments.

3. Modern Natural Treatments and Remedies

Some warts naturally disappear within a few months. Sometimes treating a virus internally actually clears up some warts without external treatment. (See *Viruses* for natural virus remedies.) However, the process of clearing up warts can be speeded up by using external applications as well. One of the best treatments is to apply 100 percent tea tree oil to the wart(s) and also soak the oil on a band-aid strip and place it on the wart for four to eight hours a day (it is easiest to do it at night and sleep with it on) until the wart lifts out or dries up. This takes between a few days to three weeks. Aloe vera gel, either directly from a plant or in a potent liquid form, can also be used, but it works more slowly than tea tree oil and may take up to a month or more to be effective.

Oil of oregano is also highly effective. Place a drop on the wart several times a day, or use the band-aid method described above for even faster results. The speed of healing varies greatly with the type and size of wart. Commercial liquid wart removers sold in most drug stores have side effects that may be dangerous for people with certain health problems.

4. Helpful Supplements and Dosages
- Take 1,000–2,000 mg vitamin C a day for body warts and 2,000–10,000 mg a day for genital warts.
- Take 10,000 IU vitamin A a day, or two or three times this amount if your doctor recommends, for a month or so while treating the wart externally.
- Take 20,000–100,000 IU beta-carotene daily, as your doctor recommends, for one or two months for multiple or persistent warts.
- Take one vitamin B50 complex two to four times a day to promote normal cell growth.
- Take 500 mg L-cysteine twice a day alone (away from food or other supplements) with water and vitamin C and B complex, to help prevent or heal warts.
- Optional but helpful: One or more cloves of fresh, raw garlic a day, chopped and not chewed, and taken as directed in the "Natural Remedies Glossary," is a great anti-viral for warts. (Use a lemon or lime juice cleanse if allergic to garlic.) You may also take high-quality garlic capsules (two to six daily), though they are typically not as beneficial as fresh garlic.
- Optional but helpful: Take 200–400 IU vitamin E daily, particularly for genital warts.

- Optional but helpful: Take 15–50 mg zinc daily to assist healing.

5. Cautions and Exceptions

Stick with one external treatment within a given time period. Follow with another method if necessary. Avoid treatments you are allergic to. Lemon or lime juice, grapefruit or citricidal should not be taken during the same time period as colloidal silver, because citrus expels and counteracts silver and some other metals. Remember that most warts are contagious. If you have genital warts, avoid intercourse and wear light-colored cotton underwear until the warts clear up. Keep warts clean and dry. Do not take anti-viral remedies with conflicting drugs. Consult your holistic doctor to avoid possible complications from herb/drug interactions. If pregnant, consult your doctor before using internal treatments.

6. Nutrition Aids and Recommended Foods

A nutrient-rich diet of mainly natural foods gets the best results and promotes healing. Avoid fried foods, junk foods, refined foods, sugar or sugar substitutes, dairy products except yogurt, too many raw foods, red meats, corn products, pasta, potatoes, tropical and sweet fruits, oranges, and other non-healing foods. Eat mainly green vegetables (at least two servings a day) and orange vegetables (carrots, winter squash and yams, six to eight servings a week), high sulfur foods (garlic, onions, horseradish, cabbage, Brussels sprouts, chili peppers, eggs, white fish and salmon, one to two servings daily), whole grains (five or more servings a week) and legumes (at least three servings a week), yogurt or kefir, miso and/or seaweed. Include a teaspoon of flax meal sprinkled on food four to six times a week or one to three teaspoons of flax oil three to five days a week.

High-sulfur foods contain nutrients that assist the healing of warts.

7. Beverage and Herbal Tea Suggestions

Herbal tea suggestions include: chamomile, fennel, fenugreek, peppermint, spearmint, ginger and raspberry leaf for general consumption, and licorice (if allowed) or senna leaves with flax for laxative effect. To aid sleep, skullcap or valerian tea is best. Taheebo tea can be beneficial for some people, if your doctor recommends it. Vegetable juices with added green food products, three to six times a week, are highly beneficial. Fresh grapefruit juice or club soda with a slice of ginger, lemon or lime can be a helpful digestive aid if taken with protein meals or between meals.

WEIGHT PROBLEMS

1. Condition and Cause
Weight problems include both weight gain and weight loss. Obesity has never been a greater problem than it is today. Sedentary living habits play a major role in our unhealthy lifestyles, and often contribute to or cause obesity. Contributing factors include the increase in desk jobs and the corresponding drop in manual labor, the rise of motorized transportation, general lack of exercise, the predominance of refined and junk foods in the diet, hours of sitting around watching TV, hours of doing computer work or playing computer games, increasing use of drugs, alcohol and tobacco. These poor living habits not only contribute to obesity, they may cause it. Health problems and disease, and increasing hereditary predisposition to weight problems, are also factors in obesity.

Underweight is less of a problem, but there are still individuals who can consume unlimited quantities of calories and are still not able to attain or maintain a desirable weight.

2. Ailment History, Signs and Early Treatments
In earlier times, only the wealthy had the means and opportunity to overeat, and to sit or lie around long enough to become overweight. In some less privileged cultures, such as in India, extra weight is considered attractive and a sign of good health. In places where poverty and malnutrition are common, extra weight is a luxury and a blessing. In North America, by contrast, we worship thinness, which promotes bulimia and anorexia. Yet, despite the seriousness of these issues, overweight problems far outstrip the problem of underweight.

3. Modern Natural Treatments and Remedies
Dieting, exercise and appetite-curbing drugs are the common prescription for overweight problems today. Proper eating is often

ignored as a major remedy for weight problems. However, even if you have a perfect diet and exercise regimen, dozens of other underlying factors can interfere with weight loss (or gain).

Individuals may not be able to lose (or gain) weight if:

1. they are overstressed due to emotional problems or overwork (extra weight can be a physical "protection" from psychological stress)
2. they have allergic reactions to food and/or the environment
3. they have Candida yeast problems
4. they have major vitamin or mineral deficiencies or overabundances
5. they have heavy metal poisoning
6. they have an underlying major health problem, organ malfunction or disease
7. they have digestive problems
8. they have an active viral infection
9. they are abusing alcohol, tobacco or drugs
10. they have thyroid problems, a chemical imbalance or genetic problems that interfere with body weight
11. they eat too many of the wrong kinds of fatty foods, or avoid fats altogether
12. they eat too many sugars and sugar substitutes
13. they binge or splurge, then starve, without eating regular, balanced meals
14. they don't know, understand or follow proper weight loss (or gain) requirements
15. they do not follow proper food combining
16. they do not chew their food properly but gulp it down
17. they rest, lie down or close their eyes after eating, which slows digestion and thus increases calorie absorption (this is only for inability to lose weight)
18. they take too many digestive aids
19. they have major parasite problems
20. they have blood sugar problems
21. they have hormone imbalances
22. they are pregnant (this is only for inability to lose weight)
23. their body is toxic and clogged with poisons
24. they do not get enough rest and quality sleep

25. their life pace is too fast
26. they eat too much meat that contains weight-gaining hormones and drugs
27. they have psychological reasons why, at some level, they do not really want to lose weight (for instance, wanting to hide behind it, being sexually frustrated or wanting to punish themselves or others).

If one or more of these factors are a problem, then weight loss or gain, even with proper diet and right exercise, may not be possible until these problems are addressed. See the nutrition aids section below for essential diet information for weight loss and gain. See your doctor for medical tests to rule out contributory problems such as those listed above.

Daily exercise, both aerobic and stretching, is essential. But if you mostly sit around, just one exercise period a day will not be enough. Walk to the store, take a walk after each meal, walk up and down stairs as much as possible throughout the day, deliver your interoffice mail and messages yourself, do your own housework and gardening, cook to exercise your arm muscles, iron (while standing), ride an exercise bike while watching TV, play with the kids. All these activities will help stimulate good digestion and a healthy metabolism. Keep moving! This is essential for weight loss.

If you want to gain weight, you need to s l o w d o w n. Fast metabolism is often to blame when one is underweight (other factors such as those listed above may also be part of the problem). It is best to lie down after eating to slow digestion and increase absorption of nutrients and calories. Close your eyes and take a nap after eating if possible.

You should not need weight-loss (or weight-gain) drugs if you get to your underlying problems with weight. You have to discover the real reasons why you cannot lose the weight—then you have to make a decision to do what is required to lose the weight.

4. Helpful Supplements and Dosages
- Take a quality, natural multivitamin every day.
- Take 500–1500 mg vitamin C a day.

- Take two to four vitamin B50 complex a day to combat stress and assist carbohydrate metabolism.
- Take a green food product every day (such as spirulina, blue-green algae, barley greens, chlorella, alfalfa). See *Toxin Overload* for information on green foods.
- Talk to your holistic doctor about supplements that may be suited to your weight program. Possibilities include: lecithin granules, liquid or capsules to provide energy and to help remove fats from the body; HCA (hydroxycitric acid) and/or calcium to break down fats; amino acids to reduce fats; GLA (gamma linolenic acid) to control fat metabolism; CoQ10 to convert fats into energy; phenylalanine or guar gum to suppress the appetite; chromium to reduce sugar cravings; digestive aids and acidophilus; ephedra (ma huang) to decrease appetite and elevate mood, which helps with obesity; and citrin to suppress cravings and hunger, block fat accumulation and promote fat loss. Health stores carry other weight loss products and combinations.

5. Cautions and Exceptions

Stay away from crash or fad diets like the grapefruit diet, bran diet, brown rice diet or fruit-only diets that limit your food intake to only specific foods. These diets are dangerous and may lead to serious health problems and actually increase your weight in the long run. People who diet incorrectly often increase their weight within 6 to 12 months. Beware too of diet pills and of drugs with harmful side effects.

6. Nutrition Aids and Recommended Foods

The good news is that you do not have to ever go hungry or starve to lose weight. You can actually lose more weight eating three meals a day than by bingeing and starving yourself! Living on raw celery and carrots alone could kill you over time, or at the very least send you into depression and frustration. *How to Lower Your Fat Thermostat*, by Dr. Dennis Remington—one of the most excellent books on weight loss—gives many important principles of dieting, the chief of which is that the brain helps regulate weight gain and loss. When eating or dieting by bingeing and then starving yourself, you send a message to the brain that occasional "famines" (starving) are occurring, which you are trying to make up for with occasional "feasting" (bingeing). The brain gets the message and raises the fat regulator or "thermostat" in the brain to a higher level so your "normal" weight will be raised higher to protect you from these "famines."

When you eat healthily—that is two to three meals a day with up to three snacks, at regular intervals—the brain notices that the "famine" is over and that you will no longer need extra weight to protect yourself. It lowers your thermostat correspondingly and your "normal" weight is lessened. This is why diets like Weight Watchers® are more successful in the long term than crash diets. Specialized, extreme fad diets help you lose weight temporarily, but you will regain the weight, and then some, after you go back to your regular eating patterns. Diets that include regular, full, meals cause you to lose weight more gradually and sustainably, and you usually will keep it off if you continue good eating habits. Such diets allow you to lose more than just water weight. So eat a variety of good foods in your overall diet.

Counting calories is essentially a waste of time! Each individual absorbs a different number of calories from the same quantity and type of food. If a 200-pound man and a 130-pound woman ate exactly the same meals, it's possible that the man might gain more weight than the woman. The difference is in how your individual body processes food. This is affected by your body metabolism and by the various factors listed in the treatments section above. Calories from wholesome foods are more beneficial than those from fats, sugars and sweets. Skipping a 1,200-calorie lunch for a 1,200-calorie candy bar can trigger the brain's "feast or famine" mechanism just like bingeing and starving can, because while the candy bar may have usable calories, it is deficient in proper nutrients that can be used to nourish the body. Calories from sugars and fats do not satisfy the body's needs for nutrients, so cravings may occur.

How you combine foods in each meal makes a major difference as well. Very healthy individuals do not need to worry about how they combine their food. But if you are not healthy, or if your digestion is impaired for any reason—which may be evidenced by the fact of having a weight problem—then food combining becomes necessary.

Food combining is not supported, or is actively opposed, by the majority of physicians, in part because of the one-sided information presented to North Americans over the last few decades. Among those holistic doctors who do accept it, the principles are widely debated and disagreed upon. There are no do-or-die rules of food combining, but if the major principles are followed, digestion improves and fewer calories are absorbed. You can prove its value to yourself by trying it. If two people of the same weight, sex, age, health and body type, who do the same amount of exercise, were to eat the same foods but in different combinations, the person who followed the food combining rules would absorb fewer calories and therefore gain less weight. Thousands of people are finding this out by following "new" protein power diets (which can cause future health problems if followed for too long, because the minimal carbohydrate intake can eventually help "starve" the brain) or high-carbohydrate diets like those of Dr. John MacDougal. Both of these vastly different diets follow food combining. The first diet is made up of protein meals and the latter (which is safer and more practical in the long run) is made up of carbohydrate meals.

There are two main tried and tested food-combining principles:

1. Eat raw fruits alone or first in a meal—never after a meal. Fruits, which are high in enzymes, are one of the easiest foods to digest, but when mixed with other foods (such as when eaten after a meal) fruit digestion is slowed, increasing calorie absorption and causing or contributing to possible fermentation of foods. (When dieting, stay away from really sweet fruits like grapes, mangoes, coconut, bananas, pineapples and oranges, especially if you have health problems like allergies, blood sugar problems and Candida.) Eating fruit after a meal increases indigestion and gas. Eat raw fruit 15 to 30 minutes *before* breakfast, if possible, or, if eating it *with* breakfast, cook the fruit to kill the enzymes so it will be digested more slowly, like a carbohydrate food. Eat raw fruit no sooner than 90 minutes after a full meal. Do not eat any raw fruit after supper or at night. Raw, dried fruit should be eaten according to the same rules as raw fresh fruit, and cooked dried fruit like cooked fresh fruit.

2. Eat heavy protein foods (like red and white meats, dairy products, and a limited quantity of nuts) and heavy carbohydrate foods (like potatoes, rice, millet, corn, wheat and other whole grains) in separate meals. Most vegetables are considered neutral and can be eaten with either a protein meal or a carbohydrate meal. Because fish and seafood are such light proteins, they can be eaten with either type of meal. Eating proteins and carbohydrates separately reduces calorie absorption and improves digestion. In a "protein meal," enjoy red or white meat such as steak, chops, chicken or turkey; a salad with creamy dressing (like yogurt); a vegetable soup (which may be creamy) and one or more vegetable side dishes (which may include cooked cheese). In a "carbohydrate meal," eat whole grains such as rice or millet (for example, in stuffed peppers), wheat or rye breads, and/or a legume/bean chili or stew; a salad with natural oil and vinegar or lemon dressing or a tasty tofu dressing; and a vegetable soup that can include whole grains, potatoes or legumes. (Those who wish to *gain* weight should not follow this second food-combining principle, but only the first one.) I explain many other minor food-combining rules in my books, especially *For the Love of Food* and *Complete Candida Yeast Guidebook*.

Other important tips for weight loss include eating a mainly whole-food, natural diet and drinking lots of pure, tested spring water throughout the day, away from meals. Avoid refined foods, junk foods, fried foods, nuts (especially roasted nuts), high-calorie foods in excess, sweet fruits, sugar, sugar substitutes, artificial sugars and additives like preservatives, shellfish, meats in excess, pork, processed meats, hard cheeses, fatty dairy products, any dairy products except in moderation, and highly processed commercial oils extracted by the solvent method.

Eating lots of nutrient-deficient foods, like junk foods, creates cravings. Do not completely exclude fats from your diet when trying to lose weight, as it triggers more cravings and body imbalances that contribute to weight gain (see *Cravings*). Eat good fats like olive oil, flaxseed oil (and ground flaxseeds sprinkled on cereal and other foods), those in fish and other natural oils found in whole foods. Eat at least four to six servings of raw and cooked vegetables a day—they are low in calories and help digestion. Eat two or three meals a day with up to three snacks.

Desserts can be eaten two or three times a week, provided they are wholesome, unrefined desserts eaten 60 to 90 minutes after a full meal. Fewer calories are actually absorbed (sometimes 15–35 percent less) if desserts are eaten this way. If you eat desserts on an empty stomach, most or all the calories are absorbed.

Many people who want to gain weight are put on high-calorie, high-fat diets by their doctors, and still fail to gain the desired weight. High-calorie/fat diets made up of refined foods, refined fats and animal fats will not help most underweight people gain weight. Switch to a balanced natural, whole-foods diet and you will, in time, gain the desired results. Chew your food very slowly, as it will increase the absorption of nutrients.

7. Beverage and Herbal Tea Suggestions
Drink lots of pure, tested spring water. Avoid alcohol and carbonated pop and soft drinks. Low- or one-calorie pops can still result in weight gain, due to the artificial additives they contain. Limit or avoid high-calorie, sweet fruit juices and enjoy nutritious, vegetable juices often. Helpful herbal teas include alfalfa, corn silk, dandelion (and dandelion "coffee"), fennel, fenugreek, ginger, organic green tea, oat straw, parsley, peppermint and spearmint.

WORMS

See *Parasites*

WOUNDS

See *Cuts and Wounds* and *Bleeding, Excessive*

WRINKLES

1. Condition and Cause
The skin is the largest organ of the body. As we age, the skin wrinkles

more and more each year. The skin begins to lose its elasticity in our twenties and, by the age of 50, the outer layers of skin have thinned out, which can cause sagging. How fast and how much you wrinkle is determined by genetics, environment, diet, exercise, sun exposure, cleanliness habits, patterns of facial expressions and other factors.

Bowel health is one of those other factors. A clean colon is usually accompanied by good digestion. Your internal health has everything to do with your external health. The lubrication, tone, clarity of complexion, softness and smoothness, and evenness of coloring of your skin are all affected by what you eat and how you digest and absorb your foods. Multiple brown age spots, or so-called liver spots, are one sign that your body needs internal cleansing. If you are beautiful on the inside, your skin will be beautiful on the outside.

2. Ailment History, Signs and Early Treatments
Cleopatra bathed in milk and cream. Mud and clay packs and baths have been employed for centuries, and still are used today, to draw out toxins and rejuvenate the skin. Facial cleanses of buttermilk, cream and lemon juice with brandy, yogurt and nutritional yeast, witch hazel, beaten egg whites, aloe vera, cucumbers, oatmeal or strawberries have been used to cleanse the face in the hope of achieving a more youthful appearance.

North American Indians were proud of their wrinkles, which were plentiful from their outdoor life in the sun. Their elders were revered and respected, and each wrinkle was like a line of wisdom. Today, Europeans have a greater tolerance for wrinkles and other signs of aging than do most North Americans, who are inundated with ads proclaiming the glory of endless youth.

Throughout the ages, people have searched for the fountain of youth and ways to retain young skin and avoid wrinkles. All manner of wonder potions, lotions, creams, drugs, herbs, and foods have been touted as miracle remedies. And still no one has found a simple answer.

3. Modern Natural Treatments and Remedies
There *are* answers to problems of aging, but none of them are simple. No matter how many treatments, surgeries, drugs, natural remedies and "miracle cures" are promoted, the secret lies within. It takes daily, conscious effort and hard work to halt or reverse the aging process.

Doing two or more internal cleanses each year helps to flush out inner body toxins that contribute to skin rashes and discoloration, dry skin, age spots and wrinkles (see *Toxin Overload* for basic cleansing techniques). Cleansing requires hard work: removing the poisons stored in the body is tiring, though rewarding in the end. It is also important to stop putting poisons *into* body! This means a diet overhaul. The diet can be gradually improved and this will result in visible signs of improvement in the outer body as you do this (see the nutrition aids listed below). Also see *Skin Problems* for methods of cleansing the skin externally to unclog pores and stimulate a healthy glow.

Aerobic exercise can also help you retain youthful skin. Exercise alone will not halt or reverse wrinkles, but various Asian cultures formulated, over thousands of years, numerous methods of rejuvenating the body and reversing the effects of aging. They include yoga, tai chi, qi gong, various martial arts and similar forms of body movements that go beyond simple vigorous exercise. I have practiced Hatha yoga for 30 years and have, according to my doctor, the skin tone of a woman in her twenties. People who regularly practice one of these methods do often look and feel 10 or 20 years younger—and more!—provided they eat well and live well too. Yoga includes facial and other exercises that prevent and erase wrinkles on the face. Making love is also considered to be great exercise, and good for the skin.

If your heating system causes your home and your skin to get dry in winter, place pans of water near radiators and heat vents, or cover them with wet cloths. Use a humidifier (or vaporizer), boil pans of water on the stove or leave the bathroom door open while you shower to keep the air moist, so your skin does not dry out and loose moisture that prevents wrinkles.

Avoid harsh soaps that dry out the skin, and always rinse soaps thoroughly from the skin. Choose natural skin moisturizing lotions if they are needed. You are less likely to need them if you follow these tips. At night, do not cover the face in creams that clog the pores and do not allow the skin to breathe. Choose natural, non-allergenic cosmetics and use as little as possible.

Finally, I will mention external preparations for erasing wrinkles. They appear last because if you ignore the rest of this information, no external applications will have any lasting effect.

The movie industry has whispered the amazing benefits of using hemorrhoid medication on crows' feet and facial wrinkles. The active ingredient in hemorrhoid medicines is shark oil, or squalane (see *Shark Oil* in the "Natural Remedies Glossary"). It is clear and non-greasy and can be applied generously on the face and the rest of the body. It actually erases wrinkles and helps prevent skin discoloration, and also softens the skin and protects it from sun damage. It has even been used successfully to prevent and help cure skin cancer (along with good diet and other treatments). Shark oil can be used under or with sun tan lotions. See *Sunburn* for more skin protection and healing methods.

Calendula creams help promote healthy skin formation. Chamomile creams and baths help sooth and soften skin, while oatmeal has an astringent effect that draws out poisons. GH 3 cream helps prevent wrinkles. See *Skin Problems* for important skin care tips. The use of collagen and/or elastin cream should be discussed with your doctor or skin care expert.

4. Helpful Supplements and Dosages
- Take a well-balanced, natural multivitamin daily.
- Take 1,000 mg or more vitamin C a day to help slow the aging process. Some experts, such as the late two-time Nobel Prize–winner Dr. Linus Pauling, recommend as much as 10,000 mg of vitamin C a day for anti-aging. Consult your holistic doctor before taking large doses, as (harmless) side effects can occur.
- Supplement needs vary widely with the individual for anti-aging and anti-wrinkling. Consult your holistic doctor about some of the following: CoQ10, evening primrose oil, vitamin A, vitamin E, zinc, selenium, calcium/magnesium, silica, pycnogenol, ginseng, royal jelly, melatonin, DHEA and SOD.

5. Cautions and Exceptions
Smoking, drinking alcohol frequently, excessive caffeine, unnecessary drugs and the use of any harmful or addictive substances contribute to speedy aging and wrinkles. Do not overuse internal and/or external skin-purging methods, as they can actually age the skin faster.

6. Nutrition Aids and Recommended Foods

A wholesome, well-balanced diet helps to slow down aging. See my other books, especially *For the Love of Food,* for complete guidelines. Avoid fatty foods, too many sugars and junk foods. Eat fish two to four times a week and add a teaspoon of ground flaxseed to cereal or other food three to five times a week to promote healthy, soft, well-lubricated skin. Use natural cold-pressed and expeller-pressed cooking oils, especially extra virgin olive oil, instead of highly processed solvent extracted oils. Avoid food additives, preservatives and artificial sweeteners.

7. Beverage and Herbal Tea Suggestions

Drink lots of water—at least four to six glasses of water a day—to help lubricate the skin and flush out body poisons. Drink eight glasses or more in hot weather. Drink healthful vegetable juices three to six times a week and protein power drinks occasionally. Stay away from carbonated pop and soft drinks, especially colas and drinks that contain artificial flavors, colors and sweeteners. Do not drink excessive fruit juices. Drink mainly lots of water!

-Y-

YEAST INFECTION, VAGINAL

For other types of yeast infection, see *Candida.* See also *Jock Itch.*

1. Condition and Cause

When there is internal yeast overgrowth, it usually manifests outwardly as well, as in vaginal yeast infections. Vaginal yeast infections can be sexually transmitted. In men, yeast infection appears as jock itch. Both partners need to treat for Candida regardless of whether they have outer symptoms or not. Two to four weeks' treatment is enough for mild cases. More severe cases may require a month or more of treatment. See *Candida* for more information.

2. Ailment History, Signs and Early Treatments

Until quite recently, yogurt was commonly inserted into the vagina to treat yeast infections. However, this method was not very effective and quite messy as well. Another messy method—douching with white vinegar or apple cider vinegar and warm water (one part vinegar to six or eight parts water) every day for a week or two—was more effective, but could actually spread infection in some instances, especially if other sexually transmitted diseases (STDs) were present. Also, too much douching has been found to be unhealthful and unnecessary for most women. Regular bathing, good cleanliness habits and wiping front to back after going to the bathroom are more beneficial.

3. Modern Natural Treatments and Remedies

Both partners must take oral supplements for Candida for between two weeks and two months—until at least a week after symptoms have completely abated. During this time, only have sex with a condom and avoid oral sex in order not to reinfect each other. Even open-mouth kissing can pass Candida back and forth.

Women can use boric acid capsules (available without prescription at any pharmacy) externally for vaginal infections. Insert one capsule high up into the vagina before sleeping. Wait at least 12 hours before engaging in any sexual activities. Use boric acid capsules daily, for one to two weeks as required. It is helpful to use a moderately heavy feminine napkin during the night and the next morning, as there is some discharge of Candida when using boric acid capsules (the capsules do dissolve completely). Vinegar douches (described above) can be used occasionally if your doctor approves, but they are not always necessary.

A large clove of garlic—skin removed and slightly peeled to expose the juices and remove the shiny outer covering—may be used instead of boric acid. It kills the yeast quite effectively, though the odor is offensive to many and there is some danger that the garlic may become lodged in the vagina and be hard to remove. Squat and bear down to remove the garlic clove.

Another effective treatment is to apply tea tree oil generously to one or two entire fingers, and insert them as high as possible into the vagina. Do this daily for a week or two. This is less acidic than the boric acid treatment, and is not harmful if ingested (though ingesting large amounts could cause a possibly intense healing reaction). One drawback is that tea tree oil tingles a little for between

10 and 30 minutes. You will feel it working but it is less messy than boric acid and better smelling than garlic.

4. Helpful Supplements and Dosages

- It is essential for most people with Candida (unless they have high stomach acid, which is unusual) to take two high-quality acidophilus capsules (may include bifidus) to replenish friendly bacteria and help digestion. Take it once or twice a day, an hour or more away from food, with six to eight ounces of pure water. Try to use a brand that includes added FOSs (fructooligosaccharides), which assist the growth of friendly bacteria. Take before and/or after breakfast and/or lunch—not after supper.
- Take digestive aids and/or laxative teas and flushing agents as needed.
- Vitamin C—especially Allergy C, Ester C or buffered C can help reduce symptoms and energize and boost the immune system. Take 500–1,000 mg one to four times a day, as needed, at least three or four hours before sleeping. Do not take chewable vitamin C. (For children, vitamin C powder can be mixed into solid food.)
- Take energizing supplements if needed. See *Energy, Low.*

5. Cautions and Exceptions

Do not take boric acid internally! Keep it in a childproof container, out of the reach of children. Stop using boric acid if the yeast infection clears or if the vagina or discharge becomes too acidic (that is, if it stings). Pregnant women should not use boric acid and should not douche. If pregnant, consult your doctor. Do not douche if you suspect you may have STDs, or if your doctor doesn't approve.

6. Nutrition Aids and Recommended Foods

A yeast-free diet without alcohol, sugar, artificial sweeteners, refined foods, junk foods, hard-to-digest foods, pork, processed meats, milk and cheese, sweet and tropical fruits, natural sweeteners, desserts, potatoes, pasta, corn, oatmeal, breads, crackers or grain flour products is essential to successfully treat Candida. Also, do not smoke during Candida treatment. Good foods to include are whole grains, legumes (brown and black beans and lentils), abundant vegetables, limited subacid (tart) fruits, yogurt, butter and some seeds and nuts (such as pumpkin, sunflower, sesame and flaxseeds, and home-roasted almonds or filberts). See my *Complete Candida Yeast Guidebook* for complete diet details. Pregnant women's diets should be doctor-approved.

7. Beverage and Herbal Tea Suggestions

Drink plenty of pure (spring or distilled) water. Helpful herbal teas include peppermint, spearmint, lemon grass, raspberry leaf, fennel seed, fenugreek seed, alfalfa seed, senna with flax and slippery elm. Some stronger teas could be harmful for pregnant women or those who are sensitive, and should only be used with your holistic physician's advice. They include burdock, comfrey, ginger, goldenseal, ginseng, eucalyptus, licorice and taheebo. Five to six glasses of vegetable juice a week can be very helpful, especially those that include carrots, beets and green food (barley green, spinach, parsley, or others, some of which require a special juicer or to be blended in water before using). See *Fresh Vegetable Juices* in the refrigerator remedies section.

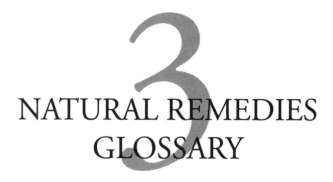

NATURAL REMEDIES GLOSSARY

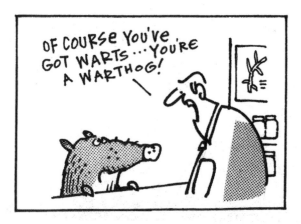

PROPERTIES, USES, DOSAGES AND STORAGE OF NATURAL REMEDIES

Not every known herb, vitamin, mineral and remedy is included in this book. A huge encyclopedia would be required to name and describe all possible treatments here. The good news is that all the most important remedies are included. Many individuals do not need the majority of remedies that have been left out of this glossary. Unless there are serious diseases involved, all practical, everyday treatments for common ailments can be found in this section.

Most of these products can be purchased at your local health food store. A few may need to be purchased through a holistic pharmacy or from your holistic medical doctor (where doctors are allowed to sell them), naturopathic physician, herbalist or apothecary. Some may be available at your local pharmacy or drug store. Whenever possible, buy organic and natural products, not synthetic or commercially prepared products. Ask your holistic doctor where to find these items if they are too difficult to locate.

This section provides information on storage requirements (shelf, cool cupboard or refrigerator) or temperatures for these products. All herbs, unless otherwise stated, should be kept in a cool cupboard, away from all light. Keep *all* products out of direct light, especially direct sunlight, out of high heat and away from stoves, heating vents and other sources of high temperatures. Do not freeze *any* remedies unless recommended here or by your holistic physician. Note the remedy bottles or packages for the acceptable length of storage or expiry date.

Dosages are included at the end of many of these remedies. The dosages are numbered from 1 to 10, the dosage 1 being for the most sensitive people and dosage 10 for the hardiest individuals.

DOSAGE 1	for very sensitive people and those severely ill individuals (and, except where otherwise specified, children from 2 to 7 years of age)
DOSAGE 3	for fairly sensitive individuals and those with less acute illnesses (and children from 7 to 12 years of age)
DOSAGE 5	for average, relatively healthy people (and children from 12 to 16)
DOSAGE 8	for fairly hardy individuals (or healthy teenagers about 16 or 17 years old)
DOSAGE 10	for very hardy individuals with a strong constitution, who are not presently ill (or healthy young adults 18 years or older)

Not every dosage from 1 to 10 is always given, especially if a product is mild and generally easily tolerated. When numbered dosages are not given, half dosages can be given to children and sensitive people. The amounts given for children are for relatively healthy children; youngsters with frequent or continued health problems may require even smaller dosages than those stated.

Important: For safety's sake, consult your holistic doctor before giving *any* remedies to children two years old and under! Dosages for herb teas are usually one to three cups daily and occasionally only spoonfuls are recommended for stronger teas. Dosages of many herbs are not given for tinctures and capsules, as potency varies product to product. Consult the package label or your doctor for amounts of herbs to take in these forms.

Those individuals with allergies are usually more on the sensitive side. Avoid any products if you are allergic to them. Often, products are available that contain several remedies in one capsule or dose. These may or may not be more beneficial. Sensitive or highly allergic individuals are sometimes better off taking individual doses of fewer different remedies and avoiding too many multiple products blended in one capsule or extract.

It is up to you, preferably in consultation with your holistic doctor, to determine the strength of dosage you require. If unsure, it is always best to start with a low dose for two or three days to see if a delayed reaction or any troublesome side effects occur. Then, if there is no reaction or only a little discomfort is experienced, move on to a higher dosage. It may be difficult to determine exact dosages. Seemingly strong individuals have complained about even small doses, while sometimes those who may appear less hardy find that only a higher dose has any noticeable effect.

Expect some discomfort when using remedies that are antiviral or cleansing or that may have a healing reaction—such as green food products and some minerals and strong herbs. Most vitamins, herbs, energizers, sleep aids and digestive aids have little or no side effects when used properly. Improper doses of *any* remedies can cause side effects and be potentially dangerous! Be on the safe side: start small and follow, first, your doctor's instructions and, second, the recommendations given here. Be aware that dosages recommended on packages often tend to be on the high side, because companies do want to sell more products. A doctor is usually not required for simple everyday health concerns that are not serious like headaches, colds, sunburn and warts, and so on.

Important: Consult your holistic physician if unsure how to proceed or if major side effects occur.

If you derive no effects (good or bad) from a certain remedy, it may be because you do not require it, because the quality is low, because the potency is too low or because you are using it incorrectly or in improper combination with other products or foods. Sometimes it may actually be working, but the effects are not immediately visible. Consult your doctor to be sure.

If you have a reaction or side effect to a remedy such as: indigestion, fatigue, nausea, anxiety, headache, depression, runny nose, aches or other discomforts, it could mean one or more of the following:

1. You could be allergic to the remedy.
2. You could be allergic to binders and fillers that accompany the remedy. Another brand may be okay for you.
3. You could be having a "healing reaction," as when using green food products or colostrum or when cleansing.
4. You may be taking too much of one remedy or too many different remedies at once.
5. You may be improperly combining treatments that should not be mixed together and may be counteracting each other (e.g., citrus fruits or citricidal and colloidal silver should not be taken during the same time period, because Citrus expels metals).
6. You may be taking too high a dosage.
7. You may be taking an inferior product, one that is not natural or organic or one that has not been properly or safely processed. Or the product could be outdated or contaminated.
8. You may be taking natural remedies and drugs too close together or during the same period (some natural remedies and drugs should not be taken simultaneously or, if they are taken in the same period, should be taken four hours or more apart).
9. If you are smoking, drinking alcohol, taking unnecessary (pleasure or prescription) drugs, eating excessive fats, sugars or non-healing foods or beverages, they may be interfering with the proper absorption and utilization of some remedies.
10. If you have serious vitamin or mineral deficiencies or overabundances, are suffering from depression, have

acute digestive problems, have a serious illness or major disease, have thyroid problems or are pregnant, these conditions may interfere with proper absorption and utilization of some remedies.

HOMEOPATHIC RESTRICTIONS

While using homeopathic remedies, do not use any of the following products internally, as a food or a beverage, as a mouthwash or toothpaste or topically in any form: coffee, peppermint, spearmint, eucalyptus, camphor, menthol, tea tree oil or similar products or derivatives.

VITAMINS AND MINERALS

Most vitamins and minerals are listed in a separate chart at the end of the alphabetically listed remedies, except for vitamin C and zinc, which are listed in both places.

Acidophilus
See also *Probiotics*
(capsules, powder, tablets, liquid)

Acidophilus or, to give its full name, Lactobacillus acidophilus (L. acidophilus) is a type of probiotic ("for life"), an anti-fungal and a beneficial or "friendly" bacteria found in the large and small intestines. Acidophilus assists in the digestion and absorption of proteins, vitamins and minerals. Friendly bacteria are destroyed by taking antibiotics or birth control pills. This disturbs the natural balance of bacteria in the intestines, weakening the immune system and allowing harmful, "unfriendly" bacteria to multiply and contribute to health problems. Acidophilus and other friendly bacteria should be taken whenever antibiotic drugs are taken and for 10 to 14 days afterwards. Take acidophilus at least four hours or preferably more away from antibiotics. Bifidus and bulgarus are other types of beneficial bacteria.

Excellent brands include DDS®, Natren®, Sisu®, Primadophilus®, Neo-Flora®, and Kyo-Dophilus®. These friendly bacteria come in a milk base or in non-dairy varieties for those with dairy allergies. They are available in capsule and powdered forms, which are generally more potent than liquid varieties because the friendly bacteria are better assimilated and implanted in the intestines. Be sure the product is refrigerated when you purchase it. Keep refrigerated but do not freeze.

Sometimes acidophilus is taken as a digestive aid with food or with other vitamin guidebook or health specialist approved natural supplements. In this case, if the acidophilus is in capsule form and coated so it breaks down only in the intestines, it is best to place it in a new gelatin or veggie capsule so it can work like a digestive aid and break down in the stomach. Individuals with high stomach acid who get upset stomachs from taking acidophilus or other friendly bacteria should take it right after or 15 minutes after eating a meal.

DOSAGES 1 (SENSITIVE) TO 10 (HARDY)
Take each dose with four or five ounces water or, for young children (under 13), one to three ounces. Take between 60 and 90 minutes away from food and at least four hours away from drugs or other supplements. For some individuals, it is best to take one type of friendly bacteria at a time. Children under the age of seven should take bifidus instead of acidophilus.

Do not take after supper or at night. In the case of acidophilus and other friendly bacteria, hardy individuals require a *smaller* rather than a larger dose. One capsule, or a quarter teaspoon of powder, should contain at least one billion organisms or more. Avoid brands with less.

Friendly bacteria can be taken for long periods, or alternated on and off, with no withdrawal or side effects. Most liquid brands are best avoided due to less effectiveness, with very few exceptions. If taking a liquid, follow bottle instructions.

1	Take 2 capsules or 1 teaspoon powder twice a day.
3	Take 2 capsules or ½–1 teaspoon powder once or twice a day.
5	Take 3 capsules or 1 teaspoon powder once a day.
8	Take 2 capsules or ½ teaspoon powder once a day.
10	Take 1 capsule or ¼ teaspoon powder once a day.

Activated Charcoal

Activated charcoal is used to treat diarrhea, and is often brought on trips to tropical areas to use for parasite treatment. See *Tormentavena®* for more information.

Aerobic Oxygen
(liquid)

There is a wide range of oxygen therapies available today. Most need to administered by a medical professional and are not available—or even legal—in some places. Aerobic (stabilized) oxygen for oral use is a relatively new treatment these last few decades and is available in some health stores, clinics and pharmacies. Oxygen promotes healing and helps destroy micro-organisms that cause disease in the body. Aerobic oxygen can be found in some bottled waters or in beverages at some specialized juice bars. Aerobic oxygen is antibacterial and energizing. It can be added to drinking water in small amounts for these properties, or may be used as an antibacterial mouthwash (use the 10 dosage). Store at room temperature. Most brands should not be put directly on skin or taken full strength (undiluted) orally. Those who are sensitive should avoid drinking aerobic oxygen at night, as it may be too energizing.

DOSAGES 1 (SENSITIVE) TO 10 (HARDY)
Can be taken for long periods of time, but do not take high doses and then quit quickly. Instead, build up to higher doses and reduce doses gradually before stopping.

1	Take 2–4 drops in 8 ounces of water once a day.
3	Take 5–6 drops in 8 ounces of water once a day.
5	Take 8–10 drops in 8 ounces of water once or twice a day.
8	Take 14–16 drops in 8 ounces of water twice a day.
10	Take 20 drops in 8 ounces of water 2–3 times a day.

For extra antibacterial protection, add 10–20 drops of aerobic oxygen to each gallon of bottled drinking water.

Alfalfa

(tablets, liquid extract, leaf or seed tea or sprouts)

Alfalfa is a mineral-rich, green food product that is high in chlorophyll, and is especially beneficial for arthritis, joint pains and muscle aches. It has an alkalizing and cleansing effect on the body. Like other green food products, it is good for bleeding gums, stomach and bowel problems and anemia. In sprout form it is high in protein and vitamin C. The dried form is higher in iron. Sprouts can be eaten five or six days each week. They should be well washed and the brown hulls washed away or cut off. Alfalfa tea can be drunk two or three times a day. For taking other forms of alfalfa, see the discussion of green food products under *Toxin Overload* in the ailments section (remember to build up green products slowly and reduce before quitting them).

DOSAGES 1 (SENSITIVE) TO 10 (HARDY)

Take for 30 to 45 days. It can be taken for longer periods if a holistic health specialist recommends it. If taking alfalfa for more than 60 days, it is best to take it only five or six days each week. Build up to higher doses and reduce doses gradually before stopping. Basically very safe and non-toxic. One of the easiest to tolerate green foods.

1	Take 2–3 tablets or ½–1 teaspoon extract once a day, preferably with meals.
3	Take 5–6 tablets or 1 teaspoon extract once a day, preferably with meals.
5	Take 10 tablets or 2 teaspoons extract once a day, preferably with meals.
8	Take 15 tablets or 2–3 teaspoons extract once or twice a day, preferably with meals.
10	Take 20 tablets or 1 tablespoon extract once or twice a day, preferably with meals.

Aloe Vera

(juice, gel, cream or fresh plant extract)

This is a green food product. See *Toxin Overload* and *Cleansing* in the ailments section for information on green foods and how to take internally. Aloe vera can also be used externally on cuts, wounds, burns and sunburn.

Amino Acids
(capsule, tablet or powder)

Amino acids are the building blocks that make up protein in the body. There are about 29 known amino acids. The names of amino acids are sometimes preceded with the letters L or D or DL (e.g., L-lysine, D cystine, DL-phenylalanine). Most individual amino acids are not legally sold in Canada. Exceptions are L-tryptophan, which is available with a prescription, and L-arginine, which can be purchased over the counter. Amino acids *are* individually available in the United States. Complete amino acids combinations are legal in both countries. Although they are not dangerous in general, indiscriminate use of individual amino acids in large amounts can cause some problems. Free-form amino acids are the purest. See the ailments section for the use of amino acids to treat some health concerns, or consult your doctor.

Anti-Flam®
See *Infla-Zyme Forte®*

Anti-Inflammatory Supplements
See the entries for these specific anti-inflammatories: Anti-Flam®, arnica, barberry, buchu, calendula, cat's claw, comfrey, echinacea, elderberry, eyebright, Flammaforce®, fenugreek, flaxseed, garlic, ginger, goldenseal, grape seed, horsetail, Infla-Zyme Forte®, licorice, MSM, myrrh, onions, primrose oil, pycnogenol, silica, slippery elm, SOD, vitamin C and yarrow.

Anti-Viral Formula®
This combination product from Natural Factors company contains echinacea, lomatium, astragalus, reishi mushrooms and licorice. As the name suggests, it is good for viruses and infections. The herbal ingredients boost the immune system and have a natural

antibiotic effect. At present this product is available only in tincture form with 40 percent alcohol, but will soon be available in gel capsules. Follow package instructions or consult your holistic doctor for dosages.

Arnica

Arnica is an herb that is generally too potent to be taken internally. It can be used in external creams and lotions frequently. However, in a homeopathic remedy, arnica can be taken internally by just about anyone—even by infants and pregnant women—for pain, inflammation, wounds, bruises and sprains, sore muscles and numerous other related injuries or health concerns. Athletes in particular can benefit from homeopathic arnica. Homeopathic dosage is 6 c to 12 c for localized pain and symptoms and 30 c for serious conditions. Doses vary, though usually three to five pellets are taken one to three times a day, or every four hours. Arnica is also available in tincture form. Take according to package directions, or consult a homeopathic doctor or pharmacy. See *Homeopathic Restrictions* at the beginning of this section.

Artichoke Extract

See also *Artichokes, Globe* in the refrigerator remedies section for major information

The extract of the globe artichoke is a potent healer for the liver and gallbladder and an aphrodisiac, and it also aids digestion and helps to reduce high cholesterol levels. The extract is safe and nontoxic. In rare instances, allergic reactions are possible.

Take according to package instructions or consult your holistic health expert.

Astragalus

Astragalus is a potent green food product that improves immune function, helps adrenal gland function and inhibits certain viruses. It increases the metabolism, induces sweating, helps heal colds and flu, fights infections, increases stamina and speeds healing. Astragalus is also beneficial for cancer, lung problems, fibromyalgia, AIDS and Alzheimer's disease. Two to three cups of astragalus tea may be drunk each day, as required. Safe if used as directed. See *Toxin Overload* for more information on how to take green food products.

Barberry

This herb is used for congestion, diarrhea, digestive problems, inflammation, skin problems and vaginal infections. It can be taken internally or used topically. Most people can drink up to two or three cups of the herbal tea a day, as needed. Sensitive individuals can make a weaker concentration of tea. Tinctures, extracts and capsules vary in their potency and should be taken as recommended by package instructions or by your doctor or herbalist. Do not use this herb for more than two weeks at a time. Use under a doctor's supervision during pregnancy and while breastfeeding. Like goldenseal, barberry is quite potent and should not be overused. Its effect is gentler when it is used in combination with other milder, balancing herbs.

Barley Green

This is a green food product. See *Toxin Overload* and *Cleansing*, in the ailments section, for information on green foods and how to take them.

Bee Pollen

See "Remedies from Your Refrigerator and Cupboard"

Bifidus

Bifidus is another strain of friendly bacteria, a probiotic like acidophilus, which is beneficial to the digestive tract and intestines. It is more beneficial than acidophilus for children seven years old and younger and for people with liver problems. Like all probiotics, make sure it is refrigerated when you purchase it. Keep refrigerated at home but do not freeze. See *Acidophilus* above for more important information.

DOSAGES 1 (SENSITIVE) TO 10 (HARDY)
Take each capsule with three or four ounces of water or, for young children or babies, one to three ounces. If in powder form, mix each dose with the above amounts of water. Take bifidus 60 to 90 minutes away from foods and at least four hours away from drugs or other supplements. For some individuals, it is best to take one type of friendly bacteria at a time.

Do not take bifidus after supper or at night. As with other friendly bacteria, hardy individuals require a *smaller* rather than a larger dose. One capsule, or one-quarter teaspoon of powder, contains a billion organisms or more. Bifidus can be taken for long periods or alternated on and off, with no withdrawal or side effects.

1	Take 2 capsules or 1 teaspoon powder twice a day.
3	Take 2 capsules or ½–1 teaspoon powder once or twice a day.
5	Take 3 capsules or 1 teaspoon powder once a day.
8	Take 2 capsules or ½ teaspoon powder once a day.
10	Take 1 capsule or ¼ teaspoon powder once a day.

Bilberry

Bilberry, also called huckleberry, is a herb related to the North American blueberry. This is an edible berry that is also dried for herbal use. It is beneficial for diabetes (its effects are similar to those of insulin), diarrhea, heart problems and eyesight problems including cataracts and night blindness. The tea or tincture can also be used as a gargle for sore throats.

Dosage: one to three cups of tea a day, away from food and on an empty stomach, as needed. Average capsule dosage is 200–400 mg a day, broken into two doses if possible, taken with water on an empty stomach. Bilberry is not recommended during pregnancy or while breastfeeding. Sensitive individuals should begin with half a cup of tea a day or 100 mg and build up gradually.

Bile Salts

For those who have no gallbladder, or have impaired liver and/or gallbladder function, bile salts supplements can be a lifesaver. If there is physical discomfort or inability to handle foods or meals high in fat content, bile salts will eliminate many side effects and assist in the assimilation of fatty foods. However, this is no reason to abuse fried foods and overindulge in fats—fats should be reduced for those with liver or gallbladder problems so the body can focus on healing. Remedies such as milk thistle (silymarin), dandelion, black radish, globe artichokes or artichoke extract can be used to purge and, in many cases, repair these organs if properly utilized.

Dosage is usually one 100 mg tablet of bile salts with each meal that contains average or above-average fat content. Take a maximum of three tablets a day, unless your doctor recommends otherwise. Consult your physician for children's doses or alternatives. No "1–10" doses are needed for bile salts. Some bile salts brands have added ingredients, which you should ensure are compatible with any allergy restrictions you may have. Trophic is a great Canadian brand.

Bio Strath®

This natural product comes in tablets or liquid and is used to boost energy and vitality, to nourish cells and tissues, to support and protect the immune system and to aid concentration and help improve the memory. It has been helpful in some cases for children with learning disabilities and/or hyperactivity. Bio Strath® is also excellent for boosting strength and endurance during athletic activities and increased or continuous physical labor. It is a "good yeast" (Saccharomyces cerevisiae) product, which also contains lecithin, B vitamins, amino acids, enzymes and trace elements. Take according to package instructions. This product is safe for most individuals with few or no side effects. Those with allergies or who are highly sensitive can usually tolerate this product, but consult your holistic doctor before taking if you are unsure. This European product is available in Canada and the U.S. from Flora Distributing.

Biotin

This B vitamin is used especially to help counteract yeast growth. Individual B vitamins should not be taken alone, so take a B complex between one and four times a day when using biotin. Take one 300–500 mcg tablet or capsule of biotin one to three times a day with meals or snacks that are very starchy or sweet. There are no side effects with B vitamins. Good for Candida problems.

Bioxy (Cleanse)®

This stabilized oxygen supplement in capsule form is used for cleansing and as a flushing agent (to prevent constipation and flush other supplements through the body) with parasite treatments, other supplements or cleansing products. Take according to package directions. It is generally safe and non-toxic with no side effects if taken as directed, though you may experience a slight aftertaste or a burp or two reminiscent of bleach. Take according to bottle directions. Store in a cool cupboard.

Black Cohosh

This herb is especially good for female health, for: inducing labor, labor pains, menstrual problems, hot flashes and menopause. It is also beneficial for arthritis, circulation, heart problems, osteoporosis, and lowering blood pressure and cholesterol levels. Do not use when pregnant or nursing without a holistic doctor's consent and supervision.

Blue-Green Algae

This is a green food product. See *Toxin Overload* and *Cleansing* in the ailments section for information on green foods and how to take them. Blue-green algae are considered one of the most potent and nutritious green food products.

Bromelain

Bromelain (or pineapple enzymes) is used as an anti-inflammatory and digestive aid, especially for protein foods. It is also used for healing, for minor injuries, asthma, arthritis, and heart problems. It should not be taken with certain drugs, particularly blood-thinning drugs. Avoid if you have certain allergies, including one to pineapple. Consult your doctor for allergy restrictions.

Buchu

This is an herbal leaf tea prized in macrobiotic circles for its potent healing qualities. It may also be spelled *bookoo*, *bucco* or *buku*. It is used especially for kidney and bladder infections, diabetes, digestive problems, gout and gas, and for inflammation of the male and female reproductive organs, the colon and the breathing passages. Take one cup of the tea once or twice a day, as needed. Avoid during pregnancy and while breastfeeding unless you have your doctor's consent.

Calendula

Calendula flowers (which are sometimes called marigolds, though they are not at all like the common North American marigold) are used most often in a topical cream or ointment for healing skin problems, rashes (including diaper rash), eczema, burns, sunburn and wounds. Calendula can also be used internally as a tea for aiding the aforementioned problems as well as stomach problems, ulcers, kidney and bladder problems, fever and some menstrual problems. Calendula is antiseptic and anti-inflammatory. It is also quite gentle and non-toxic. Two to three cups of tea can be drunk a day, as needed.

Cascara Sagrada
This strong herb, derived from the dried bark of the California buckthorn tree (also called sacred bark or Persian bark), is found growing in Pacific coast states and British Columbia. Cascara sagrada is quite potent and used primarily as a laxative and a cleansing agent. It is also used for constipation, colon problems and parasites. Alone, cascara sagrada should not be taken for more than seven days. Used in combination products with other cleansing herbs and supplements, it may be taken for up to 14 days. People with major bowel diseases, or damaged or partially removed colons or intestines, should not use this herb. If you are pregnant or breastfeeding, do not use without a doctor's consent. Cascara sagrada is generally too potent to be drunk alone as an herbal tea. The tincture or extract can be taken according to package directions or in smaller amounts than the package directs. Drink at least six glasses of water a day when using cascara sagrada in any form.

Catnip
Catnip is an excellent, mild herbal tea suitable to give to babies and children to dispel nightmares and induce sleep. Catnip also helps fight coughs, colic, colds, corns, hives and cancer, and may also be used as a mild aid for toothaches. This delightful, non-toxic, green-leaf herb tea can be drunk two or three times a day, as desired or required. *Note:* Never use pet store varieties of catnip for human consumption.

Cat's Claw
This South American herb, like devil's claw, is derived from a vine that wraps around rainforest trees in Peru. This herb is excellent for arthritis as well as for treating injuries, ulcers, tumors, cancer, some allergies, chronic fatigue and Candida, and for cleansing the intestinal tract

and bowels. It helps boost immune function and is an anti-viral, an anti-inflammatory and an antioxidant. Cat's claw is not well known in North America and is used less than many other remedies with similar properties. One to three cups of the potent tea can be drunk per day, as needed. Do not use if pregnant or breastfeeding or if you are the recipient of an organ transplant. Cat's claw has very low toxicity, but it may cause diarrhea if overused or used incorrectly.

Cayenne Pepper
See "Remedies from Your Refrigerator and Cupboard"

Chamomile
This gentle, yet very beneficial, herb tea flower is one of the most commonly used and beloved herbal remedies. Chamomile (or *camomile*, spelled the old-fashioned or European way) is a mild sleep aid, gentle digestive aid and tension-reliever excellent for babies, children and adults. It is also good for colic, skin problems (it can be used in a bath or sitz bath for skin rashes or irritations, eczema or sore muscles), stomach upset, ulcers, minor bowel problems, mouth and gum problems and as a hair rinse (to enhance the color and soothe the scalp of those with light-colored hair; rosemary works for dark hair). Chamomile flower tea is a popular pleasure tea that can be drunk several times a day, as desired. Only a few individuals with pollen allergies may have a small problem with this tea and may need to avoid it.

Chaste Berry
See *Vitex*

Chlorella
This is a green food product. See *Toxin Overload* and *Cleansing* for information on green foods and how to take them.

Chlorophyll
Chlorophyll is the green pigment in plants. All the green food products mentioned in this book are high in chlorophyll. It can also be purchased as a liquid supplement or in tablets that can be taken in or with water. Chlorophyll-rich foods and supplements improve blood

quality and help build red blood cells, which carry oxygen to the body's cells. Chlorophyll can also help boost the immune system, prevent constipation, help prevent and heal anemia, soothe and strengthen the nervous system, prevent tiredness, improve sleep quality, help heal skin and gum problems, assist cleansing (especially of the liver and other organs), dispel heavy metals, eliminate bad breath, and is good for anti-aging. Hardy individuals can take the recommended bottle or package amount of chlorophyll, and more sensitive individuals can start with one-quarter to one-half the dose (or less) and build up.

There are no significant side effects to chlorophyll, other than a possible "healing reaction" (an effect of cleansing poisons from the body with a high-chlorophyll green food) that can occur with some green foods if too much is taken too quickly. Chlorophyll is sometimes added to water as a purifying agent. (See *Toxin Overload* and *Cleansing* in the ailments section for more information on chlorophyll-rich green food products.) A quarter teaspoon of some concentrated green foods is similar or even more abundant in nutrients and chlorophyll than in a small green lettuce salad.

Citricidal

This concentrated extract of grapefruit seeds is used to fight Candida yeast infections and parasites, also for sore throats, colds and flu, and to boost the immune system. Citricidal comes in tablets, liquid and toothpaste (not recommended, see note below). The liquid is the most potent form and is best assimilated when taken in two or three ounces of very warm or hot water (use between 1 and 12 drops of citricidal) an hour or more away from meals and starchy snacks. It does taste a bit like dirty socks in water, so it is good to drink it quickly; but it may also be used as an antiseptic gargle occasionally. Fruit or yogurt may be eaten half an hour after, if desired.

Citricidal is antiseptic, antibacterial, anti-fungal, anti-viral, and anti-parasitic. Do not use near eyes or use full strength in the mouth or on the skin. It is best not to use citricidal for more than two weeks at a time unless your doctor recommends it. Prolonged use may contribute to dry skin and scalp. Citricidal is okay for use by most sensitive individuals, except those who are citrus allergic. Pregnant and breastfeeding women should consult a holistic doctor before using. Do not take during the same period as colloidal silver, and take 6 to

12 hours away from other minerals. Citricidal toothpaste may strip tooth enamel and cause teeth hypersensitivity, so it is best avoided.

DOSAGES 1 (SENSITIVE) TO 10 (HARDY)

1	Take 1–2 drops dispersed in 2–3 ounces very warm water, at the back of the throat (to avoid taste buds) if desired, once a day, every other day, for 3–7 days.
2	Take 1–2 drops dispersed in 2–3 ounces very warm water, at the back of the throat (to avoid taste buds) if desired, every other day, for 7–15 days.
3	Take 1–2 drops dispersed in 2–3 ounces very warm water, at the back of the throat (to avoid taste buds) if desired, once a day, for 3–7 days.
4	Take 1–2 drops dispersed in 2–3 ounces very warm water, at the back of the throat (to avoid taste buds) if desired, once a day, for 7–14 days.
5	Take 2–5 drops dispersed in 2–3 ounces very warm water, at the back of the throat (to avoid taste buds) if desired, once or twice a day, for 7–14 days.
6	Take 2–5 drops dispersed in 2–3 ounces very warm water, at the back of the throat (to avoid taste buds) if desired, 2–3 times a day, for 7–14 days.
7	Take 5–10 drops dispersed in 2–3 ounces very warm water, at the back of the throat (to avoid taste buds) if desired, once or twice a day, for 7–14 days.
8	Take 5–10 drops dispersed in 2–3 ounces very warm water, at the back of the throat (to avoid taste buds) if desired, 2–3 times a day, for 7–14 days.
9	Take 10–12 drops dispersed in 2–3 ounces very warm water, at the back of the throat (to avoid taste buds) if desired, once or twice a day, for 7–14 days.
10	Take 10–12 drops dispersed in 2–3 ounces very warm water, at the back of the throat (to avoid taste buds) if desired, 2–3 times a day, for 7–14 days.

Clove Oil

Clove oil is a common toothache remedy. Use a drop or two on a cotton swab to dab on infected teeth and gums. If full strength is too potent, especially for children and those who are very sensitive, dilute in water or olive oil. (See *Toothaches* in the ailments section.)

Clove oil and the spice it is derived from are also used as an antiseptic, an anti-fungal, an anti-parasitic (for intestinal worms and other parasites) and a digestive aid, as well as in cleansing products. Do not take the oil internally because it is very potent and can cause intense cleansing side effects! Clove herbal tea and tincture should be used sparingly as needed. Consult your doctor before taking for more than two or three months (for parasites or Candida) or if pregnant or nursing. Clove capsules are used for parasites.

Co Enzyme Q10 (CoQ10)

This potent antioxidant protects the body from the formation of free radicals, which cause cell damage, reduce immune function and contribute to diseases. CoQ10 is good for: circulation, heart problems, immune system, cancer, allergies, breathing problems, blood sugar problems, Candida, degenerative diseases, periodontal disease, male infertility, high blood pressure, stomach problems and anti-aging. It is better absorbed if taken with meals, especially with oil or fatty foods. It is best kept below 110°F. A supplement in oil or liquid form is preferable. Take 30 mg one to four times a day for most health needs. No troublesome side effects have been documented.

Colloidal Silver

This product was used back in the 1930s but its popularity waned because of its high price tag: $100 per ounce. Modern prices for colloidal silver are around $15–$20 a bottle. In the last decade it has experienced a renewed popularity because of its powerful yet nontoxic antibacterial, anti-fungal, anti-viral and natural antibiotic qualities. It also kills some types of parasites and is good for cleansing. Colloidal silver destroys viruses, fungi and bacteria by cutting off their oxygen supply. It kills disease-causing organisms for over 600 different diseases. It consists of silver particles suspended in distilled water, which is either yellowish or, and in the highest quality brands, clear. Some people use a special machine to make their own colloidal silver, but it is cheaper and the quality is higher if the product is purchased through a health store. Avoid brands sold in plastic containers and those with glycerin or other additives.

While standard recommended doses taken daily for up to 30 days, twice yearly, can be very beneficial, excessive amounts may cause skin damage or discoloration. As with all minerals, excessive use of silver may be harmful. Potency is measured in parts per million, from 3 or 4 ppm through 6, 10, 15, 24 and 50, and up to 500 ppm in some brands. High dosages over 50 ppm are best used only externally for wounds and skin infections. The amounts given below are for healing or cleansing, and may be also be taken for a day or two or for a week or so, especially during colds or for special short time needs. Some very sensitive people should avoid colloidal silver treatments during colds and some low-energy periods and start silver when energy levels are higher. If you are unsure of what amount to take, start with a small dose and build up, then reduce the dose if needed. Do not take during the same time period as citricidal, and take 6 to 12 hours away from all citrus fruits.

DOSAGES 1 (SENSITIVE) TO 10 (HARDY)

Take the following doses on an empty stomach followed by a few sips of water:

1	Take ¼ teaspoon 3 ppm, 4 ppm or 6 ppm silver, or ⅛ teaspoon or 8 drops 10 ppm silver, once a day, every other day for 10–20 days.
2	Take ¼ teaspoon 3 ppm, 4 ppm or 6 ppm silver, or ⅛ teaspoon or 8 drops 10 ppm silver, once a day for 10–20 days.
3	Take ½ teaspoon 3 ppm, 4 ppm or 6 ppm silver, or ¼ teaspoon 10 ppm silver, once a day for 10–20 days.
4	Take 1 teaspoon 3 ppm, 4 ppm or 6 ppm silver, or ½ teaspoon 10 ppm silver, once a day for 10–30 days.
5	Take 1 teaspoon 10 ppm silver, or ½ teaspoon 24 ppm silver, once a day for 15–30 days.
6	Take 1½ teaspoons 10 ppm silver, or ¾ teaspoon 24 ppm silver, once a day for 15–30 days.

7   Take 2 teaspoons 10 ppm silver all at once or at two different times, or 1 teaspoon 24 ppm all at once or at two different times, daily for 10–20 days.

8   Take same as dosage 7 for 30 days.

9   Take 3 teaspoons (1 tablespoon) 10 ppm silver, or 1¼ teaspoons 24 ppm silver, all at once or at two different times, daily for 15–20 days (or up to 30 days if your doctor recommends).

10   Take 3 teaspoons (1 tablespoon) 10 ppm silver twice a day, or 1¼ teaspoons 24 ppm silver twice a day, or 1 teaspoon 50 ppm silver once a day, for 10–15 days (or up to 30 days only if your doctor recommends).

Colostrum

Colostrum is the substance secreted from a mother's breasts during the first 24 to 48 hours of breastfeeding that is essential for a baby's health and immune defenses. Babies who do not drink their mother's colostrum have a 60 percent greater chance of developing allergies or other health problems in their lifetime. Children and adults who did not get adequate quantities of high-quality colostrum can make up for it by using this supplement of bovine colostrum. Colostrum is a potent cleanser and is more likely to cause reactions, flu-like symptoms and side effects (especially during the first few days) than most other cleansing products. The benefits can also be dramatic. Colostrum increases energy and endurance, assists weight loss and anti-aging, boosts the immune system, is beneficial for autoimmune diseases, is anti-fungal and anti-viral and has natural antibiotic qualities. It is not recommended for first-time cleansing.

Important: Dosages vary widely. It is best to take colostrum first thing in the morning, during the day or before supper, an hour or more before eating. Unlike other cleansing products, the dosage should *not* be decreased when having reactions, but should be continued until symptoms disappear. Colostrum is one supplement that needs to be taken regularly, every day (*never* ever other day) for a certain period of time, to avoid added, unnecessary side effects. All but the very hardy are best to consult their holistic doctor before taking colostrum.

DOSAGES 1 (SENSITIVE) TO 10 (HARDY)
(Take with water.)

1	Take 1 capsule in the morning and 1 in the afternoon, daily, for 15–30 days. Be sure to take *every* day, (never every other day).
3	Take 2 capsules in the morning and 2 in the afternoon, daily, for 30 days.
5	Take 2 capsules in the morning and 2 in the afternoon, daily, for a week. Then take 3 capsules in the morning and 3 in the afternoon, daily, for 3 to 4 weeks.
8	Take 2 capsules in the morning and 2 capsules in the afternoon, daily, for a week. Then take 3 capsules in the morning and 3 in the afternoon, daily, for 30 to 60 days.
10	Take 2 capsules in the morning and 2 in the afternoon, daily, for 3–7 days. Then take 3 capsules in the morning and 3 in the afternoon, daily, for 1 week. Then take 4 capsules in the morning and 4 in the afternoon, daily, for 3–7 weeks.

The dosage can be increased to as much as to 8 or 10 capsules twice a day (according to colostrum distributor guidelines), under a holistic doctor's supervision only.

Important: Do not decrease dosage *while experiencing* symptoms (unlike with some other cleansing products), but wait until symptoms pass before decreasing the dosage! Consult your holistic doctor *PRIOR* to taking colostrum if you are sensitive or ill! Do not take during the same time frame as drugs or other cleansing products. Do not take if pregnant or nursing, unless your doctor approves.

Despite these warnings, colostrum is not a dangerous product—but side effects *can* be troublesome.

Comfrey
Comfrey leaf, or "healing herb," is a potent green herb used in compresses, poultices and creams, especially for healing topical skin

problems, sore feet (soak in tincture), wounds (use for only one to three days on open wounds), bruises, sprains and broken bones. The root is more potent, as are Russian and prickly comfrey, and some believe these varieties may be dangerous if used internally, especially if used too long or incorrectly by sensitive individuals. The comfrey leaf is used cautiously and sparingly internally for coughs, inflammations, breathing problems, internal healing and ulcers. A tincture of comfrey root makes an excellent gargle or mouthwash, especially for sore throat or bleeding gums. Pregnant and breastfeeding mothers should not take comfrey internally. All sensitive individuals or anyone of less than sturdy constitution should consult a qualified herbalist or holistic doctor before using comfrey internally.

A generally safe dose is to prepare a cup or two of comfrey leaf tea (see "How To Make Herb Teas") and take one tablespoon of strained tea, away from food, one to four times a day. Refrigerate the remainder and take for up to 30 days, no longer, unless your doctor recommends otherwise. The dose may be reduced to as little as one teaspoon. Consult your holistic physician before altering this suggested internal dosage.

Cornsilk

Indian corn, maize jagnog and turkey corn are other names for cornsilk. The tea is used as a diuretic, for urinary tract infections, for kidney problems, to prevent bedwetting, to thin and increase the output of bile, to help lower blood pressure and cholesterol and for other heart problems. Take between one tablespoon and one-quarter cup of the tea, one to three times a day for up to 30 days or so, or take for just a few days at a time, as required. This non-toxic tea is safe for most individuals in normal dosages. (Do not make your own, especially from non-organic corn!) Avoid if you have corn allergies.

Cranberry

This food supplement is used in juice form, extract or capsule. It is used for bladder infections and incontinence as an acidifier, mainly for adults. Usually one to three glasses of unsweetened juice are taken daily, as required, until the problem improves (usually within a week or two). If capsules are taken, 400 mg of extract per capsule, taken one capsule at a time, two to four times a day, is the standard amount. Take for one to two weeks, as needed. A physician should determine children's needs for this supplement.

Dandelion

The beneficial dandelion plant originated in Greece but is now found all over the world. Young, tender, light green dandelion leaves (which contain more than five times the vitamin A of lettuce, plus vitamins B and C) can be picked from unsprayed plants (away from roadsides) before the plant buds or flowers (to avoid bitterness) and used in salads, after washing. The roots can be used as a coffee substitute. They should be washed and dried, then finely chopped or minced and spread on a flat baking pan. Bake at 200°F for one to two hours until completely dry, then remove from the oven, cool and grind in a blender, herb grinder or coffee mill. Use one or two teaspoons per cup of boiling water as a coffee substitute. Health stores also carry dandelion coffee substitutes. An herb tea made from the leaf or root can also be purchased.

The potent dandelion root is a major healing and cleansing aid for the liver, gallbladder and spleen. It is also helpful for alcohol damage and withdrawal, indigestion, constipation, water retention, skin problems, eczema and for female organs (including during pregnancy). The coffee and the dried leaf herbal tea can be drunk daily for long periods, as they are very safe and non-toxic. Drink a cup or two a day for 30 to 60 days, or three to five days a week, on a regular basis. Capsules and extracts should be taken according to package instructions, for limited periods of time if very concentrated.

Devil's Claw

This is an herb used primarily to treat arthritis. Other uses include the treatment of indigestion, heartburn, gout, joint pain and to reduce cholesterol levels. Those with high stomach acid or gallstones should avoid this remedy. Use up to 4 to 6 grams a day (take 2 grams two or three times a day) for arthritis and one-quarter that amount for other conditions. Use for up to 30 days at a time. Avoid during pregnancy or while breastfeeding. Consult your holistic physician before more extended use.

DHEA

Dehydroepiandrosterone or DHEA is a hormone produced by the adrenal glands. It helps to generate male and female sex hormones and helps heal erectile disfunction. DHEA is also good for anti-aging and osteoporosis, can increase muscle mass and decrease body fat and can be beneficial for cancer, blood sugar problems, high blood pressure, heart problems, multiple sclerosis, lupus and Alzheimer's. A synthetic form of this hormone is available in the United States, in lower doses without a prescription and in higher doses with a prescription. DHEA is not legally available in Canada. Consult your holistic physician for more information and for regulated doses of this product. It is important to take antioxidant supplements with DHEA to protect the liver.

Digestive Aids

See *HCL Betaine Hydrochloride, Glutamic Acid Hydrochloride, Plant Enzymes, Bromelain, Papain, Bile Salts, Essiac® or Flor Essence®, Swedish Bitters®, Acidophilus, Bifidus, Probiotics* and the individual entries for many herbal teas. See also *Beets, Beet Powder, Flaxseed, Grapefruit, Tomato Juice, Lemons, Limes* and *Yogurt* in "Remedies from Your Refrigerator and Cupboard." All these supplements and foods can be used as digestive aids.

DMSO

Dimethyl sulfoxide or DMSO is an industrial solvent, a byproduct of papermaking. Its benefits are still disputed and it is considered by many health experts to be toxic. This product is available in Canada only by prescription, in a liquid form for external use only. In the United States, DMSO is a non-prescription product. Never buy industrial, hardware store-grade DMSO; only purchase the superior health food store quality. DMSO is usually applied externally and is readily absorbed through the skin, along with any impurities and bacteria on the skin, so the hands and area to be applied to should be very clean. It has been used successfully to treat arthritis, minor injuries, back pain or other back problems, acne, burns, skin problems, herpes, cancer and other health problems. The use of DMSO causes an odor similar to garlic. Side effects can include headaches, light sensitivity and skin irritation among others. DMSO is not recommended for use without a holistic doctor's recommendation and supervision. It is not needed for healthy individuals and is not for use by the very sensitive or by pregnant or nursing women.

Dong Quai

Dong quai is considered the "female ginseng," as it is especially beneficial for women and, unlike some other varieties of ginseng, will not stimulate too many male hormones (with side effects including facial hair growth). Dong quai, also known as angelica, is beneficial for PMS, most menstrual problems, menopause, hot flashes, uterine bleeding, circulation, heart problems, high blood pressure and female infertility. It is not recommended for pregnant or nursing mothers. Avoid excessive sunlight while taking. Dosages vary widely depending on need: 1–2 grams, 1 to 3 times a day as required, with water. Take the larger dosages prior to (or during) painful menstruation and menopause symptoms.

Echinacea

Echinacea is an important immune system-boosting herb commonly used to treat colds, coughs, colic, flu, sore throats and infections. Also known as purple coneflower, echinacea is also beneficial for cold sores, bleeding gums, ear infections, breathing problems, Candida yeast infections, vaginal infections and some STDs (sexually transmitted diseases). It is anti-viral and anti-inflammatory. Echinacea was traditionally also used by North American Indians for snakebite. Take 1–2 grams a day, spread throughout the day, to improve immune function. Echinacea is safe and non-toxic for regular use, even (and especially) by sensitive individuals. Some doctors recommend using it intermittently for only one to three months at a time, then taking a break, to increase effectiveness. However, recent research suggests that ongoing daily use is beneficial and even more effective. Do not use echinacea with some allergies or with any autoimmune diseases such as HIV infections or for multiple sclerosis.

Elderberry and Elderflower

The flowers, leaves and—best—the unsweetened berry extract are used as herbal remedies. Elderberry builds up and purifies the blood; cleanses; boosts the immune system and is beneficial for: colds, flu, sore throats, coughs, fevers, bronchitis, asthma, infections, cold sores, inflammation, circulation, skin problems and respiratory problems.

The leaf or flower teas can be drunk up to three times a day, as needed. Never use the stems of the plant, which are toxic! Take the extract according to package directions, or use a bit less. Elderberry is basically non-toxic and highly beneficial.

Epsom Salts

One or two cups of Epsom salts (magnesium sulfate) can be added to bath water (see "Healing Aids") to remove body toxins, soothe sore muscles and reduce side effects of illness or cleansing, and as a cleansing aid. Epsom salts can also be taken internally as a flushing agent to aid cleansing or the absorption of supplements, or as a laxative. For flushing, mix 2 teaspoons of Epsom salts with 2 ounces (4 tablespoons) of hot water and drink an hour or more after taking cleansing products. The flavor is salty and not particularly pleasant. It may be followed by half a cup of orange or grapefruit juice if desired. (More pleasant flushing agents include psyllium, acidophilus or Bioxy®.) Purchase Epsom salts at any drug store or pharmacy. They may be stored indefinitely, if kept dry and clean at room temperature in a closed plastic bag or other sealed container.

Essiac® or Flor-Essence®

This exceptional herbal blend, also known by other names such as "Native Legend Tea®," is comprised of: burdock root, slippery elm, sheep sorrel, Turkish rhubarb and sometimes additional ingredients. It was originally used by North American Indians for cancer, severe illness, cleansing and healing. This mixture is high in vitamins, minerals, chlorophyll and enzymes. See *The Essiac Report*, by Richard Thomas, for detailed information on this product.

Taken twice a day in large doses, it has been used successfully as a cancer treatment. In smaller doses, it can be taken once a day as an energizer for fatigue, some allergies, healing and chronic fatigue syndrome. Take 1–2 tablespoons (the same amount each day) of liquid Essiac® or Flor-Essence® in double the amount of boiling water once a day (anytime, but around the same time each day), at least an hour before or after food. Take for 3, 6 or 12 months at a time to energize and act as a mild cleansing agent. This is one of the few cleanses that can be done for so long and that can also be combined with another cleanse during the same time period, if desired. Missing this herbal energizer for even one day will create a noticeable drop in energy for most people, so it is important to wean yourself off it before stopping. Small doses can also assist digestion and can be used occasionally as a separate digestive aid.

Too much Essiac® or Flor-Essence® can cause major cleansing and possible skin rashes, especially if you have bowel problems or your body is very toxic. It is a good remedy for most individuals, except those with the above problems or with particular allergies. Once the liquid is prepared or the bottle opened, it must be refrigerated and used within one or two months. Keep it properly covered and bacteria-free while stored. As with all cleansing products, do not smoke (anything) while using this product.

Eucalyptus
This mild, stimulating herb gives off an aromatic scent that is familiar from its use in some decongestant products, cold remedies and cough syrups. Eucalyptus is a tall, evergreen tree native to Australia. It is antiseptic and beneficial for headaches, joint aches and pains, sore muscles, swelling, arthritis, snoring, breathing problems, increasing blood flow and fevers. The oil is good for bleeding gums, burns and infections. It is tastiest and even more beneficial if mixed half-and-half with peppermint to make an herbal tea. One or two cups of this tea can be drunk a day, only as needed. Do not use excessively internally.

Eucarbon®
This is a natural brand of activated charcoal that is used to treat diarrhea. See *Tormentavena®* for more information regarding its use while traveling.

Evening Primrose Oil
See *Primrose Oil, Evening*

Eyebright
This herb is mainly grown in Europe. The whole plant except for the root is used as a remedy for hay fever; allergies; sore, swollen, strained or watery eyes (an eyewash can be used); cataracts; sinus problems; colds; and as a mouthwash or gargle (in tincture form)

for mouth, throat and respiratory tract inflammations. The tea or non-alcoholic tincture can be used externally (and if needed, should be strained to remove herb particles and sediment) as an eye compress. The tea may be taken internally—about one to three cups a day as needed. Eyebright is generally non-toxic in reasonable amounts, when used occasionally as required.

Fennel Seeds

Fennel seeds are used in cooking as a flavoring and have a mild licorice-like taste that accents bean, grain, vegetable and desert dishes. This herbal seed is used to prevent gas and assist digestion especially with foods like beans and dried peas. Add a teaspoon of ground fennel per 1–2 cups of beans at the start of the cooking time. Fennel capsules, tablets, tincture and tea can be taken for: digestion, eliminative organ function, stomach upset, heartburn, gas, flatulence, colon problems and mild stimulation; to increase the flow of nursing mothers' milk, expel mucus and to stimulate the appetite; and as a diuretic. This gentle seed or its vegetable root can be eaten frequently, as fennel is generally non-toxic. It can on rare occasions cause allergic reactions in sensitive individuals. One to three cups of fennel tea can be drunk a day, as needed.

Fenugreek

This herbal seed tea smells like chicken soup while simmering, but tastes nothing like it. Fenugreek is good for fevers, sore throats, skin irritations, asthma, digestion, constipation, blood sugar problems, sinus problems and inflammation. Use occasionally, only as needed, about one to three cups daily. Excessive use may cause stomach upset, though fenugreek is basically safe and non-toxic.

Feverfew

Feverfew is particularly used to treat headaches and migraines. It is also beneficial for internal stimulation, colic, colds, fevers, gas, flatulence, stimulating appetite, digestion, muscle tension, pain, promoting menstrual flow, alcoholic DTs and strengthening organs. A cup or two of tea can be drunk daily as required. Excessive use may cause stomach upset and jitters. Do not use while pregnant or nursing. Do not use at the same time with white willow bark.

Flammaforce®
See *Infra-Zyme Forte®*

Flaxseed
See "Remedies from Your Refrigerator and Cupboard"

FOSs
See *Probiotics* and *Acidophilus*

Flushing Agents
See *Epsom salts*

Garlic
Also see "Remedies from Your Refrigerator and Cupboard" for even more information. When buying garlic capsules, be sure to choose potent brands. Garlic is best eaten raw, minced finely, not chewed but washed down with water in the middle of a big meal, once a day. Usually one clove a day or every other day is enough. See also *Toxin Overload* in the ailments section for how to use garlic for cleansing, healing and as an anti-viral. Garlic helps to expel heavy metals from the body; it is anti-aging, antioxidant, helps balance the blood sugar and protects the liver.

Gelatin
This tasteless, odorless, clear gel is an animal-product protein, and is used to make some capsules. (Vegetarian capsules are made from vegetable gel.) Gelatin is also used as a supplement to help build strong nails and hair. Fill empty capsules with unflavored gelatin and take two to four a day with water at meals, to aid hair and nail growth and strength. Gelatin and gelatin capsules are non-toxic and can be used liberally for filling with herbs or other natural remedies such as cayenne or goldenseal.

Ginger
See also "Remedies from Your Refrigerator and Cupboard"

If using capsules, take between two and four (depending on the potency) as needed, one to three times a day, or follow package directions. It helps to take ginger a day before traveling, boating or expected motion sickness, as well as during and after travel. Excessive amounts can cause upset stomach, though ginger is basically non-toxic. Pregnant women should take minimal doses, only as needed. A small piece of fresh, peeled ginger can also be chewed on instead of taking capsules. Fresh ginger juice (one teaspoon) or ginger slices can also be added to club soda for nausea or motion sickness. Drink one to three cups of ginger tea daily, as needed.

Ginkgo Biloba

Ginkgo—known as the "smart herb"—comes from the leaves of an ornamental tree that can live as long as a thousand years. Ginkgo originated in China, but also grows in the United States today. The leaf extract and supplements are especially beneficial for anti-aging and for memory problems. Ginkgo is also used for: Alzheimer's, depression, impotence, heart problems, muscle pains, leg cramps, skin problems, loss of hearing or ringing in the ears, breathing problems, blood sugar problems, headaches, migraines, poor circulation and high blood pressure. Standard dosage is one 60 mg capsule a day. This potent antioxidant is generally safe and non-toxic. It can occasionally cause allergic or cleansing reactions including mild headache, skin rash or stomach upset. If this occurs, reduce the dosage, find a purer brand or, if side effects continue, consult your holistic doctor.

Ginseng

Ginseng root has been a popular remedy in parts of Asia for thousands of years. It has also been used by some North American Indians and is now one of the most popular herbal remedies in North America. Ginseng's potency is affected by its source, its age and its quality. Volumes of information are available on ginseng's qualities and uses. There are Chinese, Siberian, Korean and American varieties. Many doctors of Oriental medicine claim that American ginseng is more beneficial than Asian ginseng for North Americans (though it is not as potent and does not have all the same benefits). Ginseng is considered most beneficial for people over the age of 40; it is claimed to lose some of its value for individuals who begin to take it at too young an age. Ginseng is used as an energizer, a stimulant and an anti-aging herb primarily. It also is good for: endurance, stress, infection, flu, impotence, infertility, athletic performance, autoimmune diseases, blood sugar problems, immune function, circulation, breathing problems and appetite stimulation. Ginseng is a potent yet safe aphrodisiac.

Dosage will vary with quality and potency. Consult your holistic health expert or read up on ginseng and experiment, starting out with low doses. Ginseng is basically safe and non-toxic unless abused. Pregnant and nursing women should not use ginseng. Women in general are better off using dong quai instead of ginseng, to minimize stimulation of male hormones and avoid possible breast tenderness and menstrual problems that may result from taking the regular ginseng varieties mentioned here.

Glucosamine Sulfate

Glucosamine sulfate helps inhibit cartilage breakdown and promotes cartilage repair. It is good for bones and connective tissues, beneficial for all types of arthritis and excellent for osteoarthritis. Glucosamine sulfate is also beneficial for asthma, bursitis, allergies, backaches, kidney stones, vaginal infections, skin problems, minor injuries and healing. Regular dosage is 500 mg taken three times a day. Though basically safe and non-toxic, some brands may not be good for individuals on salt-restricted diets.

Glutamic Acid Hydrochloride

This product, like HCL betaine hydrochloride, is a stomach acidifier and digestive aid. It may work better for some individuals than HCL. You need to experiment—try both and see which works best for your body type. See *HCL Betaine Hydrochloride* for the benefits of these products and how to take them.

Goldenseal

This very potent herbal root is a powerful natural antibiotic, antibacterial, anti-inflammatory and anti-viral. It is used for: strengthening the immune system, respiratory infections, increasing organ function, diarrhea, digestion, stomach problems, bowel problems, menstrual regulation, vaginal infections, reducing blood pressure, cold sores, all kinds of infections and sinus problems. Goldenseal is often used in combination with echinacea to treat colds, sore throats and flu. Goldenseal is too powerful to be used for longer than 7 to 14 days, and can be toxic if abused. The powdered root makes a powerful tea or tincture, which may be used for a mouth-wash, for gargling or to treat toothaches and internal problems. Take the capsules or tablets as the package directs (usually two, taken once or twice a day), or consult your holistic doctor. Improper use may cause stomach problems or nervous reactions. Pregnant and nursing women should not use goldenseal.

Gotu Kola

This Asian-African plant now also grows in parts of Europe and is beneficial for skin problems, circulation and varicose veins, minor wounds and injuries, heart and liver problems, high blood pressure, fevers, coughs, nervous system disorders and depression, and is used to increase appetite, to stimulate energy and as an aphrodisiac. Gotu kola can be used topically for burns and some minor wounds, though it can cause skin irritation in some people when used externally. In rare instances, it may cause allergic reactions. It is generally best to avoid gotu kola while pregnant or nursing, though it may be used in some cases with a holistic doctor's approval and supervision.

Grape Seed

Grape seed is a source of OPCs (oligomeric proanthocyanidins) or PCOs (procyanidolic oligomers), which are bioflavonoids with powerful antioxidant qualities. Grape seed extract has greater antioxidant effects than vitamins C and E according to naturopathic physician Dr. Michael Murray in his *Encyclopedia of Natural Medicine.* It is beneficial for allergies, heart disease, stroke and PMS; lowers cholesterol levels; strengthens capillaries; repairs connective tissues and blood vessel and skin damage; prevents bruising and varicose veins; prevents inflammation and improves the circulation. Dosage is 100 mg one to three times a day, as required. See also *Pycnogenol.*

Green Tea

Organic green tea, unlike black teas, is beneficial for healing, mainly because of the bioflavonoids, tannins, vitamin C and other nutrients it contains. It also contains caffeine though in organic form, the caffeine in green tea is not detrimental as it is in coffee. Organic green tea is beneficial for fatigue, gum diseases, cancer, some heart problems, increased immune function and infections. This tea is basically non-toxic, but excessive amounts can cause nervousness, anxiety and insomnia.

Hawthorn Berry

The hawthorn fruit is a well-known remedy for heart problems. It is beneficial for angina, lowering cholesterol levels, normalizing blood pressure, dilating blood vessels, and restoring weakened, aging or inflamed heart muscle. The leaves and flowers of the hawthorn are also used in remedies. For hawthorn tea, soak two or three teaspoons of crushed fruit in 8 to 12 ounces (one-quarter litre or quart) of cold water and let sit for 7 or 8 hours. Then heat quickly to a boil, remove from heat, cover and allow to steep for a few minutes. Strain and drink. Drink this mixture once a day for as long as required. Hawthorn can safely be used daily for long periods by all adults. It can be used in small amounts for children and pregnant women.

Important: If taking prescription heart medications, consult a holistic doctor before taking hawthorn.

HCL Betaine Hydrochloride

This is a good stomach acidifier and digestive aid for those with low stomach acid, especially if the condition is accompanied by Candida yeast problems, impaired digestion, weakened immune system, severe illness or chronic fatigue. It is also beneficial for those who are cleansing and need additional help digesting foods, in particular heavy foods, meats, dairy products and popcorn. Added pepsin makes this an even better supplement for helping the digestion of these protein and heavier foods.

Dosage is one or two capsules, up to three times a day (with meals—never on an empty stomach). Some doctors recommend taking enough that you feel a warmth in your stomach, though this may prove too much for some individuals. One tablet a day, or only with heavy meals, may be enough for some individuals. Take only as much as you need to help your digestion. If you wake up after four or five hours of sleep, hungry, even though you have eaten well that day, you will know your dose was too high. HCL is basically safe and is not habit-forming, but excessive amounts can cause heartburn and stomach distress. Do not use if you have high stomach acid or ulcers. Do not take more than six capsules a day. See your doctor if you consistently require this amount! Glutamic acid hydrochloride, another type of digestive aid, may be better for some individuals than HCL. See *Glutamic Acid Hydrochloride.*

Hops
Hops are a major ingredient in beer making. Herb flower petals, known as hops, are used primarily to combat stress, relieve anxiety and induce sleep. Hops are also beneficial for heart problems, ulcers, shock and some STDs (sexually transmitted diseases). They are not recommended for use during Candida yeast or parasite treatment. Hops are basically non-toxic, though some may have mild allergy reactions as it is a type of flower herb.

Horsetail
Horsetail is rich in silica and increases calcium absorption and is therefore very beneficial for weak or brittle nails and dull hair, improving their strength and luster. Horsetail is also good for healthy skin and bones, healing, heart and lung problems, arthritis, inflammation, muscle cramps, kidney and gallbladder problems, urinary tract infections and edema. Be sure to use high-quality horsetail to avoid problems, and do not use if pregnant or nursing, unless your doctor recommends it and approves the brand you choose.

Hydrogen Peroxide
This product is available in three grades: drugstore grade (for external use) and two types of food grade (3 or 35 percent). They are *not* interchangeable. The drugstore remedy is used as an antiseptic and is excellent for topical use on small wounds and insect bites and stings. It is particularly healing for poison ivy, poison oak and sumac. It also dries up and quickly heals the sores from measles and chicken pox, and helps prevent scarring. Use a cotton swab to apply externally. *Warning: Never* take drug store hydrogen peroxide internally.

Food grade hydrogen peroxide (3 percent) can be used mixed with water (*never* use full strength!) as a mouthwash (see *Oral Hygiene Problems* in the ailments section) and is also used to treat Candida yeast and some other ailments. Consult your holistic doctor for internal treatments, which should be doctor-supervised because side effects from misuse are major. Do not use food grade hydrogen peroxide on the skin—it will burn! Never use 35 percent food grade hydrogen peroxide unless recommended by your holistic doctor!

Infla-Zyme Forte®
This is one of many brand-name supplements, this one an American product, from American Biologics that are helpful for chronic or acute inflammation. It is also used as a digestive aid. Anti-Flam® is a similar American product. Flammaforce®, a Canadian brand, is available from Prairie Naturals. Take these products with water, away from meals, for anti-inflammatory effects. Taken with a meal, these supplements act more as a digestive aid. See packages for directions.

Kava Kava
This Pacific island herb is known as a mild sleep aid and tension- and anxiety-reliever. It is also good for treating depression and urinary tract infections. It is safe if used only occasionally as required. Kava kava is not recommended for pregnant or nursing women. Long-term use or excessive amounts may cause allergic reactions, skin damage or hair and nail discoloration. Expect drowsiness, and do not drive after using.

Kombucha
See *Mushrooms* under "Remedies from Your Refrigerator and Cupboard"

Lemon Grass
This delightfully flavored herb has long been used in Asian cuisine, particularly in Thai cooking. Lemon grass also adds flavor to pleasure herbal tea blends and lightens the flavor of some medicinal teas. It is high in vitamin A and good for the eyesight. Lemon grass is an astringent and is beneficial for healing, fevers and stress and good for hair, nails and skin. Use the tea liberally, either on its own or blended with other herbs. The fresh or dried leaves can be used in cooking often, as they are safe and have no ill effects.

Licorice
Licorice herb grows throughout Europe and Asia and is used commonly in Oriental medicine. More recently it has become popular in North America for its long list of healing uses. The herbal tea is used as a mild laxative. The tincture or powdered herb is beneficial for: colic, ulcers,

liver problems, bowel problems and colon cleansing, muscle spasms, allergies, asthma, eczema, depression, chronic fatigue, fibromyalgia, stomach problems, colitis, shingles, fever, viruses, hypoglycemia, PMS, menopause, cold sores, HIV and inflammations.

Important: Licorice can be detrimental for individuals with diabetes, glaucoma, heart problems, high blood pressure, edema, menstrual disorders, or a history of stroke. (For some of these disorders, deglycyrrhizinated licorice is not detrimental.) Consult your holistic doctor before using licorice as a remedy, to be sure it is okay for you. Increase your potassium intake if you take licorice for extended periods. Do not take while pregnant or nursing.

Lobelia
Herbalists have used this powerful herb for centuries to induce vomiting. However, it also has other uses for infections, colds, coughs, flu, viruses, asthma, heart problems, panic attacks, painful cramps and seizures. Do not take too much or for extended periods. It is best to use lobelia only under your holistic doctor's supervision. Do not use if pregnant or nursing, and do not give to young children. Lobelia is used occasionally in the "Ailments and Remedies" section as a healing tea with small doses of one or more spoonfuls at a time.

Lysine or L-lysine
This singular amino acid is used primarily for treating cold sores and herpes. L-lysine also assists calcium absorption and is essential for growth and maintaining a nitrogen balance in the body. It is legally available as a separate amino acid supplement in the United States, but not legally in Canada. Between 1,000 and 3,000 mg may be taken each day as required, for limited periods. Excessive use could contribute to high cholesterol, cramping, diarrhea and other problems. Consult a holistic doctor before using.

Melatonin
This synthetic hormone is used primarily as a sleep aid and to avoid jet lag. It is also beneficial for glaucoma, ringing in the ears, protecting body cells, helping to repair cell damage and anti-aging. It is not legal in Canada, but is inexpensive in the United States. The sublingual form is the more readily absorbed type of mela-

tonin. Melatonin capsules are better than most tablets, and are most effective when taken with a digestive aid like an acidophilus capsule (uncoated so it will break down in the stomach rather than in the intestines, or placed in a new gelatin or veggie capsule before taking with melatonin). Melatonin works best on an empty stomach at least an hour away from eating foods. Taken close to foods, it may actually cause elevated energy, sleeplessness or restless sleep with many wakeful periods. Use only occasionally, as needed. Excessive amounts can cause morning grogginess. Do not use for depression or schizophrenia. Not for use by pregnant or nursing women. Consult your holistic doctor for more information.

Milk Thistle

Milk thistle is sometimes called silymarin, though silymarin is actually a component of milk thistle. It is one of the most beneficial liver-cleansing and healing herbs known. This powerful antioxidant is potent enough to help reverse liver damage, by regenerating liver cells injured by alcohol abuse and drug use. It is effective for cirrhosis, jaundice and hepatitis and also helps prevent gallstones. Milk thistle is also good for the kidneys and bowel disorders, and boosts the immune system and provides adrenal support. The usual treatment is about 400 mg of silymarin a day, for two to four months. There are no side effects except possibly minor ones from the toxins eliminated by milk thistle's cleansing properties.

MSM

Methylsulfonylmethane (MSM) is a naturally occurring organic sulfur compound, and a dietary derivitave of DMSO. It is present in a variety of foods including fruits, vegetables, milk, meat, seafood and some whole grains, but is easily destroyed by food processing and cooking. MSM is beneficial for low blood sugar, muscle soreness, backaches, athletic injuries, arthritis, fibromyalgia, gout, pain, inflammation, wound healing, PMS, headaches, migraines, hangovers, circulation, allergies, parasites, asthma, acne, eczema and other skin problems, and for cleansing and healing. MSM comes in eye drops, lotions, liquid and supplements. Suggested dosage is one 1,000 mg capsule taken one to three times a day (Dr. Earl Mindell recommends 2,000–6,000 mg a day) or as directed by your holistic doctor. It is very safe and non-toxic, as the body flushes unused, excess MSM after about 12 hours. MSM is more effective when taken with vitamin C.

Myrrh

Myrrh was one of the precious gifts given by the three wise men to the baby Jesus in the Christian nativity story. It was also used for preserving mummies. Today it is used, often in combination with goldenseal, to treat gum disease, toothaches and bad breath; for teething babies; and as an antiseptic and antibacterial mouthwash. Myrrh is also good for cold sores, canker sores, skin problems, athlete's foot, ulcers, colds, coughs, sore throats, mouth and throat inflammations, wounds, sores, asthma and breathing problems. Myrrh can be taken internally or applied topically in a cream or ointment or as a non-alcoholic tincture. It is also used in scented candles, oils and incense. Though it is safe and non-toxic, drink only a few teaspoons of myrrh tea a day, as required, or mix a tiny amount with other pleasure teas.

Neem

Neem is an ancient East India remedy used for cleaning the teeth. Gandhi used this marvelous antibacterial cleaning tool from what is known as the "miracle tree." Many people in India still use a stick from the neem tree to clean their teeth. Neem powder can be mixed with baking soda (six to eight parts baking soda to one part neem) for a wonderful natural tooth powder. Two 500 mg neem powder capsules can be taken daily for dental problems. About 500–1,000 mg of neem powder can be mixed with 6–8 ounces of water for an excellent antibacterial mouthwash and gargle. Neem is safe and non-toxic when used as directed.

Olive Leaf Extract

This is not, as you might think, an oil product, but a dried, powdered extract of olive leaves. Olive leaf extract is a powerful healing and cleansing agent and is antibacterial, anti-fungal, anti-parasitic and anti-viral. It protects and strengthens the immune system and is beneficial for: flu, colds, sore throats, herpes, HIV, AIDS, heart problems, infections, arthritis, Epstein-Barr virus, chronic fatigue syndrome, heart problems, skin diseases, and some STDs (sexually transmitted diseases). For more detailed information see the book *Olive Leaf Extract*, by Dr. Morton Walker.

Because olive leaf has strong cleansing effects, many individuals may experience some side effects, especially during the first couple of weeks of use, so varied dosage is provided here. However, to effectively heal some infections, viruses and STDs, you should take it for 30 days or longer at dosage 7 or stronger. There is no guarantee of healing, and it is essential to consult with your holistic doctor and have him or her supervise all use of olive leaf extract *for infectious diseases.* Prescription antibiotics may also be required. The doses below are also potent for cleansing and eliminating toxins.

DOSAGES 1 (SENSITIVE) TO 10 (HARDY)

Take the following doses on an empty stomach, an hour away from food, with one-half to one glass of water:

1	Take 1 capsule a day for 15 days.
2	Take 1 capsule once or twice a day, for 15 to 30 days.
3	Take 1 capsule in the morning and one capsule in the afternoon, daily, for 30 days.
4	Take 2 capsules in the morning and 1 capsule in the afternoon, daily, for 30 days.
5	Take 2 capsules in the morning and 2 capsules in the afternoon, daily, for 30 days.
6	Take 3 capsules in the morning and 2 capsules in the afternoon, daily, for 30 days.
7	Take 3 capsules in the morning and 3 capsules in the afternoon, daily, for 30–45 days.
8	Take 2 capsules, 3 times a day, for 30–45 days; or take 1 teaspoon 10 ppm colloidal silver once a day followed by a few sips of water and, separately, 2 capsules olive leaf extract twice a day, for 30–45 days.
9	Take 4 capsules in the morning and 3 capsules in the afternoon, daily, for 30 days, then reduce amount and take for 15–30 days more.
10	Take 4–5 capsules in the morning and 4–5 capsules in the afternoon, daily, for 30 days, then reduce amount and take for 15–30 days more.

Oregano Oil

Oil of oregano is a potent antiseptic, antibacterial, anti-fungal and anti-viral. The purest forms come in a base of extra virgin olive oil and nothing else. Oregano is rich in vitamin C and a variety of minerals. It is beneficial for colds, flu, coughs, congestion, breathing problems, cleansing, infections and joint aches and pains. It can be used topically on cuts, wounds, skin problems and warts. Do not apply directly (it needs further dilution—one drop or a few can be diluted in a tablespoon of extra virgin olive oil or pure water) to sensitive areas of skin, such as near the genital area, or use on a baby's skin, as it can sting on sensitive places.

Some people add a few drops to shampoo or soap, but unless you rinse it off thoroughly, you may end up smelling like a salad or pizza. A few drops can also be added to water as a mouthwash. It is not recommended, though, as the flavor is strong, and it may sting or leave an aftertaste. Oregano oil does wonders for the hair, skin and nails. Skin and hair feel softer after as little as three days of use, and nails become very strong and healthy after taking oil of oregano internally for 30 days.

DOSAGES 1 (SENSITIVE) TO 10 (HARDY)

Take the following doses on an empty stomach and follow with a few sips of water:

1	Take 1 drop dispersed in 1 tablespoon water, at the back of the throat (to avoid taste buds) if desired, once a day, every other day, for 10–20 days.
2	Take 1 drop dispersed in 1 tablespoon water, at the back of the throat (to avoid taste buds) if desired, once a day for 10–20 days.
3	Take 1 drop dispersed in 1 tablespoon water, at the back of the throat (to avoid taste buds) if desired, once a day for 20–60 days.
4	Take 2 drops dispersed in 1 tablespoon water, at the back of the throat (to avoid taste buds) if desired, once a day for 10–30 days.
5	Take 2 drops dispersed in 1 tablespoon water, at the back of the throat (to avoid taste buds) if desired, once a day for 20–60 days.

6	Take 3 drops dispersed in 1 tablespoon water, at the back of the throat (to avoid taste buds) if desired, once a day for 15–60 days.
7	Take 2 drops dispersed in 1 tablespoon water, at the back of the throat (to avoid taste buds) if desired, twice a day for 15–30 days.
8	Take 3 drops dispersed in 1 tablespoon water, at the back of the throat (to avoid taste buds) if desired, twice a day for 30 days.
9	Take 1–3 drops directly under the tongue, once or twice a day, for 15–30 days.
10	Take 3–6 drops directly under the tongue, once or twice a day, for 15–30 days.

Papain

Papain (papaya enzyme) is used mainly as a digestive aid for proteins. Avoid if you have related allergies.

Passion Flower

This beautiful flower, as well as the leaves and stem are dried for use as a mild sedative and sleep aid that also lessens anxiety. The tea can be drunk as required. It is best not to use it during pregnancy and nursing, unless your doctor recommends it and supervises the treatment. Do not use with antidepressant drugs. Use catnip or chamomile for children instead.

Pau d'Arco

See *Taheebo*

Peelu

Peelu is a potent yet gentle healing herb that is particularly beneficial for mouth and gum protection (it is used in toothpastes and mouthwashes) and infections. It is antibacterial and anti-fungal. The liquid extract can be placed directly on the gums and swished around the mouth. Spit out the remainder, as it may have some cleansing effects if swallowed. Basically non-toxic and safe if used as directed.

Peppermint

Peppermint leaf tea is a long-time favorite and definitely the most well-known and loved herbal tea in North America. It can be used daily and is beneficial for digestion, mild nausea, vomiting, colic, colds, chills, dizziness, headaches, energy, stimulation, increased appetite, gum disease, diarrhea and bowel problems. It is frequently mixed with other pleasure and medicinal teas to improve their flavor and increase the absorption of their nutrients—and thus enhance their medicinal properties.

A drop or two or peppermint oil can be dabbed on the wrists to increase energy or as a mild stimulant to help keep you awake. The oil can also be applied to the temples to alleviate mild headaches for adults. Do not apply the oil around the face or nose, as it is too strong, especially for children. Do not take the oil internally without a doctor's consent and supervision.

Pine Bark

See *Pycnogenol*

Plant (Pancreatic) Enzymes

Plant enzymes are also just as frequently called pancreatic enzymes. These helpful digestive aids are best if taken 15 minutes (or right before if forgotten) before meals to stimulate natural digestive enzymes in the body. Plant enzymes include protease, amylase, lipase, lactase and cellulose. They assist the breakdown of proteins, fats and carbohydrates. If plant enzymes are combined with HCL betaine hydrochloride, bile salts or other stronger digestive aids, do not take them *before* a meal, as the mixture may be too acidic for an empty stomach. Have plant enzymes *with* your meal if these strong digestive aids are included in these tablets or capsules. (If acidophilus, bifidus, papain (papaya enzyme) or bromelain (pineapple enzyme) is added, plant enzymes may be taken before the meal.) Use as directed by package. Good for vegetarians and vegans.

Primrose Oil, Evening

Evening primrose oil (EPO) contains gamma linolenic acid (GLA), a fatty acid that converts to a substance that is anti-inflammatory and particularly beneficial for heart problems, PMS, menopause, arthritis and diabetes. Other uses are for: eczema, breast cancer, alcohol withdrawal, attention deficit disorder (A.D.D.), multiple sclerosis, bowel problems and lowering cholesterol levels. A multivitamin taken with evening primrose oil helps to increase absorption. Take 1,000 mg one to three times a day or as directed by your holistic doctor. Other high sources of essential fatty acids and GLA are flaxseed oil, borage oil and blackcurrant seed oil. Unless you have trouble digesting oils, this product is easy to assimilate and has no known side effects.

Probiotics

Probiotics are "friendly bacteria" that are beneficial for the body. They counter the effects of other bacteria that have harmful effects on the body. Probiotic means "for life." Probiotics help protect health and are fed by FOSs (fructooligosaccharides), sometimes called "pre-biotics." Jerusalem artichokes are the major food source of FOSs. Other sources include garlic, onions, asparagus and bananas. Probiotics include acidophilus, bifidus and bulgarus. See *Acidophilus* and *Bifidus*. All probiotics require refrigeration.

Propolis

This marvelous bee product, known as "nature's penicillin," is collected by bees from the resins beneath the bark of certain trees, and used as a sealant for the hive. Propolis is antibacterial, anti-fungal, anti-microbial, anti-viral and a natural antibiotic. Propolis contains active bioflavonoids, which inhibit the cellular enzymes that release viruses. Like royal jelly, this product is loaded with vitamins, minerals and enzymes, particularly B and C vitamins, calcium, iron, zinc and bioflavonoids, and is more than 10 percent protein. It is beneficial for: healing, energy, colds, flu, mouth and throat infections, gum disease, skin cancer, depression, bowel problems, lowering high blood pressure and heart problems. For mouth and throat problems, use with water as a gargle and mouthwash and use propolis powder, chew tablets or open capsules in the mouth for better effectiveness. Take 300 mg a day as required. Safe and non-toxic with normal use.

Psyllium

These seed husks are fiber—"bulking agents"—used as a laxative, especially when constipated and while cleansing. Frequent or unnecessary use may actually have the opposite effect. David Webster, colon specialist, warns about abusing psyllium in his excellent book: *Achieve Maximum Health.*

Psyllium is "a lubricating, mucilaginous, fibrous herb, with cleansing and laxative properties. Acts as a 'colon broom' for chronic constipation; effective for diverticulitus; a lubricant for ulcerous intestinal tract tissue," according to *Healthy Healing* by Linda Rector Page, N.D. Use 1–3 teaspoons in a glass of water, or as directed, between meals. Also found in Experience®, a flushing agent for use with Clear®, a parasite cleanse from Awareness Products (see *Parasites* in the ailments section). Though basically safe and non-toxic, use psyllium sparingly, and only as required. Use alternative laxatives when possible.

Pycnogenol
This is one source of OPCs (oligomeric proanthocyanidins) or PCOs (procyanidolic oligomers), which are bioflavonoids with powerful antioxidant qualities. In his *Encyclopedia of Natural Medicine*, naturopathic physician Dr. Michael Murray claims that pycnogenol (pine bark extract) has greater antioxidant effects than vitamins C and E. Pine bark is beneficial for: allergies, heart disease, and stroke; lowering cholesterol levels; strengthening capillaries; repairing connective tissues blood vessel and skin damage; preventing bruising, varicose veins, PMS, and inflammation; and improving the circulation. Dosage is 100 mg one to three times a day, as required. See also *Grape Seed.*

Raspberry Leaves
The young leaves of the organically grown raspberry bush are most potent when picked before the plant flowers and berries appear. The leaves are high in vitamin C and stimulate female hormones. The herb is used for female health—for lessening PMS, menstrual problems; preventing miscarriage, morning sickness; increasing mothers' milk supply and reducing labor pains. Raspberry leaves are also beneficial for nausea, diarrhea, canker sores and spasms, and can be used as an astringent or a very mild laxative. This mild yet potent tea can be drunk quite frequently, even daily, as a pleasure tea for women and an occasional tea for men. When mixed in

equal proportions with alfalfa tea, raspberry leaf tea tastes like a regular caffeinated tea, though it is caffeine-free.

Rescue Remedy®

This Bach Flower Remedy favorite is composed of five herbs given here with their properties: star of Bethlehem for shock, rock rose for terror and panic, impatiens for mental stress and tension, cherry plum for desperation and clematis for the faraway, out-of-body feeling that precedes fainting or loss of consciousness. This potent combination is obviously used for shock, trauma and severe upset, after accidents, injuries or other traumatic situations.

Add three drops of Rescue Remedy® to a glass of water and sip frequently. When calmer, take a few sips every 15 minutes, then every half-hour until calm. If a person is not able to drink, rub it on their lips, gums, behind the ears and on the wrists. The remedy can also be applied externally, diluted or full strength, a drop or two at a time on insect bites and stings, injuries, wounds and skin irritations. It may also be used in compresses and poultices. Rescue Remedy® is sometimes available as an ointment.

Rose Hips

This is one of the most common pleasure herb teas. Unlike most other herbals, this tea comes from the base—the "hips" or receptacle—of the petals of the wild rose bush. The dried, crushed red base and its seeds are used for this very high-vitamin C tea. In Europe, the red-skinned hips of the rose (usually picked after the first frost, when they have turned from green to red) are also made into a nutritious soup, good for colds and flu. (Be sure to remove the hard seeds if you want to make your own soup from wild rose hips—and never use cultivated roses!) Sometimes candies are made from the rose hip "skins." Syrups and rose petal honey jams are sometimes made from the rose petals. Rose hips are added to many vitamin C supplements—especially the chewable variety. Rose hips make a gentle yet beneficial herbal tea, though they are not good for Candida yeast and certain allergies. Enjoy rose hips tea frequently, many times a day, especially when colds, flu, sore throats and coughs arise. Safe and non-toxic for all ages.

Royal Jelly

Royal jelly is the food that is fed to the queen bee, that makes her the queen bee and the only bee in the hive capable of laying eggs—about 500 a day, or up to 250,000 a year during her eight-year life span. Royal jelly is a mixture of pollen and the glandular enzymes of "nursing" bees. It contains between 18 and 22 amino acids, including all the essential ones, and is packed with an array of vitamins and minerals, notably B5 and other B vitamins; vitamins A, D, E and K; 16 minerals; and enzymes, lecithin and essential fatty acids. In humans, royal jelly increases stamina, endurance, energy and fertility, and enhances sexual performance. It is anti-bacterial and is good for PMS, menstrual problems, menopause, athletic performance, wound healing, lowering high cholesterol, stomach and liver problems, skin disorders and strengthening the immune system.

This potent yet gentle energizer is best if taken only a few days a week, or if limited to one to three months at a time, followed by a break, to be sure it is effectively utilized. Take one (or up to three for special needs) 300–500 mg capsules of high-quality royal jelly (Montana brands are among the best, especially: Premier One® and Big Sky®) during the day, an hour or so before sex, or about two to four hours before sleeping. This product is safe, with reasonable use, except for a very small number of individuals with specific allergies to royal jelly or bee products.

Saw Palmetto

This berry is particularly used for prostate problems, cancer and healing specifically for men. Its secondary uses are for urinary problems, colds, flu, asthma, bronchitis, congestion, increasing appetite and aphrodisiac properties. Consult your holistic doctor for appropriate treatments for male health.

St. John's Wort

This powerful herb is sometimes called hypericum, which is its Latin name. The main use of St. John's wort is for depression. Naturopathic physician Dr. Michael Murray, in his book *Natural Alternatives to Prozac,* calls St. John's wort "the most thoroughly researched natural anti-depressant." It is also beneficial for stress, anxiety, upset, shock, trauma, minor injuries and wound healing, nerve pain and viral infections like herpes and HIV.

Standard dosage is one to three 300 mg capsules (or tablets or tincture equivalent), each containing 0.3 percent hypericin, daily. St. John's wort can also have a calming effect that induces sleep, but it should not be used as a sleep aid unless there is anxiety or if other sleep remedies fail. Excessive use may cause daytime drowsiness and fatigue. It cannot be used with certain prescription drugs. Do not use St. John's wort to replace antidepressants or other drugs unless suggested and supervised by a holistic doctor! Large doses can cause sun sensitivity, especially in fair-haired people. Pregnant and nursing women should take St. John's wort only if a doctor recommends and supervises the treatment. Consult your holistic doctor before using St. John's wort if you are taking *any* drugs.

Senna Leaves

Senna leaf herb is used mainly mixed half-and-half with flaxseed as a potent laxative. It is also used in combination with other herbs for parasites and as a mouthwash. Use during pregnancy and while nursing only with a doctor's approval and supervision. Senna leaf should be used sparingly, only as needed.

Shark Oil

Shark liver oil or *squalane* is used topically on: skin rashes, sunburn, skin eruptions, brown liver spots, skin cancer, wounds, frostbite and roughness from shaving. It is also used in some cosmetics. It softens, lubricates, protects and helps to heal skin. The clear, light oil is non-greasy, and can be applied either lightly or generously and used under makeup or suntan lotions.

The *squalene* variation is used internally to treat cancer—strengthen the immune system and for diabetes and tuberculosis. Dosage is one to three 450 mg capsules a day for 30 days or more. It is best to check with your holistic doctor before taking shark oil internally, especially if you are sensitive, have allergy problems or have trouble absorbing oils and fats. If you are allergic to fish, consult your doctor before using this product in *any* form.

Silica
See *Horsetail*

Silymarin
See *Milk Thistle*

Skullcap
Skullcap leaves and stems are used primarily as a sedative and sleep aid. Skullcap herb may be mixed with peppermint and sometimes also with hops for a potent sleep tea that is safe and non-toxic. It is also beneficial taken alone, as a diuretic and for: circulation, some heart problems, muscle cramps, menstrual problems, pain, spasms, anxiety, nervous conditions, excitability and restlessness. Drink a cup or two of the tea, as required. Use catnip or chamomile for children.

Slippery Elm
Slippery elm bark herb is usually ground and used in teas, capsules and tinctures. It is excellent for colds, flu, sore throats, stomach upset, ulcers, diarrhea, inflamed mucus membranes and bowel problems. The tea can be drunk as frequently as needed. The powder is commonly used in sore throat herbal remedies. Safe and non-toxic.

SOD
Superoxide dismutase is an enzyme that vitalizes body cells, neutralizes free radicals and reduces cell destruction. SOD can be purchased in the United States as a supplement, but is not legally available in Canada. It is also found naturally in green food products such as barley green and wheat grass, as well as in green vegetables and plants like broccoli, asparagus and Brussels sprouts and green herbs. Consult your holistic doctor or pharmacist for more information.

Spearmint
Spearmint leaf herbal tea has nearly identical properties to those of peppermint. It is good for digestion, gas, colic, mild nausea, vomiting, spasms, painful urinating, bowel problems, and for inflammation of the kidneys and bladder. Spearmint can be used frequently as a pleasure tea, alone, or mixed with other herb teas. It is totally safe for daily use by adults, children and pregnant women.

Spirulina

Spirulina is a green food product. See *Toxin Overload* and *Cleansing* in the ailments section for information on green foods and how to take them.

Squalane or *Squalene*

See *Shark Oil*

Swedish Bitters®

This European remedy was popularized in North America by an Austrian, Maria Treben, in her book *Health Through God's Pharmacy*. This combination of many herbs—including aloe vera, angelica, myrrh, senna and rhubarb—is used to improve digestive function. It increases stomach acid and the absorption of protein and nutrients, and has a laxative effect. As the name implies, it does have a bitter flavor. Avoid if you have diarrhea, ulcers or high stomach acid. See package instructions for amounts to take for digestive aid.

Taheebo

Taheebo (also known as pau d'arco or lapacho) is a potent herb from the bark of a South American rainforest tree. It is antibacterial, antifungal and anti-viral. It is used in cancer treatment and is also beneficial for heart problems, lupus, AIDS, allergies, ulcers, tumors, Candida yeast, infections, blood purifying, bowel problems and rheumatism. See the recipe for the tea in "Herbal Teas, Tinctures and Treatments." It is not legally available in some forms in Canada. It is freely available in the United States. Use the whole bark for the best results and safety. Using excessive amounts may cause dangerous side effects. Not for use by pregnant and nursing women.

Tea Tree Oil

Tea tree oil is a potent, clear oil from the leaves of an Australian evergreen tree. Its aroma is similar to that of eucalyptus. Tea tree oil in its pure form is antiseptic, antibacterial, anti-fungal and anti-viral. This wonderful, gentle, natural remedy is nothing short of magical for quick healing of burns, cuts, scrapes, wounds, bruises, warts, scars, athlete's foot, herpes, insect bites and stings, blemishes, acne and skin problems, for preventing scarring and for hundreds of other healing uses. Tea tree oil stings when applied full strength on wounds, but the stinging is part of the action that promotes and expedites healing. The more it stings, the more it is healing. Potent tea tree oil shampoos and kits are available for the treatment of head lice, and tea tree oil is also an effective treatment for crabs or body lice.

While tea tree oil is mainly used externally, a drop or two taken internally promotes internal healing and is a powerful treatment for: Candida yeast, vaginal infections, parasites, infections, viruses, sore throats (it makes a good gargle and mouthwash), colds, flu and many other ailments. It is best if diluted in water before internal use.

Do not overuse tea tree oil, especially internally, or a healing reaction and side effects may occur which, though not harmful, can be uncomfortable. *Warning:* Do not use more than one or two drops a day internally! Similarly, frequent external application (several times a day) to a large area of skin can cause a healing reaction for sensitive people, and may cause tiredness. Do not use on staph infections and some other contagious skin infections. Do not apply to third or fourth degree burns or major wounds or injuries until partial healing and wound closure has already occurred! Do not use it near the eyes. For more information, see *The Tea Tree Oil Bible*, by Dr. Elvis Ali, Dr. George Grant, Dr. Selim Nakla, Don Patel and Ken Vegotsky.

Tormentavena®

This herbal extract from European herbalist Alfred Vogel of Bioforce® is used (especially when traveling in tropical countries) as a parasite killer. If diarrhea and signs of parasites become obvious, take this preparation immediately, along with natural activated charcoal (Eucarbon® or another natural brand) to counteract parasites before they multiply and cause more serious problems. Some tropical parasites can cause severe illness and, in rare instances, even death, within two months. See your doctor or visit a tropical disease clinic immediately upon returning home for follow-up parasite treatment. It is best to always travel with Tormentavena® and Eucarbon®.

Traumeel®

This homeopathic combination contains arnica, calendula, echinacea, chamomile, St. John's wort and several other herbal homeopathic preparations blended for use for: trauma, shock, accident and serious upset. Take as directed on package label. This is a marvelous combination for calming and healing when used as directed. See "Homeopathic Restrictions," at the beginning of this section.

Valerian

Valerian is a potent herbal root with an overpowering smell of old, dirty socks—so it is better to take in tablets or capsules rather than to brew the smelly tea. It is used mainly as a strong sleep aid and is also good for stress and anxiety. Although strong, it is safe and non-toxic, does not cause drowsiness and can still be used occasionally during pregnancy and while nursing. Valerian is also beneficial for: high blood pressure, bowel problems, ulcers, cramps, spasms, measles, colic, low fevers, hysteria, trauma, and nervous disorders.

Vitamin C

This remarkable vitamin and antioxidant is briefly explained in the vitamin chart at the end of this section and used throughout the ailments section because it is a major vitamin for healing and support-ing the immune system. Vitamin C is antibacterial, anti-fungal and anti-viral. One of many ways to eliminate the discomfort of cleans-ing—such as gas, stomach upset, nausea, fatigue and headaches—is to do a vitamin C flush. Dr. Linus Pauling, a two-time Nobel prize winner who lived into his late nineties, proved the value and safety of mega doses of vitamin C for anti-aging and healing.

VITAMIN C FLUSH   Take one-quarter to one teaspoon of buffered vitamin C powder (the amount depends on the potency of the vita-min C and your personal tolerance; you can start small and build up the amount if needed) in one-quarter to one-half a glass of water or apple, apricot, pear or peach juice. Repeat every half-hour until watery diarrhea occurs. Begin taking the vitamin C about an hour or so after breakfast (or skip breakfast), or take after lunch if preferred. Then alter and lower the amount of vitamin C to a comfortable daily dose.

Vitex

Vitex, or chaste berry, is used for female problems like PMS, menstrual difficulties, infertility, breast diseases, hot flashes and menopause. It is also beneficial for acne and pituitary function. A regular daily dose is about 30 mg, taken as required. Do not use during pregnancy or while nursing unless your doctor recommends it and supervises the treatment.

White Willow Bark

This herb is used as a diuretic and for headaches, backaches, fever, arthritis, rheumatism, diarrhea, nosebleed, bleeding wounds, bee stings, burns, poison ivy, pain, heartburn, eczema and cancer. Do not use for children's fevers without a doctor's consent and supervision. Safe if used only occasionally, as required. Do not use at the same time with feverfew.

Witch Hazel

Witch hazel is not recommended for internal use. It is used externally as an astringent and for skin problems, eczema, itching, varicose veins and minor wounds and injuries. Can be applied a couple of times a day in warm compresses, poultices and in creams and ointments.

Wormwood

This herb is used particularly to treat worms and other parasites, and also to aid digestion, to increase appetite and to treat heartburn, fevers, diarrhea, and some liver problems. Only use for limited periods of time or stomach problems and other side effects may result. Do not use while pregnant or nursing. Consult a holistic doctor immediately if severe side effects occur from improper use. Never take with or near alcohol.

Yarrow

Yarrow is a potent healing herb, which helps stop excessive bleeding by improving blood clotting. It is also an astringent and a diuretic and is good for: digestion, heartburn, inflammation, ulcers, fistulas, measles, colic, menstruation problems, PMS, fevers, viruses, colds and sore throats. Drink two to three cups of yarrow tea a day, when required, for limited periods. Yarrow may aggravate some allergies and should not be used externally on large, open wounds.

Yucca

This desert herb is used mainly as an arthritis treatment and as a blood purifier and anti-inflammatory. About three cups of tea can be drunk a day. It can be used safely for up to two or three months at a time.

Zinc

Zinc is a very important mineral for healing and boosting the immune system. Zinc is not only essential for colds, flu and sore throats, it speeds the healing of wounds, injuries, operations, infections and viruses. This essential mineral is also required for proper growth and functioning of the reproductive organs and to protect the body from damage by free radicals. Zinc supplementation is beneficial for: impotence, infertility, energy levels, memory functioning, anti-aging, protein synthesis and the absorption of other vitamins and minerals. Zinc picolinate is the most absorbable form. Zinc gluconate is the first choice in Canada, where zinc picolinate is not legal for sale.

Potent food sources of zinc include: oysters, pumpkin seeds, sunflower seeds, pecans, meats, fish, soy lecithin, soybeans, legumes, whole grains, brewer's yeast, torula yeast and parsley. Do not take zinc supplements during fevers. Do not take with or near citrus fruits or juices, as they diminish zinc's effectiveness.

VITAMIN AND MINERAL USE

This is a very general section listing the basic benefits and food sources of major vitamins and minerals. Only the most important nutrients are included. Consult one of the many vitamin and mineral supplement books in "Recommended Reading" for more detailed information.

VITAMINS (In alphabetical order)

Vitamin A (fat soluble)

Functions: prevents night blindness and respiratory infections; essential for normal growth and teeth formation

Sources: orange vegetables—especially carrots, orange yams (a type of sweet potatoes), winter squash—bright green and yellow vegetables, sprouts, pumpkins, papayas, mangoes, peaches, apricots, fish oil, dairy products, and egg yolks

B Vitamins (B1–B12) (water soluble)
Functions: promotes normal growth and functioning of the nervous system, proper digestion and utilization of nutrients, regulates weight and stabilizes emotions, promotes healthy skin and eyes and stable blood sugar (B6 especially helps edema and hangover; B12 prevents anemia)

Sources: whole grains, legumes, vegetables, fruits, citrus fruit, green food products, sprouts, nutritional yeast, nuts, dairy products, and meats

Vitamin C (water soluble)
Functions: promotes healing and resistance to disease and infections, healthy bones and teeth and gums, fights colds and viruses

Sources: citrus fruit, papayas, mangoes, strawberries, blackcurrants, tomatoes, cantaloupes, broccoli, cauliflower, bell peppers and other produce

Vitamin D (fat soluble)
Functions: promotes calcium and phosphorus absorption, normal growth and development of the body and formation of teeth and bones, protects heart and muscles

Sources: sunlight, fish, fish liver oils, dairy products, eggs yolks, sunflower seeds

Vitamin E (heat and fat soluble)
Functions: improves oxygen efficiency of the muscles, aids heart functions, strengthens reproductive system, promotes internal and external healing and normal blood clotting

Sources: dark green leafy vegetables, natural oils (especially flax and pumpkin), beets, nuts, seeds, oranges, molasses, eggs, whole grains and legumes

Vitamin K

Functions: needed for blood clotting and bone formation and repair; helps convert glucose to glycogen, enhances liver function, has anti-aging properties

Sources: seafood, seaweeds, dark green leafy vegetables, sprouts, broccoli, cabbage, Brussels sprouts, cauliflower, blackstrap molasses, soybeans, oats and egg yolks

Vitamin P (bioflavonoids)

Functions: has an antibacterial effect, promotes circulation, preserves capillary structure, stimulates bile production, lowers cholesterol, helps cataracts, aids healing

Sources: citrus fruit inner peels, bell peppers, prunes, apricots, cherries, rose hips, elderberries, hawthorn and green food products

MINERALS (In alphabetical order)

Calcium

Functions: promotes strong bones and teeth and healthy gums, helps balance minerals in body tissues, helps regulate heartbeat, promotes normal blood clotting, assists nerve impulses

Sources: dark leafy greens, dairy products, soybeans, black beans, chickpeas, pinto and kidney beans, tofu, sesame seeds, tahini, molasses, broccoli, carob, filberts and almonds

Chromium

Functions: helps metabolize glucose, helps synthesize cholesterol and fats and protein, maintains stable blood sugar, aids the heart, helps prevent anxiety and fatigue

Sources: millet, brown rice, other whole grains, brewer's yeast, legumes, cheese, meat and blackstrap molasses

Iodine
Functions: promotes proper growth and development, regulates food use by the body, prevents goiter and enlargement of the thyroid gland

Sources: kelp, dulse, other seaweeds, iodized salt, saltwater fish, garlic and dark leafy greens

Iron
Functions: helps form hemoglobin in red blood cells, transports oxygen to the blood cells, helps prevent anemia

Sources: dark green leafy vegetables, molasses (especially black-strap), dried fruit, legumes, whole grains, meats, almonds and egg yolks

Magnesium
Functions: relaxes nerves, helps digestion, promotes new cell growth, aids calcium and potassium absorption, aids transmission of nerve and muscle impulses

Sources: whole grains, citrus fruits, dairy products, meat, fish, seafood, blackstrap molasses, brown rice, brewer's yeast, bananas, apples, apricots and avocados

Manganese
Functions: essential for forming blood cells, helps improve memory, benefits the pancreas, assists protein and fat metabolism, for normal bone growth and reproduction

Sources: avocados, whole grains, legumes, brewer's yeast, bonemeal, egg yolk, green leafy vegetables, blueberries and pineapples

Phosphorus
Functions: promotes strong bones and teeth, assists waste removal and food absorption, important for cell growth and contraction of heart muscle, assists nutrient utilization

Sources: bran, brewer's yeast, meat, fish, poultry, legumes, whole grains, dried fruit, asparagus, garlic, corn, nuts and seeds

Potassium
Functions: regulates the weight, good for nerves and muscles, important for heart rhythm, with sodium helps control body's water balance

Sources: blackstrap molasses, dried fruit, whole grains, legumes, dark leafy greens, winter squash, yams, bananas, apricots and avocados

Selenium
Functions: inhibits oxidation of fats, protects the immune system by preventing formation of free radicals, prevents tumor formation, helps produce antibodies

Sources: whole grains, meats, salmon, seafood, Brazil nuts, nutritional yeast, garlic, broccoli and other vegetables

Zinc
Functions: increases blood volume, promotes healing and proper growth, assists protein synthesis and collagen formation, assists growth and functioning of reproductive organs

Sources: legumes, whole grains, meats, liver, fish, seafood, oysters, pecans, pumpkin seeds, sunflower seeds, soybeans, nutritional yeast, alfalfa and cayenne

REMEDIES FROM YOUR REFRIGERATOR AND CUPBOARD

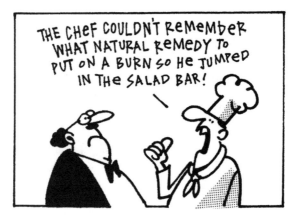

THE CHEF COULDN'T REMEMBER WHAT NATURAL REMEDY TO PUT ON A BURN SO HE JUMPED IN THE SALAD BAR!

FANTASTIC FOODS FOR HEALTH

Artichokes, Globe

Artichokes are members of the thistle family, a European delicacy favored by royalty. Ancient Egyptians, Romans and Greeks also prized these tasty vegetables. These are considered a "pungent" vegetable although their flavor is mild and delicate. They have similar healing properties to other pungent vegetables like garlic and onions. Globe artichokes are high in potassium and other trace minerals. They enhance the flavors of other foods and are powerfully healing for the liver, both in their cooked form—eaten warm, and as an herbal extract. The cold, marinated ones, however, are no friend to the liver or the rest of the digestive tract. Artichokes are among the most popular of aphrodisiacs, probably because they help stimulate good digestion and make you feel good from the inside out! See recipe following. Refrigerate for up to two or three weeks. Why not share them with a loved one? (See also *Artichoke Extract* in the "Natural Remedies Glossary.")

Artichokes, Jerusalem

Their other name, sunchokes, is more true to their nature as they are not from Jerusalem nor are they really artichokes! Sunchokes are tubers that grow underground from a variety of sunflower. Originally, some people thought they tasted similar to artichokes, hence the name. They were first discovered and eaten by North American Indians. Jerusalem artichokes look like ginger roots only rounder and mainly white with brown ribbing. These are particularly good for blood sugar problems as they are one of the highest sources of FOSs (fructooligosaccharides) and natural insulin. They can be eaten raw, grated into salads or cooked (never in aluminum) like potatoes or as a substitute for them. Sunchokes also make a tasty and nutritious pasta flour. Like globe artichokes, sunchokes have a limited availability. They are high in A and B vitamins, iron, calcium, magnesium and potassium. Refrigerate for up to one month, however they are more beneficial if eaten sooner.

Bee Pollen

Honeybees collect a yellowish/orange substance (from the anthers of stamens) within male seed flowers and mix it with their own secretions to form pollen granules.

Bee pollen is a "superfood" rich in zinc, magnesium, calcium, iron, potassium, C and B vitamins, protein and unsaturated essential fatty acids. It is excellent for: male prostate problems (possibly due to its sex hormone content), lowering blood pressure and cholesterol, respiratory problems, anti-aging and some allergies, especially as a treatment and cure for some hay fever problems. Pollen also helps balance the endocrine system and aids some menstrual problems. Bee pollen is a potent energizer used by worldwide athletes. Local, unsprayed bee pollen is the most beneficial. It can be eaten sprinkled on foods and in protein blender drinks. Start with a small amount and build up. Keep in a sealed container in a cool, dry cupboard.

Beet Powder

Beet root powder has anti-fungal properties, is a good digestive aid, helps alleviate constipation and aids the liver. It is high in most minerals, especially iron, vitamin C, folic acid and carotenes. It enriches the blood and is a great tonic for general use. The powder can be purchased in health stores and sprinkled on foods or concentrated capsules can be bought and taken with meals. Keep in an airtight container in a cool, dry cupboard. See also *Beets* following.

Beets

In the Roman Empire, beets were used medicinally as a cure for toothaches and headaches. Beet greens were eaten young and raw or cooked long before the beet roots were eaten. The greens (and dried beet powder) are higher in iron and some minerals than the beets themselves. Today one-third of the world's sugar comes from sugar beets. Low in calories, fresh beets are high in vitamin C, calcium, phosphorus and potassium. Although most people are familiar with cooked or pickled beets, they are especially nutritious eaten raw or juiced. Use them often as a digestive aid, grated into salads. See the recipes following for digestive and energy drinks and liver aids.

Carob

Carob is also called honey locust or St. John's bread, as St. John the Baptist was said to have lived on it in the desert. It grows throughout the Mediterranean in pods on a large tree and is a member of the legume family. Carob is a much-maligned chocolate substitute containing no caffeine or oxalic acid (which hinders calcium absorption) and one-tenth the fat of chocolate. Unfortunately most people, even those in the health industries, do not always seem to know how to use it correctly. It can be used in recipes to mimic chocolate so effectively, only an expert would know the difference, however, few experts know how to do this. It is delicious, low in calories, low in fat and is usually non-allergenic and a mild digestive aid. Carob contains trace B vitamins, phosphorus, calcium, and traces of iron. The roasted carob powder can be used just like cocoa powder, and by adding sweetening and a teaspoon or two of coffee substitute powder per recipe, it can be made to taste like chocolate. The raw carob powder has a more fruity flavor. The carob pods (not seeds) can be eaten as is or washed and baked (around 350°F) for 5 minutes for a toasty flavor. They are rarely found in health stores, more often in specialty food markets. Store, wrapped in plastic or in a container, in a cool, dry cupboard.

Cayenne Pepper

The healing power of cayenne comes from capsicum, its active healing ingredient. Cayenne is anti-fungal and anti-viral. It helps break down cholesterol deposits in the body and helps the circulation. Cayenne is very beneficial for ulcers, Candida yeast, heart problems, colds, flu and sore throats. It can be sprinkled in herbal teas to help break up mucus and can be used externally to stimulate warmth to cold hands and feet (See *Circulation Problems*). Although it tastes fiery to many, it has a cleansing and purging effect on the body and is an excellent expeller of poisons and toxins. Unlike black and white pepper, which are spices, cayenne is a therapeutic vegetable. See Dr. John Christopher's excellent book *Capsicum* for more information. Store in a cool, dry place, out of sunlight.

Flaxseed

Flax plants are cultivated in Europe and Asia to produce linen for clothing and to make fine paper as well. North American flax is used mainly for oil. Flax seeds and oil are anti-fungal, anti-inflammatory, a good digestive aid/laxative and an important source of omega 3 and omega 6 essential fatty acids. Flax seeds and the raw, unrefined oil (expeller pressed) are beneficial for cancer, shiny hair and strong nails, blood sugar problems, PMS, allergies, skin problems, heart problems and lowering cholesterol and triglyceride levels. Flax, also called linseed, is a good source of zinc, magnesium, potassium, fiber and protein.

The raw, unrefined flax oil is used like a medicine for people deficient in essential fatty acids but some doctors feel it is better to eat the seeds regularly, not only for their fiber but because they are better digested and assimilated than the oil and are in a form naturally more beneficial for human digestion. The brown seeds can be ground, a quarter cup or so at a time, in a blender and sprinkled on cereals, yogurt, cooked whole grains and other foods, as well as used in blender drinks. Keep the ground seeds in a jar in the refrigerator for a few weeks or more. The whole seeds may be used in cooking, however, eaten raw they tend to pass through the system undigested and their nutrients unutilized. Store the whole seeds in a plastic bag, tin or jar in a dry cupboard.

Garlic

Ancient Greeks, Romans and Egyptians ate garlic regularly for strength and endurance. In Egypt, a male slave could be bought for 15 pounds of garlic and garlic was fed to the builders of the pyramids. It has also been mentioned in Biblical records. The "stinking rose" has been used to ward off evil spirits and fight off plague, disease and infection. Not to forget, it wards off vampires as well! It was used in early World War I on wounds as a natural antiseptic and antibacterial when medical supplies were short. Garlic is a powerful natural antibiotic. It is also anti-fungal (great for Candida yeast problems), anti-viral, anti-parasitic and an aphrodisiac. It is excellent for colds, flu, fevers, digestion, circulation, cleansing, balancing blood sugar, lowering blood pressure and cholesterol, heart problems, herpes and for other viral infections. Regular (not elephant) garlic can be chewed raw for mouth and throat problems or taken internally without chewing (see Cleansing in *Toxin Overload*) for internal benefits. Garlic capsules can also be employed although many are not as potent as taking garlic internally, the way it is outlined in Cleansing. Always use organic garlic for therapeutic purposes. Even cooked garlic has benefits. Store in a cool, dry cupboard in the open air. See also *Garlic* in the "Natural Remedies Glossary," and under *Toxin Overload* in the Ailments section.

Ginger

Popularized by Asian cooking, ginger is now a commonly used vegetable in North American recipes as well, particularly for stir-fries and desserts. Asians use ginger for colds, congestion, diarrhea, stomach problems, nausea, muscle aches and nervous conditions. Ginger is a warming food that kills parasites; that is why the pickled variety is so often served with sushi to assist digestion and counteract bacteria and parasites in the raw fish along with horseradish that performs a similar purpose. Ginger contains potassium and a variety of trace minerals. It is beneficial for nausea, morning sickness and motion sickness, colds, congestion, circulation, diarrhea, bowel problems, stomachache, gas and flatulence, prevention of headaches, ringing in the ears, digestion, cleansing, lowering cholesterol, cancer, joint aches, infections and nervous diseases. It is also a natural antibiotic and anti-inflammatory. Store ginger roots, like garlic, in a cool, dry cupboard in the open air. Ginger tea, capsules and extract are also available. See also the "Natural Remedies Glossary."

Grapefruits and Grapefruit Juice

Grapefruits were so named because they grow in clusters like grapes. Ponce de Leon first brought the grapefruit to Florida according to legend. The U.S. is now the leading producer of grapefruit in the world. Grapefruit was once considered too sour for eating but the fruit has lost much of its original tartness due to cultivation. The tarter varieties, such as the white grapefruit, are more therapeutic than the pink or red, and are used as: a digestive aid, especially for proteins; an anti-fungal for Candida yeast infections and an anti-bacterial for colds and flu. The pink and red varieties are high in beta-carotene and some lycopene. The most potent form is grapefruit seed extract or citricidal used for the above and also in treatment of parasites. See the "Natural Remedies Glossary" for citricidal use. One-half to one glass of grapefruit juice, or one-half of a fresh grapefruit can be helpful for digestion of heavy meat meals or other protein meals especially if digestion is impaired. Grapefruit are high in vitamin C, bioflavonoids, potassium, pectin, fiber and trace vitamins and minerals. Keep refrigerated. Best eaten at room temperature. *Important:* Grapefruit or grapefruit juice (not other citrus) can intensify the effects of some drugs. It must be totally avoided with some prescription medications! Check with your doctor or a knowledgeable pharmacist to find out which medications require avoiding grapefruit and grapefruit juice.

Honey

It takes more than 500 honeybees, traveling a combined distance equal to once around the world or more, to produce one pound of honey. Flower nectar mixed with bee enzymes are the ingredients of this natural sweetener. Varieties of honey take their names from main flower sources where the bees gather nectar from and include clover, alfalfa, buckwheat (a strong-flavored honey), fireweed, orange blossom, wild flower and tupelo. The latter is especially good for people with blood sugar problems, though it must still be used sparingly like other sweets. Raw, unfiltered honey or honeycomb is preferable and higher in nutrients, however, the bacteria it naturally contains is considered to be detrimental for infants under two years old who should only be given pasteurized honey.

Quality honey is a source of protein, carbohydrates and trace vitamins and minerals, and is an energy food. It has some antibiotic qualities and tranquilizing effects (provided there are no blood sugar problems) and is used for sore throats, colds and energizing and protein drinks. Unfortunately, some beekeepers feed their bees sugar water, which detracts from the medicinal values and nutrients of the honey. For therapeutic use, buy quality, local honey from a respected beekeeper, whenever possible.

Store in a cool, dry cupboard, away from heat and cold. Place a honey jar in a bowl of hot water to melt if needed. Do not cook, in order to preserve nutrients and enzymes, unless needed for recipes.

Horseradish

"Horseradish was one of the five bitter herbs of the Passover Seder dinner, along with coriander, nettle, horehound and lettuce," says Sylvia Rosenthal in *Fresh Food*, an excellent food resource book. Horseradish, or German mustard, has a long history throughout the world, in Egypt, Greece, Europe and especially Japan and all of Asia. It is a type of "hot" radish, in the mustard family. Dried, ground horseradish, "wasabi" or "wasabiko" is popularly served with Japanese foods, even here in North America. The dried cream-colored powder is mixed with water to form a light green, thick paste that is served alongside pickled ginger to enhance the flavor of food and counteract bacteria and parasites found in sushi. Horseradish contains only trace minerals.

This pungent vegetable is a cruciferous vegetable good for cancer prevention and treatment. It is also an excellent substitute for onions and/or garlic. Half a teaspoon of prepared horseradish is equal to the flavor of an onion in cooking; or use one to two teaspoons for one very large onion (or about two cups chopped onion). One-quarter teaspoon or less prepared horseradish can be used instead of each clove of garlic. Horseradish is an excellent substitute for onions and garlic for those who are allergic or avoiding these for religious reasons. The fresh root can be grated raw and eaten with vegetables and other foods. "Horseradish is a decongestant and expectorant. The root vegetable is also antibacterial, and increases metabolism, which burns calories," say Gayla and John Kirschmann in the *Nutrition Almanac.* It is also anti-parasitic. Store the fresh roots like garlic and onions in a cool, dry cupboard, in the open air.

Kelp, Sea
This beneficial seaweed is found in fresh, dried, ground, and powdered form and in tablets. Kelp contains calcium, magnesium, phosphorus, potassium, iron, sodium, folic acid and trace A and B vitamins and is especially high in iodine. It is used as a supplement, to help the thyroid (provided it does not conflict with certain medications), in some weight loss diets and to expel heavy metals. Brown kelp, or laminaria, is antibacterial and anti-viral; lowers cholesterol; and helps constipation, nerve problems, ulcers, herpes and cancer. See Cleansing under *Toxin Overload* for more information. It can be sprinkled on food or cooked into recipes to add flavor and depth to sauces, stews, soups, casseroles and other main dishes. Use it frequently, in small amounts on food, especially if you are not using iodized salt. Store in an airtight jar or tin, in a cool, dry cupboard. Keep some handy in a shaker bottle as well.

Lecithin
Soybeans are the main source of lecithin granules, liquid, powder and capsules. Eggs, brewer's yeast, whole grains, legumes and fish are other sources. Lecithin is also found naturally in large concentrations in the body, in cells, nerves and especially in the brain. Among its many benefits, lecithin helps to break up cholesterol deposits in the body, aids the liver and kidneys, prevents some heart problems, energizes the body and brain and assists the digestion and absorption of dietary fats. A tablespoon or so of lecithin granules can be sprinkled on food several times a week, or the liquid (or granules) can be used in protein and energy drinks. The liquid is more readily assimilated and contains vitamin J, which is not found in other types of lecithin. The liquid is also a great addition to baked goods as it improves the texture of breads and desserts (add three or four teaspoons per recipe) and acts as a natural preservative.

Refrigerate all forms of lecithin except the bottled liquid which can be stored on a shelf until opened, then refrigerated.

Lemons

Lemons are a tropical fruit first cultivated in Asia and today in the U.S., Europe and South America. Lemons (and limes) were once a necessary protection against scurvy. Lemon juice is a potent astringent, antibacterial, anti-viral and natural antibiotic, healing food. The sour juice also helps expel heavy metals and is good for colds, flu, sore throats, digestion and cleansing. Lemons add a refreshing zest (and digestive enzymes) to beverages and foods, especially fish and seafood. It can be used instead of vinegar or salt in some recipes. Keep refrigerated. See Cleansing in *Toxin Overload* for more information.

Limes

Limes are believed to have originated in Tahiti but now are cultivated in California and Florida. British sailors were nicknamed "limeys" in the 18th and 19th centuries because of their use of limes to prevent scurvy on sea voyages. Limes have all the same healing attributes of lemons. Use them interchangeably with lemons for remedies. Keep refrigerated. See *Lemons*.

Millet

Millet is a staple in Asia, China and India. Ground millet is made into flatbreads called *roti* in India and in Ethiopia they are called *injera*. Millet is considered a more nutritious grain than the ever-popular (brown) rice. Macrobiotics places a high value on millet and it is claimed to be the most alkaline of all grains. It is higher in B vitamins, copper, iron and especially chromium, than other grains. It is possible to raise chromium levels in the body effectively by eating millet three or more times weekly for several months. Millet is mild on the stomach, good for babies, the elderly and those with allergies, blood sugar problems and stomach problems. The color of millet ranges from white to yellow to golden (light) brown, the highest quality being the golden brown. Whole millet stores safely in a cool, dry cupboard, crushed or ground millet is best if frozen (never refrigerate or it will taste musty). Cooked millet keeps seven or eight days if refrigerated. See my cookbooks for many millet recipes.

Miso

Miso originated in Japan. East Asian cultures have thrived on miso and other soy products and used them for healing (as in macrobiotic cooking, for instance). Macrobiotic healing, discussed by Annemarie Colbin in *Food and Healing*, suggests that excessive amounts of ingested sugar can be neutralized with miso and/or tamari.

Miso is a fermented bean paste usually made from soybeans, sometimes chickpeas and a grain such as rice or barley. It is more beneficial if not boiled. However, some health specialists feel that the high enzymes in miso make it a perfect healing food. Natural miso assists digestion and is high in many amino acids (7 percent to 18 percent protein, depending on the type of miso) and also very high in minerals, including calcium, magnesium, manganese, phosphorus, potassium, iron, zinc, and sodium. It is usually more beneficial heated and if kept just under a boil. Use it in soups and sauces by first mixing it in a little hot water or broth with a fork, adding to the recipe near the end of its cooking time and simmering in recipes for 5 to 10 minutes maximum. Miso is beneficial for digestive problems, cancer and some allergies. Miso is high in sodium so not good for heart problems. A diet high in vegetables, whole grains and legumes allows more tolerance for the salt in miso and tamari. Keep it properly wrapped and refrigerated for up to a year or more.

Mushrooms

Egyptians considered mushrooms a royal food. The French were the first to cultivate them in the 17th century, in caves. Mushrooms are a fungus with attributes and detriments. Many varieties are nutritious foods, while others are poisonous. Many mushrooms are high in protein and B vitamins, including niacin. They also contain some potassium, copper, iron and other trace minerals. Shiitake mushrooms are high in germanium, a high-oxygen food that assists healing, viruses, lowering blood pressure and cholesterol and is used especially for tumors and cancer treatment. Kombucha homegrown mushrooms are claimed to help digestion, eliminate toxins and support the immune system, however, they are not beneficial for some individuals. Most raw mushrooms are detrimental for Candida yeast problems and parasites. The common button mushroom may contain many toxic additives. Like other produce, fresh mushrooms are much more nutritious and beneficial than canned mushrooms. Keep unwashed, refrigerated, for one week or so. (Washing first makes them go moldy faster!)

Natural Oils

Oils pressed without solvents, like most supermarket or commercial oils, are cold-pressed or expeller-pressed oils made without chemicals or additives. Commercial oils have toxic additives. Natural oils are beneficial for scalp, hair and skin problems, cancer and most major health concerns. See *Flaxseed* for the benefits of raw flax oil and *Pumpkin Seeds* for the benefits of raw pumpkin oil (especially for prostate problems) in this section. Extra virgin olive oil is the most beneficial oil to use for cooking.

Important: Keep all natural oils refrigerated after opening! Discard after date on label or after three to six months stored in the refrigerator. Shelf storage length is usually printed on the bottle. Do not let perspiration, saliva, or bacteria get into the oil bottle and do not let it sit out of the fridge too long, especially on a hot day. Once oil is poured out of its bottle, never pour it back into the bottle, as it may easily collect bacteria or dust once poured. Oil poisoning is very painful and dangerous!

Oatmeal

Oats have been cultivated for thousands of years, for livestock. Outside of some European countries, it has only gained popularity as a human food in the last two centuries. Oatmeal has been eaten as porridge for most of these years as a favorite oat recipe. It was more beneficial then, than today, as it is now preserved, processed and depleted in nutrients in most forms available on your store shelves. Better forms of hot oat cereals are Scotch or steel-cut oats. These contain all the beneficial oat bran layers usually removed from most oatmeal and are quick cooking, more digestible (properly cooked), more nutritious and have more healing properties. The term "feeling your oats" came from jests made regarding the use of (young, green) oats as an aphrodisiac. Even today, health stores carry an array of libido enhancers made from oats. Oats are slowly increasing in popularity for recipes like breads, cakes, muffins, date squares, apple crisp and other desserts. In folklore, oats are used in bathwater and soaps as an astringent to draw out toxins. It is relaxing and soothing for the skin to soak in a bathtub with a cup or two of oatmeal swished in it. (It is more beneficial if the oatmeal is blended, with a blender, in water before adding to the bath.) This bath is also helpful for eczema, multiple bee stings or insect bites, sore muscles, and cleansing as well. Oats have one and a half times more protein than some types of wheat and two times more protein than brown rice. Oats are high in phosphorus, potassium, manganese and iron, also good amounts of vitamin E, folacin, copper and zinc. Store in a cool, dry cupboard. Oats that are not whole can also be stored in the refrigerator or freezer.

Onions

One of the earliest foods, since pre-historic times, is onions. Ancient Egyptians, Romans and Greeks enjoyed them regularly. Egyptians worshipped onions as they thought of them as symbols of eternity, with their layers of spheres within spheres. They paid huge amounts of gold to buy them, as they were believed to prevent evil. They were fed to the builders of the pyramids along with garlic for strength and endurance. Onions are antibacterial, antibiotic, anti-viral and anti-inflammatory. "Kitchen lilies," another name for onions, contain dozens of different anti-carcinogens. They were used in folklore to apply to burns, bee stings, wounds, as a cure for baldness and to kill infections. They are also good antioxidants and beneficial for lowering blood pressure and cholesterol, heart problems, bronchitis, asthma, thinning the blood, preventing blood clots and for cancer. "Onions contain a substance called quercetin (a bioflavonoid) that quells allergic reactions [and is helpful for hay fever]," say Gayla and John Kirschmann in the *Nutrition Almanac*. "Onions defend cells against damage by oxidizing agents and heavy metals," according to Linda Rector Page, N.D., in *Healthy Healing*.

Onions are low in calories and contain high potassium, some folic acid, calcium, magnesium, phosphorus, and trace minerals. Taken improperly (raw for some people or on an empty stomach), they may cause stomach upset or gas. Some religions consider them a taboo food (as well as garlic) as they are an aphrodisiac and may "stimulate the lower passions," or block a person's spiritual connection to God. Store like garlic and ginger in a cool, dry cupboard in the open air.

Pumpkin Seeds

Pumpkin seeds have been enjoyed in Mexico for centuries, but only recently have Canadians and Americans discovered the pleasures and nutrients of these pungent treats. Unhulled (white) pumpkin seeds are extremely hard to digest. Only those with very strong stomachs should roast and eat the seeds from a fresh pumpkin. The hulls are easy to crack with the teeth and discard. The hulled (greenish) pumpkin seeds, or pepitas as they are also called, are much more palatable and digestible. Pumpkin seeds are higher in protein than all other nuts and seeds (except peanuts which are not really a nut or a seed) as well as very high in zinc, which make them a great aphrodisiac and good for expelling parasites. They are also very high in essential fatty acids, magnesium, phosphorus, potassium and iron with a variety of other trace vitamins and minerals. Raw pumpkin seeds and oil are also excellent for preventing and healing prostate problems. Store seeds in an airtight container in a cool, dry cupboard. The oil must be refrigerated.

Sea Salt

Salt, or sodium chloride, has been used to flavor foods for thousands of years. Sea salt is derived from vacuum-dried seawater, without artificial or industrial processing. Real sea salt is dried in the wind and the sun. It contains all the natural minerals found in salt that are usually refined out of "earth salt," or regular table salt. Table salt is harder to digest and usually contains sugar, in the form of dextrose (corn sugar), and additives to help preserve it, keep its color, and retard moisture. Sea salt has none of these unnecessary extras and is more easily digested. Also, it does not cause the body to retain as much water as earth salt. Most sea salt should be iodized or used with sea kelp and other seaweeds to provide iodine. Excess salt in the diet can upset potassium and calcium levels and contribute to heart problems and other health concerns. People who eat lots of vegetables, whole grains and legumes in their diet require, and can more properly utilize, larger amounts of salt in their diets. Athletes may also need more salt. Sea salt has a natural antiseptic quality and can be used with warm water to swish in the mouth as a mouthwash and kill bacteria that may lead to dental problems. Always store in a cool, dry place, out of sunlight.

Celtic sea salt (which is light gray) is the best of all sea salts, and contains 84 sea minerals while refined table salt contains only two of these. "The daily use of natural gray Celtic sea salt protects the user by neutralizing fallout radiation exposure because it supplies organic iodine to the entire glandular network," says Jacques de Langre, Ph.D., in his book *Sea Salt's Hidden Powers*. He claims it assists normal sexual functioning and benefits the kidneys, among other attributes. Use Celtic sea salt above all other sea salts as many so-called sea salts have not been in the sea for billions of years and are not truly "sea salts."

Tamari Soy Sauce

Real tamari soy sauce is a great deal different than the quickly processed soy sauces found in many supermarket and many Asian markets and restaurants these days. Commercial versions are made from caramel coloring and flavoring, preservatives and sometimes MSG and other harmful additives. Real tamari soy sauce is naturally fermented six months to two years, usually in wood, and made with natural ingredients that complement good health. All tamaris are soy sauces, but not all soy sauces are real tamaris. Always use real tamari soy sauce and accept no inferior soy sauces on healing diets especially. The best brands include San-j®, Eden® and Amano®. Tamari soy sauce can be used in a variety of main dishes and vegetable dishes. It is best if kept refrigerated after opening. See *Miso* for more information.

Tofu

Asians have thrived on tofu for centuries. Many North Americans cringe at the mention of tofu as a food. The beauty of tofu is that it absorbs and complements flavors used with it in cooking. It actually enhances other flavors when used correctly. Tofu is a processed soy product that looks like white feta cheese but tastes bland alone. It is a good meat or dairy substitute that is high in protein, calcium, phosphorus, potassium and iron. Tofu is more digestible than some types of legumes. It is better if cooked (or steamed 5 minutes for most "raw" recipes) rather than eaten raw for healing diets to avoid bacteria that can easily grow on most processed foods. Store completely covered in pure water in a jar. Keeps for up to two to three weeks refrigerated, if water is changed every few days or so. Plain tofu is fresh as long as it retains its milky white color and has no scent or taste. If the tofu smells a bit, rinse it thoroughly. If no smell remains, it can be used if cooked well. Soft (silken), medium, firm/regular, extra firm, or pressed tofu varieties are available. Avoid the dessert varieties that contain sugar.

Tomatoes and Tomato Juice

Tomatoes originated in South America and were first brought to North America and Europe in the 15ᵗʰ century. They were not popularized in North America until about 150 years ago. The tomato has been known as the "apple of the Moors," the "apple of gold" and, in Europe, where it had a reputation as an aphrodisiac and a poison, the "love apple." In truth, the tomato is a member of the "deadly nightshade" food family today and is slightly poisonous. While not harmful to healthy individuals, it may be detrimental to the very sensitive, those with allergies and severe illness. In recent years, it was thought to hinder healing and be bad for cancer, now due to the recognition of lycopene, a phytochemical—the red substance in tomatoes and other red fruits and vegetables, they are touted as great for cancer prevention. Their antioxidant agents fight free radicals.

Tomatoes are mainly red, but also available in the so-called "acidless" yellow varieties. Tomatoes are an acid fruit, actually a type of berry, though they are more often treated as a vegetable. They should not be eaten with fruit but are excellent for assisting vegetable digestion. Fresh summer field tomatoes are far more nutritious than pasty, winter hothouse varieties. Ripen most winter tomatoes by storing in an open plastic bag on a countertop until ripened, then refrigerate. All lettuces, which happen to be difficult to digest, are better digested when tomatoes (or citrus) are added to a salad. Meat and protein meals are also better digested with the addition of tomatoes or tomato juice with a meal. Tomatoes are high in vitamin A, beta-carotene, vitamin C, calcium, magnesium, potassium and phosphorus. Keep refrigerated for up to two weeks or more.

Vinegar, Apple Cider

Authors, such as D. C. Jarvis, M. Hanssen, and C. Scott, have written a great deal about the therapeutic effects of ingesting apple cider vinegar. Apple cider vinegar is made by fermenting the juice of whole, fresh apples. It is high in calcium, potassium, sodium, phosphorus, and other trace minerals. It has an average acetic acid content of 5 percent and has been used as a food and a medicine. Published research indicates that apple cider vinegar inhibits diarrhea due to its astringent property; it helps oxygenate the blood, increases metabolic rate, improves digestion, fights tooth decay and intestinal parasites, and improves blood-clotting ability. It also seems to help bad breath. Many people over age 40 suffer from a lack of stomach acid. Supplementation of one or two tablespoons of apple cider vinegar with each meal aids in protein digestion and prevents many vitamin and mineral deficiencies. Apple cider vinegar can be used as a mouthwash and throat gargle for antiseptic purposes. It has no significant side effects, is safe for people with diabetes, and, despite its sodium content, is suitable for those on low-sodium diets.

A long list of conditions can benefit from apple cider vinegar supplementation, including obesity and weight loss problems, infections, allergies, arthritis, fatigue, circulatory disorders, and thinning hair. It is true that apple cider vinegar can increase the body's acidity, but in many individuals this produces a beneficial effect, especially for those with Candida yeast problems who often have too low stomach acid. In others, the excess acidity makes their symptoms worse. Some people are allergic to it, and in some cases apple cider vinegar has no effect whatsoever. It's a matter of biochemical individuality. Its low toxicity and potentially spectacular health effects make it worth trying. Store natural vinegars in a cool cupboard or in the refrigerator if desired.

Yogurt, Plain

Less than 50 years ago, North Americans considered yogurt a food fit only for health fanatics. Asians and Europeans have enjoyed yogurt for centuries. Yogurt has long been associated with good health and longevity. Cultured milk or yogurt is made of curdled milk with a bacteria culture added and is one of the most digestible dairy products that can be eaten. Real, plain, natural yogurt contains live or active cultures and enzymes that are created by "friendly bacteria" which help counteract unfriendly bacteria and Candida yeast growth in the body. There are different types of bacterial cultures that can be used to make yogurt and kefir—which is a more liquid type of friendly culture.

Unfortunately, not all yogurts are natural or contain active or live cultures or enzymes. "In some types of yogurt, the bacteria survive the processing; in other cases, the milk is pasteurized again after the cultures are added, and the bacteria are destroyed" says *The Wellness Encyclopedia of Food and Nutrition*, by Sheldon Margen, M.D., and associates.

Choose a type of yogurt that can be used to make yogurt from itself. These are the only true yogurts. Once fruit is commercially mixed with yogurt, the live enzymes are no more. In picking real yogurts, note if the fruited variety has yogurt mixed with fruit or fruit on the bottom. If fruit is on the bottom, usually the yogurt will be "real" and contain live enzymes or "active/living yogurt cultures." Avoid all yogurt brands that contain sugar (or other sweeteners) as these nullify the healing properties of the yogurt. Many people who are allergic to other dairy products can tolerate real, plain yogurt (and kefir), even some who are lactose intolerant. Plain, low-fat yogurt is the most beneficial and nutritious. It contains high amounts of calcium, magnesium, phosphorus, potassium and folic acid, as well as trace B vitamins and zinc. Yogurt is also good for the immune system, bacterial infections, anti-aging, cancer, diarrhea, constipation, yeast infections, bad breath, liver diseases, cancer and skin problems. It is superior to milk in many nutrients, more digestible and more beneficial for combating health problems.

Eaten with certain other foods, yogurt helps to break them down and make them more digestible. Yogurt is especially beneficial when eaten with protein foods (meats or other dairy products) or with cooked, dried peas and beans. It also helps digestion of vegetables, especially lettuce and salads which are hard to digest. Yogurt may be eaten occasionally with fruits.

REMEDY RECIPES FOR HEALTH

Beneficial Beverages
FRESH VEGETABLE JUICES   Most non-starchy vegetables (starchy include: yams, winter squash, turnips, parsnips) may be juiced and drunk, provided no more than 8 to 12 ounces total are enjoyed

daily, five to six days per week maximum, unless your doctor suggests otherwise. (Or drink two glasses every other day, eight hours apart.) The body was not meant to "drink" dozens of vegetables in one day. Humans cannot digest and properly assimilate too many juices, too often. Each sip of vegetable juice should be savored. Swish the juices in the mouth so they can absorb more digestive enzymes in the saliva and drink them slowly. It should take at least 20 minutes to drink one glass of vegetable juice. Put it in a wine glass if that helps to slow your drinking down; it adds a bit of fun and elegance as well. Some raw vegetable juices like Brussels sprouts, cabbage, and green peppers contribute to gas for certain people, so should be avoided. Drink gassy vegetables sparingly or in combination with complementary vegetables that counteract flatulence (such as tomato or beet).

Fresh-squeezed vegetable juices are the most beneficial. However, some bottled or canned juices can be enjoyed, though they are not nearly as nutritious. Fresh-squeezed juices that are not drunk immediately should be refrigerated immediately, and preferably enjoyed up to four to eight hours later. Use organic vegetables (from natural food stores) as a first choice for juicing, if available. Enjoy the vegetable juice combinations that follow below and see the juicer books in the "Recommended Reading" section for more ideas. (*Note:* Do not swish citrus juices in the mouth as they strip tooth enamel!)

CARROT AND BEET JUICE

  4 to 5 medium organic carrots, scrubbed, with tips cut off
  1 small or medium beet, scrubbed, with tips cut off

Use chilled carrots from the refrigerator. Wash and cut the vegetables into sections that will fit into your juicer. Cold vegetables retain more vitamins while being juiced and they taste better juiced as well. If you are constipated, increase the beet to 2 small or 1 large. If your bowels are too loose, substitute the beet for celery or another green vegetable. (Maximum 5 to 6 glasses per week total for vegetable juices of any kind or combination, unless your doctor recommends otherwise for special health problems.)

VEGETABLE JUICE COMBINATIONS

1. ½ part carrot, ¼ part beet, ¼ part celery
2. ½ part carrot, ¼ part celery, ¼ part zucchini
3. ½ part carrot, ¼ part celery or zucchini, ¼ part red bell pepper
   Optional: 1 small garlic clove.
4. ¾ part green or Savoy cabbage juice, ¼ part beet, optional: 1 wedge onion.
5. ⅓ part carrot, ⅓ part broccoli or Brussels sprouts, ⅓ part beet. (This combo can be gassy for some, but the beet helps make it more digestible.)
6. ½ part carrot, ¼ part beet, ¼ part apple.

Create your own combinations with no more than three or four vegetables. Do not mix fruits with vegetables, except occasionally with apples.

Try adding 1 to 2 tablespoons wheat grass juice or barley green juice (or ¼–½ teaspoon of wheat grass powder, barley green powder, spirulina powder or other green food product) to any of the previous above combinations if these are available and approved by your health specialist. It requires a special kind of juicer to make wheat grass or barley green juice.

SALAD-IN-A-GLASS

3–5 carrots
½–1 small beet
1 stalk celery
½ bell pepper (red, yellow, orange or purple—green is gassy)
¼ cucumber or zucchini
Optional: ½–1 small Jerusalem artichoke
Optional: ¼ teaspoon powdered green food product

Juice all the vegetables together and enjoy. Use chilled vegetables if possible so the juice is not too warm and more nutrients are preserved.

VEGETABLE JUICE AND YOGURT SMOOTHIE
(juicer and blender required)
½–¾ cup (4–6 ounces) plain yogurt, cold

½–¾ cup (4–6 ounces) organic carrot juice or vegetable juice
  combination
Optional: 1–2 tablespoons wheat grass juice or barley green
  juice (or ¼ teaspoon green food powder)

Whiz the ingredients together lightly in a blender, drink slowly and
enjoy. Do not store. (Blender will take the chill off the yogurt and
keep the drink from being warm.)

GREEN POWER DRINK
(juicer and blender required)
  ½ cup water, carrot or carrot/beet juice
  ½ cup green cabbage, broccoli, alfalfa sprout or Brussels
    sprouts juice
  1 stalk celery, juiced
  2–4 sprigs parsley, stems removed
  4–6 spinach leaves, stems removed
  ¼ teaspoon green powder (barley green, wheat grass, green
    kamut, alfalfa, chlorella or spirulina)

Use all organic vegetables if possible. Juice the carrots/beets if any,
the celery and other green vegetables. Use a blender (unless you
have a special wheat grass juicer) to blend the water or carrot (beet)
juice with the parsley, spinach and green powder. Add the juicer
juices to the blended mixture in the blender and whiz for 30
seconds to mix. Drink slowly, savor and enjoy. Use one ice cube
instead of some of the water (or juice) for a slightly cooler drink
if desired.

EASY GREEN POWER DRINK

  1 cup water or plain yogurt
  2–4 sprigs parsley, stems removed
  6–8 leaves spinach, without stems, or ¼ cup or bit less alfalfa
    sprouts—brown seed hulls cut off first
  ½–1 teaspoon green food powder (barley green, wheat grass,
    green kamut, alfalfa, chlorella or spirulina)
  Optional: 1 small clove garlic (for the daring!)

Optional: ¼–½ peeled apple, finely chopped

Use a blender to blend all ingredients thoroughly. Drink slowly, savor and enjoy. Use one ice cube instead of some of the water for a slightly cooler drink if desired. Some hardy individuals like to increase the green food powder to 1 tablespoon. This is not recommended for everyone, only those who build up to this amount!

COLD CLASSIC

> 1 cup freshly squeezed orange juice or grapefruit juice
> 2–3 tablespoons fresh lemon or lime juice
> **Optional:** a dash of cayenne pepper (to break up mucus, soothe inflammation)
> **Optional:** 1 teaspoon honey (for soothing throat)

Mix everything together with a spoon. Drink this sore throat and cold, vitamin C booster slowly. Savor and enjoy. Add ginger (like the following recipe) if desired, or ½–1 teaspoon of fresh, pressed garlic juice if you dare! Melt the honey in a little water (3–4 teaspoons) over low heat before adding so it mixes with the juice.

WARM COLD CLASSIC

> 1 cup rose hips herbal tea (add chamomile at nighttime)
> 2–3 teaspoons fresh lemon or lime juice
> ¼–½ teaspoon freshly squeezed ginger juice or several thin slices peeled ginger
> **Optional:** a dash of cayenne pepper (to break up mucus, soothe inflammation)
> **Optional:** 1 teaspoon honey (for soothing throat)

Use bulk or loose tea rather than teabags if you want to receive the full benefits of this cold, flu and sore throat beverage. Steep the tea and add the other ingredients. Drink very warm, sip slowly and enjoy. (See "How To Make Herb Teas")

VITAMIN C MAGIC

> 1 small or ½ large papaya, peeled and seeded
> ½–⅔ cup orange or grapefruit juice
> 2–3 teaspoons lemon or lime juice
> **Optional:** ½ cup (4–6) strawberries

One papaya has nearly three times as much vitamin C as an orange! One orange has nearly one-and-a-half times the vitamin C as ½ grapefruit, however, a serving of grapefruit is given as an option for those allergic to oranges or unable to have them for other health problems like Candida. Strawberries are another very potent vitamin C source. Blend this delightful combination and drink slowly and enjoy. (In case you are wondering, 1 cup cut cantaloupe is equal to one orange in vitamin C content.)

BETA-CAROTENE BOOST
(serves 2)

> 1 small or ½ medium mango, peeled and cut into pieces, or 1
>   small or ½ medium papaya, peeled and seeded
> 1 cup cut cantaloupe
> 3–4 apricots, pitted and chopped
> ½–1 cup apricot or peach juice

One small apricot has five times the beta-carotene as one peach. One mango has more than 15 times, a papaya more than 12 times, and one cup cut cantaloupe has more than 10 times the beta-carotene as one peach, and a peach is high in beta-carotene among many other fruits. Blend and share this drink with a friend. For beta-carotene in a vegetable drink, choose or create a drink with mainly carrot juice.

DIGEST AID DRINK 1
(for protein meals)

> 1 cup fresh grapefruit juice or tomato juice
> 2–3 teaspoons fresh lemon or lime juice
> **Optional:** ¼ teaspoon fresh squeezed ginger juice or 3–4 slices
>   thinly sliced, peeled ginger

Drink this a little before or during a protein or meat meal with vegetables (preferably without starches). If using ginger slices, stir them into the beverage well and discard after drinking. They can be chewed on and spit out or swallowed if desired. See *Food Combining*. Tomato (a fruit!), grapefruit, lemon and lime juices help with the digestion of protein foods. (It is best not to use tomato and grapefruit juices together.)

DIGEST AID DRINK 2
(for any meal)
> 4–5 large carrots
> 1 large or 2 small beets
> 1 stalk celery
> **Optional (but helpful):** 1–2 teaspoons fresh lemon or lime juice
> **Optional:** 1 clove garlic (for the daring!)

Juice all ingredients, except the citrus juice. Stir the juice in last. Drink a little before or during a meal. This helps digestion of any meal.

DIGEST AID DRINK 3
(for any meal)
> ½ cup (4 ounces) plain yogurt
> 1–2 teaspoons lemon or lime juice OR apple cider vinegar
>   OR ½ teaspoon fresh ginger juice
> ¼–½ teaspoon dark miso
> **Optional:** 1 teaspoon ground flaxseed

Whiz all ingredients lightly in the blender and take with a meal. This helps digestion of any meal. A dash of cayenne is optional.

DIGEST AID DRINK 4
(good for any meal, especially protein meals)
> 1 cup club soda
> 2–3 teaspoons fresh lemon or lime juice
> **Optional:** ¼ teaspoon fresh squeezed ginger juice or 3–4 slices
>   thinly sliced, peeled ginger

Drink this a little before or during a meal. If using ginger slices, stir them into the beverage well and discard after drinking. They can be chewed on and spit out or swallowed if desired. Lemon and lime juice help with the digestion of protein foods, fatty foods and heavy foods.

HAY FEVER HELPER

¾ cup soymilk or apple juice (or peach or pear juice)
1 small banana OR ½ medium papaya or mango OR 4 apricots OR 2 medium-sized sweet peaches
2–3 teaspoons quality local bee pollen
2 teaspoons quality local raw honey
Optional: 5–7 medium strawberries or other berries

Use the soymilk if you want added protein; low-fat soymilk is fine but DO NOT use real milk in this recipe. The bee pollen and the honey are what help you to build up resistance to the flower pollen, and it is important to only use very fresh, *local* pollen and honey for this remedy to work. This recipe must be drunk, every day, beginning three months before hay fever season begins in order for it to be successful. This is a kind of homeopathic way to end hay fever problems that is effective for most people if done as directed. Use half the recipe for children and very sensitive people. Do *not* use this recipe for children under three years old and not for those under eight years old without your doctor's approval.

This drink can be had as a breakfast or between-meal snack, but not taken with a meal or after supper at night. (Don't worry if you forget and end up skipping 2–3 days a month, it will still work.) Take 500–1,000 mg vitamin C with this drink if possible to assist absorption and diminish any possible small reaction, especially if you are very sensitive. The strawberries provide extra vitamin C and flavor, and should be included if possible.

BLOOD SUGAR BALANCER

5–7 large carrots
1 small or medium beet
1 small Jerusalem artichoke (2–4 1-inch chunks)*

1 clove garlic
Optional: ¼–½ teaspoon green food powder

Use a juicer to juice all ingredients except the green food powder.
Stir in the green food powder, if any.

*If Jerusalem artichokes are out of season, one stalk of celery can be used
instead, however, the drink will not be nearly as beneficial for the blood
sugar. Garlic may also be eliminated if desired, however, it is extremely
good for blood sugar balancing. Be sure to use artichoke or garlic and/or
green food powder to be effective. Drink slowly, savor and enjoy.

HANGOVER HELPER 1

1 cup tomato juice
2 sprigs parsley, without stems
1 teaspoon vitamin C powder/crystals (or take about 2,000
    mg in capsules with drink)
¼–½ teaspoon green food powder
¼–½ teaspoon dark miso and/or ⅛–¼ teaspoon ginseng extract
Optional: ½ cup yogurt
Optional but helpful: dash of cayenne pepper

Use a blender to mix all ingredients thoroughly. Drink slowly, savor
and enjoy. For the morning after!

HANGOVER HELPER 2

5–7 large carrots
1 small or medium beet
1 stalk celery
¼–½ teaspoon green food powder
¼–½ teaspoon dark miso and/or ⅛–¼ teaspoon ginseng extract
Optional: 1 clove garlic and/or 1 small Jerusalem artichoke
    (2–4 1-inch chunks), to help blood sugar
Optional but helpful: dash of cayenne pepper

Juice all the vegetables and stir in, beat in or blend in the green powder, miso and/or ginseng. Drink slowly, savor and enjoy. For the morning after! Take with about 2,000 mg vitamin C in capsules, if possible.

MOTION SICKNESS MIRACLE (FOR NAUSEA)

    1 cup club soda, chilled or room temperature
    ½–1 teaspoon ginger juice, freshly squeezed
    2–4 thin slices peeled ginger

Mix and drink slowly. This is better than ginger ale, as the sweeteners in ginger ale are not helpful. Break open a vitamin C capsule and add it to 1–2 ounces of the soda, especially if swallowing pills is not tolerated during nausea. Do not use ice, and avoid water.

If possible before stomach gets upset, OR after it calms down, eat a warm-cooked, well-cooked starchy food, like yams, winter squash, real mashed potatoes (not French fries!), tender rice or millet. Make sure to chew extremely well and eat slowly. Eat one-half to one cup, or more as desired, and avoid other foods except plain yogurt until stomach is completely settled. Sometimes whole grain crackers or bread will do if cooked food is unavailable.

PROTEIN POWER DRINK 1

    4 ounces (110 grams) soft or silken tofu
    ½ cup (4 ounces, 110 ml) soymilk, unsweetened is best
    1 of the following: banana, ripe peach or pear, small mango,
        3–4 apricots, ¾ cup pineapple or ⅔ cup unsweetened fruit
        juice (naturally sweet variety)
    1 tablespoon protein powder (from health store)
    1–2 teaspoons edible (good-tasting) nutritional yeast or bee
        pollen granules
    Optional: 1–2 teaspoons liquid lecithin (or granular if liquid
        unavailable)
    Optional: 2–3 teaspoons or more honey, maple syrup or other
        natural sweetener

Blend all ingredients in a blender until smooth, and enjoy. Add an ice cube or two for a colder, lighter drink. Drink slowly and savor to help assimilate all the nutrients.

PROTEIN POWER SHAKE

1 cup milk or soymilk
1 of the following: banana, ripe peach or pear, small mango, 3–4 apricots, ¾ cup pineapple or ⅔ cup unsweetened fruit juice (naturally sweet variety)
1 scoop natural vanilla ice cream or vanilla soy ice cream
3–4 teaspoons roasted carob powder
1 tablespoon protein powder (from health store)
Optional: 1 teaspoon dandelion coffee (for herbal benefits and added chocolatey flavor) or other coffee substitute
Optional: 1–2 teaspoons liquid lecithin (or granular if liquid unavailable) for energy

Blend all ingredients in a blender until smooth and enjoy.

POWER PROTEIN DRINK 2

5–7 large carrots
1 small or medium beet
¼ cup or 1 handful parsley, stems removed
2–3 teaspoons bee pollen granules
Optional: ¼–½ teaspoon green food product
Optional: 1–2 teaspoons liquid lecithin (or granular if liquid unavailable)
Optional: 1 small clove garlic (for the daring!)

A juicer and blender are required for this recipe. Juice the carrots and beet, then whiz in the blender with the remaining ingredients until the parsley is fully blended. Use organic vegetables whenever possible. Honey or other natural sweetening can be added if desired.

POWER PROTEIN DRINK 3

  5–7 large carrots
  1 small or medium beet
  1 stalk celery
  1–2 teaspoons edible (good tasting) nutritional yeast or
    protein powder (from health store)
  ¼–½ teaspoon green food product
  Optional: 1–2 teaspoons liquid lecithin (or granular if liquid
    unavailable) for energy

A juicer and blender are required for this recipe. Juice the carrots,
beet and celery, then whiz in the blender with the remaining ingredients until fully blended. Use organic vegetables whenever possible. Honey or other natural sweetening can be added if desired.

RASPBERRY PASSION FOR TWO
(aphrodisiac)
  2 cups fresh or frozen raspberries*
  1½ cups sparkling white grape juice (or 1⅓ cup club soda and
    2 tablespoons honey)
  2 vials royal jelly or 2 teaspoons royal jelly extract (if
    unavailable, take with 500 mg royal jelly capsules
    for each)**
  2–3 ice cubes

Use a blender to blend until ice is crushed. Savor and enjoy.

*Strawberries or blueberries can be used instead.
**If royal jelly is unavailable take 1,000–2,000 mg vitamin C each.

PURPLE PASSION FOR TWO
(aphrodisiac)
  2 cups fresh or frozen blackberries or dark sweet cherries
  1 cup sparkling water or club soda
  ½–¾ cup purple (Concord) grape juice
  ½ teaspoon ginseng extract or 2 vials royal jelly or 2 teaspoons

royal jelly extract (if unavailable take with 500 mg royal
jelly capsules for each)*

Optional: 2 teaspoons honey or maple syrup (or other natural
sweetener)

Use a blender to blend until ice is crushed. Savor and enjoy.

*If royal jelly is unavailable take 1,000–2,000 mg vitamin C each.

NECTAR OF THE GODS FOR TWO
(aphrodisiac)

2 cups unsweetened pineapple juice (½–1 cup of this can be
crushed pineapple)

2 cups sparkling water or club soda

1 cup fresh or frozen strawberries

½ cup fresh squeezed lemon juice

2–3 tablespoons honey or maple syrup (or other natural
sweetener)

2 vials royal jelly or 2 teaspoons royal jelly extract (if
unavailable take with 500 mg royal jelly capsules for each)*

Use a blender to blend until ice is crushed. Savor and enjoy.

*If royal jelly is unavailable take 1,000–2,000 mg vitamin C each.

VITAL ENERGY FOR TWO
(aphrodisiac)

Double any of the power drink recipes and enjoy! Use soymilk or
oat milk instead of cows' milk for a more dynamic, sensuous energy
boost. Add royal jelly (or ginseng if over 40) or take with vitamin
C if desired. Aphrodisiac drinks are more potent when enjoyed at
least 30 minutes before making love, however they can be enjoyed
during the day for extra energy leading up to a night of passion!

Vivacious Vegetables

PULP POWER Wondering what to do with leftover vegetable pulp
from your juicer? If it is mainly carrot, with no beet, it can be used

in carrot cakes. With or without beet, use it in the Veggie Bean Burgers given in this vegetable section or add it to soups, stews and casseroles and create your own recipes or enhance other recipes.

CITRUS BEET TREAT
(serves 1 to 2)
    1 medium or large fresh beet, finely grated
    3–4 teaspoons fresh lemon or lime juice

Choose fresh, bright red beets, preferably ones purchased with beet green tops rather that old, slightly moldy storage beets.

    Mix the beet and citrus juice together and enjoy. The citrus makes the beet taste very sweet. This is a nutritious and healthful treat for the taste buds, digestion and the liver. Serve as a snack, side dish, or instead of a salad. Do not store. (Do not use old storage beets!)

GLOBE ARTICHOKES

    1 artichoke per person
    butter and/or fresh lemon juice

Choose firm, uniformly green, unwrinkled artichokes (no purple or "fuzz") with preferably pointy rather than rounded leaves. With each artichoke, wash and cut off the entire stem or stalk. Pull off and discard the first row or two of leaves around the stalk. With a sharp, serrated knife, trim ¾ to 1 inch off the tip of the artichoke and discard. Snip ¼ to ½ inch off the tip of each remaining leaf, with a scissors or knife. Place the vegetables upside down (top down, stalk up) in a vegetable steamer over medium boiling water and steam for 45 to 55 minutes or until very tender. When a knife slides in and out easily, it is done.

    Starting with the bottom row of leaves nearest the stalk end, pull off one leaf at a time and dip in melted butter and/or fresh lemon juice the part that was attached to the artichoke. With the inner part of the leaf facing upwards, pull the base of the leaf between your teeth, pulling off all tender, easy-to-chew parts. (These are the edible parts.) Discard the rest of each leaf. As you get closer to the center, you can eat more of each leaf, as they get progressively more tender. When you reach the "choke," scrape off the stringy, prickly part and discard. What's left is entirely edible! Dip it in the sauce and enjoy the best part—the heart, a delectable treat. Savor the delicious, stimulating aftertaste of the artichoke in your mouth. Artichokes are very healing for the liver and a sensuous aphrodisiac.

ROASTED GARLIC
(serves 1–4 people with each bulb)

    4–12 bulbs of regular garlic, preferably organic
    Extra virgin olive oil
    Parsley flakes, dried
    Rosemary, crushed
    Oregano
    Basil
    Dill weed
    Optional: sea salt

Peel the extra layers of garlic skin off each bulb, leaving each bulb in one piece. (Leave the skins on each individual clove within each bulb.) Slice the top tips, about ¼ inch or less, off each of the garlic cloves in each bulb and place the bulbs in a 2-inch deep baking dish, cut side up. Pour olive oil generously over each bulb, using at least 2 tablespoons on each bulb. Sprinkle each bulb generously with dried parsley flakes. Crush ⅛ teaspoon rosemary over each bulb. Then sprinkle about ⅛ teaspoon each of oregano and basil over each one. Add a pinch of dill weed on each, and sea salt if desired. Cover the baking dish tightly with aluminum foil, and bake in a preheated oven at about 300–350°F for about one hour, or until the garlic is completely tender and the aroma of the herbs fills the air.

    Use this soft, mellow-tasting garlic as a spread instead of butter on breads, on vegetables, and in all kinds of recipes for special flavor. Make a large batch and keep leftovers refrigerated. Reheat with other recipes or by baking alone in foil. This recipe is a delicious, nutritious, healing addition to foods that gently discourages fungus.

MASHED ORANGE YAMS OR SQUASH
(serves 2)

    2 medium orange yams, or ½ butternut or buttercup squash

Several dashes sea salt or cinnamon
Optional: ⅛ to ¼ cup milk or milk substitute
Optional: 1–3 teaspoons butter or 1–2 teaspoons natural oil
Bake the squash the quick and easy method (recipe follows), boil it whole for 45-60 minutes or steam the peeled squash or yams sprinkled with the cinnamon (if any) until very tender. Mash the very tender vegetables with a small-holed hand masher or use a food mill or food processor. Add milk or substitute and/or butter or oil to the mashed vegetables for a lighter consistency if desired. Keeps refrigerated for up to 4 to 5 days and can be baked to reheat. Do not freeze. (Good for grounding, balancing female hormones, settling upset stomach and high in beta-carotene.)

QUICK AND EASY BAKED WINTER SQUASH
(serves 2 to 4)

1 medium or large acorn, turban, spaghetti, butternut,
    buttercup, or other medium winter squash, or 2 large
    pieces cut Hubbard or other large winter squash
Optional: sea salt
Optional: butter or natural oil

Preheat the oven to 400°F. Cut the squash in half lengthwise or from top to bottom, and scoop out the seeds and pulp.

Place the pieces cut-side down on a lightly oiled, flat metal sheet and bake for 25 to 40 minutes, until tender and a knife passes through easily. The skin should be only slightly browned or wrinkled. This is one of the fastest ways to prepare large pieces of winter squash. Serve with sea salt and butter or natural oil as desired. Refrigerate for up to 4 to 5 days and steam to reheat. Do not freeze. (Good for grounding, balancing female hormones, settling upset stomach and high in beta-carotene.)

CINNAMON BAKED SQUASH
(serves 2 to 4)

1 medium butternut or buttercup squash
Water
Cinnamon

Preheat the oven to 400°F. Use a sharp knife to cut the squash in half from top to bottom. Scoop out the seeds and pulp and discard. Fill the hollowed-out section of each half with water and sprinkle the entire cut section generously with cinnamon. Place the squash halves in a low (about 2-inch deep) baking dish with ¾ to 1 inch water around the bottom of each squash in the pan. Bake for 50 to 65 minutes, or until a knife moves in and out of the squash easily and it is very tender. Cut and serve hot. Keeps refrigerated for 3 to 4 days and may be reheated by baking, steaming, or placing the scooped-out squash in a little water in a covered saucepan and simmering. (Good for grounding, balancing female hormones, settling upset stomach and high in beta-carotene.)

HONEY BAKED SQUASH
Follow the directions for Cinnamon Baked Squash preceding but, instead of water, fill the hollowed-out opening in the squash with honey and butter. When the squash is fully cooked, baste the squash with the honey oil mixture. Optional sea salt can be sprinkled on the squash with or instead of cinnamon.

VEGGIE BEAN BURGERS

1 cup cooked, mashed beans (pinto, kidney, adzuki or black beans)
1 cup vegetable pulp from a juicer, or finely chopped steamed vegetables (carrots, celery, beets, peppers, and/or broccoli or others)
½ cup ground raw sunflower seeds, almonds or filberts
1 tablespoon raw flaxseeds or hulled pumpkin seeds, ground
½–¾ cup soy flour or amaranth flour
½ cup finely chopped onion
3 teaspoons dried parsley
2–3 teaspoons soy sauce or 1 bouillon cube, mashed
½ teaspoon each: basil and dill weed
¼–½ teaspoon sea salt
Several dashes cayenne red pepper
Optional: few dashes cumin powder

See the Power Protein Soup for how to cook beans if needed. Mix the mashed beans with the rest of the ingredients. Mix well, using extra flour if mixture is too wet. Shape the mixture into 6 medium burgers about ½ inch thick and 4 inches in diameter. The burgers can be broiled on a wire grill or oiled, flat surface for 8–10 minutes on the first side and 5–8 minutes on the other side, or the burgers can be baked at about 375°F for 25–30 minutes. Serve with ketchup and mustard, a homemade sauce or gravy with whole grains and other vegetables for a complete meal. Cooked burgers keep 3–5 days refrigerated, or may be frozen. These burgers are high in protein, with added flax and cumin for good digestion.

Super Soups

EASY MISO SOUP

1 teaspoon toasted (or regular) sesame oil
2–3 green onions, chopped small
4 cups water, broth or stock
¼ cup dark miso
1 tablespoon tamari soy sauce or substitute
⅛ teaspoon sea kelp
Cayenne red pepper to taste
2–3 ounces (50–80 grams) tofu, diced in ¼–½ inch cubes
2–3 strips kombu or wakame dried seaweed, rinsed and
    chopped small*

Sauté the green onion in the oil, then add all the remaining ingredients except for the tofu. Use a wire whisk to help mix in the miso while stirring over medium-low heat. When the miso is dissolved, add the tofu, cover and let everything simmer on low heat for 8 to 12 minutes until the flavors mingle and the seaweed is tender. Correct seasonings as desired. Do not allow the soup to boil at any time, especially if reheating. Serve hot.

* In a pinch, substitute 12 to 16 spinach leaves for the seaweed, however, the soup will lose some of its healing abilities and flavor. Keeps 3–6 days refrigerated. Do not freeze.

DIGEST-AID MEAL-IN-A-SOUP

(serves 1)

- ½ cup cooked beans: brown, red, or black beans (pinto, kidney, Romano, chickpeas, adzuki, red beans OR black [turtle] beans)
- ½ cup cooked whole grains (brown rice, wild rice, millet, buckwheat, kasha, quinoa, brown pot barley OR especially millet)
- ½ cup cooked green vegetables (asparagus, artichoke hearts packed in water/drained, broccoli, kohlrabi, zucchini, kale, chard, spinach OR other cookable green)
- ½ cup cooked orange, yellow or white vegetable (carrots, orange yam, winter squash, yellow summer squash, cauliflower, Jerusalem artichokes OR occasionally parsnips)
- 1½ cups liquid (stock, broth, water, soymilk or other milk substitute, tomato juice OR yogurt)

Seasonings #1

- 1–2 chopped green onions, or 2 cloves garlic, minced, or ¼ teaspoon prepared horseradish
- 2–3 teaspoons butter or natural oil, or 3–4 teaspoons tamari soy sauce
- Sea salt or salt substitute and cayenne to taste

Seasonings #2

- 2–3 teaspoons finely chopped onion and 1 small clove garlic, or ¼ teaspoon prepared horseradish
- 1 tablespoon finely chopped fresh parsley, or 1 teaspoon dried parsley
- ½ teaspoon each basil and dill weed
- ¼ teaspoon each thyme and marjoram
- 2–3 teaspoons butter or natural oil
- Sea salt or potassium chloride or another salt substitute to taste
- Few dashes each sea kelp and cayenne

Seasonings #3

- 2–3 teaspoons finely chopped onion and 1 small clove garlic, or ¼ teaspoon prepared horseradish
- 3–4 teaspoons tamari soy sauce or substitute

1 teaspoon vegetable broth powder, or ½–1 vegetable bouillon cube
Sea salt or potassium chloride or another salt substitute to taste
Few dashes each sea kelp and cayenne
Optional: 1–2 teaspoons sesame salt (gomashio)

Seasonings #4
¼ cup chives or green onion tops (green part only), chopped
1 teaspoon vegetable broth powder, or ½–1 vegetable bouillon
  cube
1 tablespoon finely chopped fresh parsley, or 1 teaspoon
  dried parsley
½–1 teaspoon basil or dill weed
¼ teaspoon each thyme and marjoram
2–3 teaspoons butter or natural oil
Sea salt or potassium chloride or another salt substitute to taste
Few dashes each sea kelp and cayenne

Use cooked beans (see Power Protein Soup for bean cooking tips), and whole grains with fresh vegetables steamed together. Use a blender to blend the beans, whole grains, vegetables, and liquid with one of the four seasoning recipes, or create your own seasoning mixture according to your taste and diet requirements. Bring the mixture up to a boil on medium heat, then simmer on a low bubble (low to medium simmer) for 20 to 25 minutes, or until the sharp edge is off the pungent vegetables, it is hot throughout, and the flavors mingle. Correct seasonings as desired.

This soup can be made quickly and simply and adjusted for those with digestive troubles or food allergies. This is a complete meal in itself. Keeps for 3 to 5 days refrigerated and may be frozen.

PERFECT PARSLEY SOUP
(serves 4 to 6)
4 cups chopped potatoes (rinsed) or cauliflower
1 large bunch spinach leaves
1 cup water, stock, broth or bouillon (unsalted)
1½ cups soymilk or other milk substitute
1 packed cup coarsely chopped fresh parsley
1–2 tablespoons natural oil or butter

2 vegetable bouillon cubes or 3 teaspoons vegetable broth
   powder
2–3 tablespoons tamari soy sauce or substitute
3 teaspoons finely chopped onion
1 clove garlic, minced
1 teaspoon each paprika and basil
Sea salt and cayenne to taste
1 cup very finely chopped parsley (chopped 2 to 3 times as
   fine as other cup parsley)

Steam the potatoes or cauliflower for 4 minutes over 1–2 cups of
water or stock. Add the washed spinach leaves on top of them and
continue cooking for another 6 to 8 minutes, until both are very
tender. Blend the steamed vegetables with all the other ingredients
except the 1 cup finely chopped parsley. Put the blended soup
mixture in a medium saucepan and stir in the finely chopped parsley. Bring the mixture just up to a boil and let it simmer on low heat
for 14 to 20 minutes as the flavors mingle. Correct the seasonings
as desired. Serve garnished with extra sprigs of parsley or chopped
green onion tops (green part only). This soup is high in chlorophyll and iron. Keeps fresh for 3 to 6 days refrigerated. Do not freeze.

HEALING GARLIC SPINACH SOUP
(serves 4)
   2 tablespoons butter or natural oil
   12 medium-large cloves garlic, peeled and sliced
   4 cups water, stock, bouillon or broth (unsalted)
   6 medium cloves garlic, pressed
   5–6 green onions, finely chopped
   2 large bunches fresh spinach leaves, chopped
   ¼ cup tomato juice or fresh lemon juice
   ¼ cup fresh finely chopped parsley
   1 vegetable bouillon cube or 1 teaspoon vegetable broth powder
   ½–¾ teaspoon sea salt
   1 teaspoon each basil and oregano
   ½ teaspoon sea kelp
   3 tablespoons tamari soy sauce or substitute

Version 1

Heat the butter or oil on low to medium heat and sauté the garlic slices in the oil or butter until thoroughly browned (more than 10 minutes), stirring frequently. Remove and discard the garlic. Add the liquid and the remaining ingredients to the garlic butter or oil. Simmer covered for 20 to 25 minutes. This robust yet light soup is very healing and strengthening. This soup is great for Candida diets, and especially good for flu, colds and infections. Best eaten within 2 to 4 days. Do not freeze.

Version 2

Steam the spinach until totally tender. Heat the butter or oil on low to medium heat and sauté the garlic slices in the oil or butter until lightly browned (5 minutes or more), stirring frequently. Use a blender to blend the spinach and garlic (use all or half the garlic if squeamish) with the remaining ingredients and simmer covered for 15 to 20 minutes. This soup is great for Candida diets, and especially good for flu, colds and infections. Best eaten within 2 to 4 days. Do not freeze.

HEALING GREENS SOUP
(serves 2 to 3)

 5–6 bunches mixed greens: spinach, beet greens, chard, kale and/or mustard greens (3–3½ cups cooked)
 2–3 green onions, chopped small
 1 small clove garlic, minced
 1 cup bouillon, stock, broth, soymilk or milk substitute (do not use real milk)
 1 teaspoon each basil and dill weed
 ½–¾ teaspoon sea salt
 ½ teaspoon each marjoram and thyme
 2 teaspoons vegetable broth powder or 1 vegetable bouillon cube
 2–3 dashes powdered ginger or ¼ teaspoon fresh squeezed ginger juice
 Several dashes sea kelp and cayenne
 Optional: 1–2 teaspoons honey or maple syrup or other natural sweetener (to balance flavors)

Choose firm bright or dark green leaves. Remove any blemishes. Wash the greens and chop lightly. Steam the greens until tender. In a blender, blend the cooked greens with all the remaining ingredients. Simmer on medium-low heat for 15 to 20 minutes, until hot throughout and the flavors have mingled. Enjoy hot with whole grains and/or legumes. A salad is optional. This hearty soup is rich in iron and minerals. Keeps for 1 to 2 days refrigerated. Do not freeze.

ORANGE YAM OR CARROT SOUP
(serves 4)

- 4 cups orange yams, chopped and rinsed 2 to 3 times (peeled or unpeeled), or 4 cups chopped carrots
- 1¾–2 cups milk, soy milk or milk substitute, stock or broth (unsalted)
- 2–3 tablespoons butter or 1–2 tablespoons natural oil
- 2–3 vegetable bouillon cubes or 2 tablespoons tamari soy sauce or substitute
- 2 teaspoons finely chopped onion
- 4 teaspoons finely chopped fresh parsley or 2 teaspoons dried parsley
- 2 teaspoons dill weed or tarragon, crushed
- ½ teaspoon sea salt
- Several dashes sea kelp
- Cayenne to taste
- **Optional:** ¼–½ teaspoon crushed, dried mint leaves (can be peppermint or spearmint tea)
- **Garnish:** chopped chives or green onion tops, or chopped, fresh parsley

Steam the orange vegetable until tender. Liquefy all ingredients until smooth in a blender or food processor. Heat the soup in a saucepan on low to medium heat just up to boiling and simmer for 10 minutes. Do not boil. Serve hot, garnished with chopped chives, green onions, or chopped fresh parsley if desired. Serve with a salad and/or green vegetable with whole grains and legumes or other main dishes. (Good for grounding, balancing female hormones, settling upset stomach, and high in beta-carotene.)

Keeps refrigerated for 2 to 5 days. Best if not frozen.

POWER PROTEIN SOUP
(serves 8 to 10)

⅔ cup dry pinto, Romano or adzuki beans, soaked

⅔ cup dry chick peas or soy beans, soaked

⅔ cup dry black beans, soaked

(or instead of above beans: 2 cups of any 1 bean, soaked)

1 cup asparagus or broccoli, chopped OR 2 bunches fresh
  spinach (or 1 package frozen spinach), chopped small

7 cups water, stock or bouillon (make 4 cups of this liquid soy
  milk for added protein)

5–6 large tomatoes, or 1 (28 ounce, 796 ml) can tomatoes,
  cored and chopped with the juice

1 cup chopped orange yams or winter squash, rinsed

1 large onion (about 1½ cups), chopped*

2 cloves garlic, minced*

½–1 cup fresh chopped parsley, or 3–6 tablespoons dried parsley

2 vegetable bouillon cubes

3 teaspoons vegetable broth powder

1–2 tablespoons natural oil (preferably extra virgin olive)
  or butter

2 tablespoons tamari soy sauce or substitute

2–4 teaspoons honey or other natural sweetener
  (to balance flavors)

1–1½ teaspoons sea salt

1 teaspoon each dill weed and basil

½ teaspoon oregano

¼ teaspoon sea kelp

Cayenne to taste

Optional: 2 Jerusalem artichokes, chopped

Optional garnish: fresh parsley, chives or green onions,
  chopped

Optional topping: sesame salt (Gomashio)

* Instead of onions and garlic, ½ (up to 1 if you like it pungent) teaspoon
of prepared horseradish may be added to the blender.

All the beans can be soaked together for 12 to 24 hours in 8 cups
of water after sorting and removing broken, spoiled beans or debris.

Use any one or two types of beans alone if desired. After soaking, rinse the beans several times with fresh water, add fresh water, enough to cover the beans with one inch of water, and bring to a boil on high heat, uncovered. Scoop off any white froth when it boils and discard. Turn heat to a low bubble and cook the beans until very tender, about 1½ to 2 hours.

In the interim, steam the green and orange vegetables for 5 to 6 minutes until semi-tender. Then measure the water with the fully cooked beans and add or subtract water (stock, bouillon and/or soymilk) until it equals the recipe amount of 7 cups, as required. Add all the remaining ingredients to the pot and cook on low heat (low bubble) for 25 to 35 minutes until everything is tender. Then use a blender to blend the soup bit by bit until thoroughly lique-fied. Return the soup to the pot and simmer again for 10 to 15 minutes or so until flavors have completely mingled. Serve hot and garnish with chopped parsley, chives or green onion tops and sesame salt if desired. This is a very thick, rich, healing soup that is very grounding. Do not eat more than two bowls at a sitting. Keeps for 4 to 6 days refrigerated, or may be frozen.

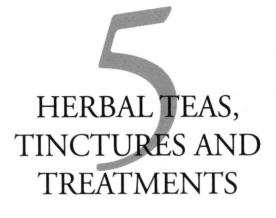

HERBAL TEAS, TINCTURES AND TREATMENTS

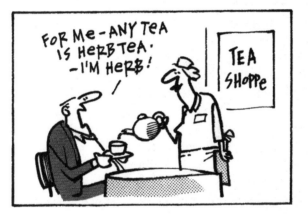

About Water

Water is the elixir of life. It is essential to the health and well-being of every human being and animal on planet earth. Water can bring health and vitality, or carry viruses and disease. In the contaminated age we live in, city tap water has been found to carry algae, parasites, bacteria, sewage, detergents, chlorine, lime, asbestos, sulfates, fluorine, aluminum chloride, toxic copper and lead, as well as a multitude of other impurities. These various impurities can contribute to allergies, joint pains, fatigue, cancer, Candida, parasites, heart problems, senility and sterility, among other problems.

For most individuals, it is preferable to drink pure, tested spring water on an ongoing, day-to-day basis (as I recommend in my encyclopedic natural cookbook *For the Love of Food*) and to drink distilled (steam or demineralized) water, preferably ozonated, *only* when cleansing and during treatments for Candida, cancer, and other major health problems. Distilled water should be drunk for limited periods of time only, preferably no more than a few weeks or a maximum of a few months. (Do not drink distilled water when fasting!)

Purchasing spring or distilled water in plastic 1-gallon, 2½-gallon or 5-gallon jugs is costly and requires time-consuming pick-up or delivery. Plastic containers must be kept out of the sun and away from warm places such as heating ducts, because heat may cause vinyl chlorides and other contaminants to leach from the plastic into the water, which will readily absorb them. As an alternative, some companies deliver water in glass bottles.

A variety of water filtration systems is available, including reverse-osmosis and charcoal filter models. Most of these are not effective in eliminating parasites, while some are not sturdy or do not ensure bacteria-free water. Higher-quality models of reverse-osmosis water filters provide testing kits to check water purity. A home water distiller is another option for safe drinking water, but should be used only for short periods of time while cleansing. A range of sizes and varieties of water filtration systems are available, from countertop units to complete household water tanks. Choose a stainless steel model, rather than plastic, for optimum-quality drinking water.

It is also possible, after filtering or distilling water, to magnetize it or change the pH by adding a few tablespoons of lemon or lime juice per gallon of water. Some health experts recommend using apple cider vinegar as an alternative to lemon or lime juice. Check with a holistic health expert or doctor to see what type of water is best for your particular body type and health, and how long you should use it for. Pure water (with nothing added) should represent 75 percent or more of all the beverages you consume.

Bottled Water Tips

1. Keep bottled water cool, and out of heat and sun.
2. Use sterile, covered containers to store home-filtered or distilled water.
3. Refrigerate water if possible, but drink it at room temperature. Water stores well in a basement or cool garage.

4. Drink a minimum of four glasses a day in cool weather, and six or more in hot weather, as well as additional beverages such as herb tea. Drink liquids away from meals and drink slowly. Have water with meals only for sipping.

5. Never drink out of the bottle, because bacteria are then introduced into the whole bottle. Pour water into a clean glass or pitcher. Keep fingers (and children) out of water containers.

6. In some areas, water that is not really distilled or from a spring is labeled as such and sold. Never buy water that is not in a sealed container. If you doubt the quality of any water, have it analyzed at a local laboratory or try water from another company.

7. If you are unable to obtain spring or distilled water at home, you can ensure safe water by boiling it for five minutes or more (boil for 20 minutes if parasites are suspected), allowing it to cool completely, and running it through a water purifier like the Brita®, Jamieson®, or Water Boy® filtration systems. Be sure to change the filter monthly or more often for large families. Store the water purifier in the refrigerator at all times to prevent bacteria growth, and bring a glass to room temperature for 10 minutes or so before drinking. Boiling kills bacteria, and the filter removes heavy metals and other impurities. Never run warm or hot water through a water filter.

8. For very questionable water that may contain parasites— as when traveling—boil for 10–20 minutes, cool and filter it before drinking.

9. Add a few teaspoons of fresh lemon or lime juice or apple cider vinegar to a glass of water, if doctor approved, to adjust pH levels and kill many kinds of bacteria. Water can be magnetized as well, if desired. If purity is still questionable, add 10 to 20 drops of aerobic oxygen per gallon to counteract impurities.

HEALING HERBAL TEAS

High-quality water is important in making beneficial, healing, herbal teas for remedies. Commercial (supermarket or restaurant) caffeinated green and black teas and coffee are not healthful for many individuals. While some healthy people can tolerate them and even benefit from these beverages, the majority of people are better off avoiding them. Some health experts believe even herbal teas should be avoided, because of possible mold content. Mold can be found on anything, including vegetables. However, herbal teas are not detrimental for most individuals if precautions are taken. (Consult your holistic health specialist for advice on this subject if you are sensitive, have allergies or Candida.)

First, when choosing herbal teas for their medicinal value, avoid most commercial brands of tea bags. They can hide inferior teas and mold. Second, choose bulk or loose teas that are prepackaged and sold in airtight bags or boxes. The kinds that are not pre-packaged and are found in jars or are bagged in stores are more likely to pick up bacteria and dirt, or to become moldy in damp weather or wet store conditions. Third, inspect your teas before preparing and discard or return any that appear moldy or inferior or that have a scent that is not typical for a particular tea. (Get experienced advice on teas if you are not sure how to tell if they are good.) Fourth, heat teas properly so that minor bacteria are killed in the boiling water. Use spring water for the most beneficial teas.

When in doubt about the purity of a tea, such as if it is made with questionable water, serve with a teaspoon of fresh lemon or lime juice. Then you can rest assured that your tea will not be affected by mold and it is as pure as any cooked food can be. The best-quality herb teas are organic and can be purchased through health food stores. Follow the directions in the next sections for making tea, and avoid all teas not mentioned here, unless they are recommended by your doctor or health specialist! Never heat water for herbal teas, or simmer herbal teas, in a microwave. Microwaves destroy the healing properties of herbs.

Pleasure Teas for Enjoyment, Health Benefits and Frequent Use

Enjoy these pleasure teas often.

HERBAL TEAS	ATTRIBUTES
Alfalfa (leaves or seeds) Catnip (natural)	High in chlorophyll, good for arthritis
Chamomile (flowers)	Children's sleep aid, prevents nightmares
Green tea (organic, caffeinated)	Mild digestive aid, mild sleep aid/relaxant
Fennel seeds	Good for pleasure, digestion and healing
Fenugreek seeds	Good for digestion, relieves gas
Lemon grass	Good for internal healing/intestines
Peppermint leaves	High in vitamin A, good for eyesight
Raspberry leaves	Good digestive aid, very mild stimulant
Rose hips (powder)	High in vitamin C, good for female organs
Spearmint leaves	High in vitamin C
Strawberry leaves	Good digestive aid
	High in vitamin C

Medicinal Teas for Healing Purposes and Occasional Use

These are potent teas, and should be used only as directed. Consult your holistic physician if you experience any reactions or side effects from any of these teas. Use sparingly, only as needed. Drink a maximum of three cups of medicinal tea a day unless otherwise directed by your holistic health specialist. See individual herbs in the "Natural Remedies Glossary" for cautions about some of these! Do not try to use all, or even most, of the medicinal teas listed. Usually one or two, plus pleasure teas, are sufficient for an ailment. For additional herbal teas, and more information on their uses, see the ailments section and the "Natural Remedies Glossary." Always try to buy organic teas for medicinal purposes, if available. They are higher quality, more potent and have better healing attributes.

Use a non-metal pot for preparing medicinal teas. Any metal pot, including stainless steel, is claimed by holistic and herbal experts to interfere with the medicinal qualities of most herbal teas. Therefore, if possible, use a Corningware® or uncracked enamel pot (preferably not glass, because of possible lead content) to simmer these teas. Avoid black or speckled enamel pots. *Never* use a microwave to heat water for herbal teas, because it destroys valuable elements in the water and tea. Microwaving any food or beverage is detrimental to health.

HERBAL TEAS	ATTRIBUTES
Burdock root	Blood purifier, detoxifier
Comfrey leaves	Strong internal and external healer (use internally only on doctor's recommendation)
Ginger root	Stimulant and mild digestive aid, helps circulation, warms body, good for nausea and motion sickness
Goldenseal	Antibacterial, anti-viral, for cleansing and healing (not for use by pregnant/lactating women or people with heart problems or glaucoma)
Ginseng	Stimulant/energizer for people over 40, enhances immune function, strengthens glands, good for stress and digestion
Hops	Sleep-inducing tea
Eucalyptus	Antiseptic, for congestion, swelling, coughs, colds, respiratory problems
Licorice root	Mild digestive aid, good for PMS, low blood sugar, stomach and bowel problems (not for use by people with diabetes, heart disease or high blood pressure, or during pregnancy)

HERBAL TEAS	ATTRIBUTES
Taheebo or Pau d'Arco	Helps kill Candida/parasites, good for cleansing (this is a strong tea)
Senna leaves	Good laxative (not for everyday use)
Skullcap	Sleep-inducing tea (not as ominous as it sounds!)
Slippery elm powder	Good for sore throats, colds, flu

How to Make Herbal Teas

LEAF TEAS

Use 1 teaspoon of loose tea per cup. Steep only—boiling makes leaf tea bitter and also kills valuable vitamins and enzymes. To steep: Boil the water. When it comes to a rolling boil, remove from the heat (put in a teapot if desired), add the tea to the water, stir and cover. Let it steep for 8 to 12 minutes. Strain and drink. A tea ball may be used for leaf teas. Leftovers can be refrigerated for up to five days and should be heated just up to boiling to serve again. Reheat only once.

SEED OR TWIG TEAS

Use ¼ to ½ teaspoon loose tea per cup. Bring water and tea to a boil together and let it boil on a low bubble for 5 to 10 minutes. Let it steep, covered, off the heat for another 10 minutes. Strain and drink. Leftovers can be refrigerated for up to five days and should be heated just up to boiling to serve again. Reheat only once.

ROOT OR BARK TEA

Use ¼ to ½ teaspoon root or bark, broken or chopped into small pieces, per cup. Make sure tea is broken up as much as possible. Bring the water and tea to a boil together and keep at a low bubble for 15 to 20 minutes. Steep off the heat for another 10 minutes. Strain and drink. Leftovers can be refrigerated for up to five days and should be heated just up to boiling to serve again. Reheat only once.

POWDERED ROOT OR POWDERED BARK TEA

Use ⅒ to ⅛ teaspoon of powdered tea per cup (unless your health care specialist recommends differently). Mix the tea well in the water before heating. Then bring it to a boil and keep it on a low bubble for 20 to 30 minutes. No steeping or straining is required. Leftovers can be refrigerated for up to 7 or 8 days and should be heated up to boiling and simmered a few minutes before serving again. Reheat only once.

HERBAL TEA BAGS

Use high-quality, natural tea bags that do not use dyes or additives. Boil water, pour in a cup or teapot, add teabag and let steep for about five minutes until the tea is as strong as you like it (but remove bag before tea becomes bitter). Swish tea bag in the tea before removing. One tea bag makes enough tea for two cups. Do not save a used teabag for later use, because bacteria can form on the wet bag if it is left sitting for more than a few minutes. Use teabags for pleasure teas only—medicinal teas are more potent and beneficial when loose or bulk tea is used. For pleasure tea drinking, buy organic tea bags whenever possible.

MEDICINAL HERBAL TEA CAPSULES

When taking medicinal herbal supplements in capsule or tablet form, it is more effective if you take the herbs on an empty stomach (unless instructed otherwise by the package or your doctor) with 2 to 4 ounces (about one-quarter cup) of water and follow three to five minutes later with a cup of hot water or a complementary pleasure tea. This way, the medicinal tea capsules are more effectively absorbed and utilized by the body.

How to Make Herbal Tea Combinations

When making an herbal tea combination, special care must be taken not to overcook the teas. For example, leaf tea should never be boiled, so when making a combination of twig and leaf tea, do not boil the leaf tea with the twig tea or the tea will become bitter and lose vitamins. The twig tea should be low-boiled by itself and the leaf tea should be added to the boiled twig tea during the steeping time only. Pleasure teas can be poured over fresh mint leaves, lemon or lime wedges, dried orange peels or other dried citrus peels, cinnamon, cloves or other spices.

SAMPLE PLEASURE TEA COMBINATIONS

Use equal parts of each of the following:

1. Peppermint and alfalfa
2. Spearmint and strawberry or raspberry leaves
3. Peppermint, alfalfa and lemon grass (a popular blend)
4. Raspberry leaf and alfalfa leaf tea poured over fresh lemon rounds (tastes like regular caffeinated tea)
5. Fennel seeds and alfalfa leaves (optional: stir with a cinnamon stick)
6. Fenugreek seeds and mint leaves
7. Peppermint and slippery elm powder
8. Chamomile flowers and lemon grass
9. Chamomile flowers and rose hips
10. Create your own combinations with two to four pleasure teas.

Caution: For frequent use, stick with the pleasure teas mentioned here or use those recommended by your holistic doctor or herbal health specialist. Some herbal teas have strong medicinal powers and can cause stomach upset, headaches or nausea if used incorrectly.

SAMPLE MEDICINAL TEA COMBINATIONS
Caution: Use the medicinal teas mentioned below sparingly, only as needed and if your holistic doctor approves.

Use equal parts of each of the following:

1. Senna and flaxseed	Potent, yet gentle laxative blend
2. Goldenseal and myrrh	Toothache remedy and antibacterial mouthwash blend
3. Rosehips, ginger and eucalyptus	Cold and flu blend
4. Licorice and fennel	Digestive aid blend
5. Chamomile and hops	Sleep aid blend
6. Spearmint and skullcap	Sleep aid blend (peppermint can be used instead of spearmint)
7. Peppermint, ginseng and ginger	Energizer, circulation aid blend
8. Rose hips and slippery elm with dash of cayenne and honey	Sore throat aid blend
9. Rosehips, raspberry or strawberry leaves with ginger/lemon	Vitamin C booster blend, cold and flu aid blend
10. Mint, ginger and fennel (can use licorice or senna instead of fennel)	Upset stomach blend

It is best not to make your own blends unless you have authoritative advice from your holistic doctor or herbalist. Some combinations can be detrimental if improperly used. See the caution above.

Taheebo or Pau d'Arco Tea

2 teaspoons taheebo tea (measure loose tea or tea taken from
  tea bags)
2½ cups water

Use a non-metal pot. Any metal pot, including stainless steel, is claimed by holistic and herbal experts to interfere with the medicinal qualities of certain herbal teas, especially this one. Use a Corningware® or uncracked enamel pot (preferably not glass, because of possible lead content). Avoid black or speckled enamel pots. Bring water and tea to a boil together and keep on a low bubble for 25 to 30 minutes. Strain and drink. Drink about 1 cup a day or as directed by health specialist. Keeps refrigerated for 2 days and may be reheated to serve. Purchase taheebo tea at health food stores or holistic pharmacies that carry natural remedies.

TINCTURES, COMPRESSES, POULTICES, OINTMENTS, CREAMS AND PASTES

Tinctures

Tinctures are concentrated herbal teas or blends of medicinal teas, and are used internally like a medicine or as a gargle or applied externally. Tinctures are usually used at room temperature. Many purchased brands contain alcohol and I do not recommend them. Tinctures can be prepared at home preferably with the advice of your holistic doctor or herbalist (who may also sell some tinctures) or with the use of this book.

TINCTURE PREPARATION Make a strong tea of one herbal tea or a blend of teas, increasing the strength by 4 to 10 times (i.e., use more herb per cup of water). Follow the tea preparation instructions above. Strain the tea and cool to room temperature for use. Most herbal tinctures can be kept refrigerated for up to a week. Do not keep longer as they do not stay fresh and safe beyond this time.

One popular tincture is made with goldenseal and myrrh medicinal teas, and is used for toothaches. It is administered as a gargle or mouthwash for adults and applied with a cotton swab to the gums of teething babies. Other tinctures can be prepared from the various medicinal tea combinations mentioned in this chapter.

Compresses

Hot or cold compresses can be prepared by soaking a cotton, linen, muslin or other soft, natural cloth in a tincture. First place the cloth in hot or cold water, wring it out and then soak one side of the cloth with the tincture. Apply the cloth to the forehead, stomach or other area of distress for 15 to 20 minutes, and then repeat the process if needed. Holistic health experts have various methods of using compresses and should be consulted for all extreme pain or discomfort. Do not use a compress as a substitute for a doctor's advice and care.

Poultices

A poultice is similar to a compress, except that dried and fresh herbs are used (rather than tinctures) and it usually covers a larger area of the body. They are moistened and often spread directly on the skin over a larger area and then covered with a larger, moistened cloth. It is best if the person receiving the treatment lies in bed during this process. Powdered or leaf herbs can be moistened or made into a paste with an equal amount of cornstarch, baking soda or arrowroot powder, plus water. (Do not use twig or seed herbs unless ground first.) Use as much water as needed to make an easy-to-apply paste for the ailing body part. Apply the herbs to the body and cover completely with a thick, moistened cloth (hot or cold), then plastic, and then cover the person with a warm blanket, especially if the poultice covers a large area of the body such as the whole back or chest. Leave on for 15 to 20 minutes or longer, as needed. Remoisten the cloth every 20 minutes or so. Follow with a hot/cold shower or bath (see "Healing Aids") or a hot/cold sponge bath if the ailing person is bedridden. Sheets may need to be changed afterwards with certain herbs, if sweating is profuse.

OINTMENTS Use ground herbs only and prepare a strong tincture, using 10 times the amount of herb that you would use to make a tea per one cup of water. Prepare a two-cup recipe. Add the finished tincture to 8 to 12 ounces of extra virgin olive oil and simmer just under a boil (in an uncovered non-metal pot) until excess water is evaporated. A little beeswax can be added if desired, to get a firmer consistency. Store in a tightly sealed glass jar. Keep refrigerated for up to one month or so. The ointment can be used on sore muscles and joints, for stomach complaints, or on other body parts, depending on the herbs used and the health concern it was made for. For the greatest benefit, remove a little of the ointment at a time and let sit at room temperature before applying. For external use only.

Creams and Pastes

Creams are best if prepared by your herbalist. However, pastes can be prepared from some powdered herbs at home, by adding just a little pure spring water. Apply the paste to the afflicted area. A common paste, used for some skin rashes, is made with goldenseal powder or ground comfrey leaves.

Note: See the "Recommended Reading" section for a list of excellent herb books that provide more information on herbs and their uses. See the "Healing Aids" section for hot/cold treatments and other beneficial healing methods that can be used comfortably by anyone to ease the discomfort of certain ailments and, often, to bring soothing relief from minor, unpleasant side effects.

Important: Remember that herbal teas and treatments should never be substituted for a doctor's care. Consult your holistic physician if *major* health problems or side effects occur.

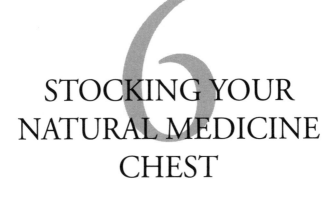

6

STOCKING YOUR NATURAL MEDICINE CHEST

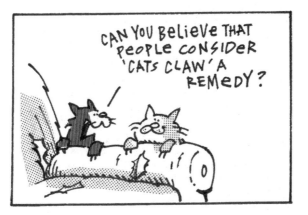

Note: Items are presented in alphabetical order within each list.

A. The Basic Starter Natural Medicine Kit

Remedies (in alphabetical order)

1. **Acidophilus capsules (keep refrigerated)**—digestive aid; contain friendly bacteria to counteract effects of antibiotic drugs; Candida and parasites; immune system aid.
2. **Colloidal silver, 10 or 24 ppm (parts per million)**— antibacterial and anti-viral; for earache and toothache; small wounds, used as mouthwash.

3. **Epsom salts**—internal flushing agent; used externally as a body soak for soothing and drawing out toxins and for minor muscle aches and as skin cleanser.
4. **Royal jelly**—energizer and aphrodisiac; increases strength and endurance; for sports, PMS and menopause.
5. **Tea tree oil**—antibacterial, anti-viral and antiseptic; for cuts, burns, sunburn, small wounds, insect stings and bites and to relieve toothache; used as mouthwash.
6. **Valerian capsules or tablets**—adult sleep aid and relaxant; helps ease anxiety.
7. **Vitamin B50 complex**—immune system aid and healing aid, for stress and for calming; energizing for some.
8. **Vitamin C**—antibacterial, anti-viral, energizer, immune system booster, acidifier and healing aid; used to relieve stress.

Herbal Teas

9. **Chamomile tea**—mild sleep aid for adults and children; mild digestive aid; for children's nightmares; used for calming and soothing, and externally as a body soak.
10. **Goldenseal root powder/tea**—antiviral; for infections, toothache and some skin problems; used as mouthwash.
11. **Peppermint tea**—mild stimulant and digestive aid; used to help relieve headaches and colic.

Kitchen Aids

12. **Cayenne pepper**—antibacterial for stomachaches and ulcers, for circulation, to soothe sore throats and to help break up mucus.
13. **Flaxseeds**—digestive aid and laxative; provide essential fatty acids and fiber.
14. **Fresh lemons**—astringent, antibacterial and anti-viral; for colds and sore throats, to purge heavy metals; used for cleansing.
15. **Organic garlic**—antibacterial and anti-viral; for earaches, infections, Candida and parasites; used for cleansing.

B. Intermediate Natural Medicine Chest

Add the following items to the Basic Starter Natural Medicine Kit for an expanded Medicine Chest.

Remedies (in alphabetical order)
1. **Aloe vera (keep juices and gels refrigerated)**—astringent, for mild sunburn or damaged skin, for blisters and warts, for some stomach problems like ulcers, and as a healing aid and for cleansing.
2. **Calcium and magnesium**—used for calming and soothing, for strong teeth and bones and as a healing aid.
3. **Echinacea**—immune system booster and healing aid; for colds, for infection.
4. **Feverfew or white willow bark**—for headaches, migraines and fevers.
5. **Oil of oregano**—antiviral; used for warts, to strengthen hair and nails, and as a general healing aid and for cleansing.
6. **Plant (pancreatic) enzymes**—to stimulate good digestion, and especially as a vegetarian digestive aid.
7. **Propolis**—for bad breath and sore throat; an immune system enhancer and healing aid, mouthwash.
8. **St. John's wort**—for stress or trauma, as a strong adult sleep aid and to aid depression and healing.
9. **Shark oil (squalane)**—for wrinkles, sun damaged skin, for some skin infections and rashes and skin cancer (usually for external use).
10. **Vegetable or gelatin capsules, empty**—may be filled with cayenne, goldenseal, or other herbs to be taken internally.

Herbal Teas
11. **Alfalfa (may also be taken in tablet form)**—a green food product that is high in chlorophyll; helps ease joint pain; promotes healing of some types of arthritis and may reduce symptoms.
12. **Lemon grass tea**—high in vitamin A; for eyesight.

13. **Raspberry leaf tea**—high in vitamin C; for stimulating female hormones; for PMS; helps prevent miscarriage.
14. **Rose hips tea**—high in vitamin C; good for flu, colds and sore throats.
15. **Skullcap tea**—adult sleep aid; relieves anxiety; is calming and soothing.

Kitchen Aids

16. **Beets**—digestive aid, laxative and cleansing aid.
17. **Ginger (vegetable or tea)**—stimulant and digestive aid; for nausea and motion sickness, for circulation, and as a healing aid and cleansing aid.
18. **Honey**—for sore throats, for bee stings, and as an energizer and hay fever remedy.
19. **Tomato juice or grapefruit juice**—mild digestive aids for proteins; tomatoes and red grapefruit are a source of lycopene.
20. **Yogurt**—digestive aid; source of friendly bacteria for stomach and intestines.

C. Advanced Natural Medicine Chest

Add some or all of the following items to the Basic Starter Natural Medicine Kit and the Intermediate Natural Medicine Chest for an expanded, more complete Medicine Chest.

Remedies (in alphabetical order)

1. **Aerobic oxygen**—for antibacterial use, mouthwash and to purify beverages.
2. **Arnica (homeopathic)**—used to relieve pain and sore muscles, for minor injuries, for wound healing.
3. **Barley green, blue-green algae, chlorella or spirulina**—green food products high in enzymes, chlorophyll and protein; used to aid digestion and enhance energy.
4. **Biotin (B vitamin)**—anti-fungal for blood sugar problems, for healthy scalp and nails.
5. **Chromium**—used to counteract sugar effects, to help balance blood sugar and as a heart aid.

6. **Citricidal**—antibacterial, anti-fungal, anti-viral; good for Candida yeast, for some infections and for colds and flu.
7. **Clove oil**—for toothaches, parasites; as a mouthwash and for indigestion.
8. **CoQ10**—antioxidant; oxygenates the body; used to slow the aging process, as a heart aid and for fatigue.
9. **Dong quai**—ginseng for females; used as an energizer, to tone female organs and to aid menstrual problems and menopause.
10. **Ginger capsules**—for nausea and motion sickness, used as a digestive aid and as an antibacterial.
11. **Ginkgo biloba**—used as an energizer and a memory aid, for mental clarity while aging and to counter depression and impotence.
12. **Ginseng**—antifungal; used as an energizer, to counteract the effects of aging and to stimulate the immune system.
13. **HCL betaine hydrochloride**—digestive aid for heavy meals or while cleansing; for digestive problems.
14. **Melatonin**—hormonal sleep aid; for anti-aging, for jet lag, for glaucoma and ringing in the ears.
15. **Milk thistle**—liver healer, cleansing aid, antioxidant and immune system booster.
16. **Multiple vitamins**—for basic vitamin and mineral needs; for general health maintenance.
17. **Olive leaf extract**—natural antibiotic, anti-viral and cleansing aid; for healing/infections.
18. **Rescue Remedy®**—for trauma and shock, for severe stress and anxiety, and for calming.
19. **Witch hazel**—for skin problems, for hemorrhoids and varicose veins, and to promote healing—externally.
20. **Zinc**—for healing and immune system protection, to fight colds; and as an aphrodisiac and a fertility aid.

Herbal Teas
21. **Catnip tea**—mild sleep aid for babies and children; good for soaking sore muscles.
22. **Cornsilk tea**—diuretic; used to help prevent bedwetting; helps to heal all bladder problems and used as an intestinal aid.

23. **Dandelion tea or "coffee"**—liver aid; increases bile production and cleanses the blood.
24. **Fennel seed**—digestive aid; for gas and flatulence; helps organs function.
25. **Green tea, organic**—for fatigue, to fight infections, to help fight cancer, as a heart aid, to boost immune function, and for gum problems.
26. **Kava kava**—used as a mild adult sleep aid, for stress or anxiety, for urinary infections.
27. **Licorice tea**—used as a digestive aid, for PMS, for low blood sugar and for digestive and bowel problems.
28. **Myrrh powder tea**—antiseptic and antibacterial; for bad breath and skin problems; as mouthwash with goldenseal.
29. **Senna leaf tea**—used as a digestive aid and laxative, for worms and to fight bad breath. (Use with other herbs rather than alone for more effectiveness.)
30. **Slippery elm bark powder tea**—for sore throats, to expel mucus; for diarrhea and for inflammation.

Kitchen Aids
31. **Apple cider vinegar**—used as a digestive aid, for weight control, as an astringent and to oxygenate the blood.
32. **Cranberry juice (unsweetened)**—for bladder problems, as an acidifier, and as a digestive aid for proteins.
33. **Lecithin**—helps control cholesterol levels; aids liver, kidneys and heart.
34. **Pumpkin seeds**—anti-parasitic, high in zinc; also used for male prostate problems.
35. **Sea kelp powder**—expels heavy metals; helps heal some thyroid problems; provides iodine; aids digestion.

D. MASTER NATURAL MEDICINE CABINET

Add most or all of the following items to the Basic Starter Natural Medicine Kit, the Intermediate Natural Medicine Chest and some of the items in the Advanced Natural Medicine Chest for an expanded, more comprehensive Medicine Chest.

Remedies (in alphabetical order)

1. **Activated charcoal**—for diarrhea, used for travel and parasite problems.
2. **Amino acids**—protein for healing, helps prevent bone loss, for blood sugar or alcohol problems.
3. **B6**—for calming, for nausea and hangover symptoms and for edema.
4. **B12**—sleep aid, for vitamin deficiency especially if vegetarian.
5. **Bile salts**—for gall bladder and liver problems, to help break down fats and as a digestive aid.
6. **Bio Strath® extract or tablets**—energizer, healing aid and nutrient supplement.
7. **Cat's claw, devil's claw, green-lipped mussel or yucca**—to promote healing of arthritis.
8. **Chlorophyll**—provides green nutrients, aids digestion and internal healing (including ulcers and internal injuries).
9. **Colostrum**—for cleansing and anti-viral; used to help heal some allergies and promote general healing.
10. **Cranberry extract capsules**— acidifier; used for bladder problems.
11. **DHEA**—hormone for anti-aging, for sexual problems, and for improved immune function.
12. **Essiac ® or Flor-Essence®**—used to promote healing, for cleansing, as an energizer (if used in small amounts) and for cancer.
13. **Evening primrose oil**—for PMS and menopause, for essential fatty acids and to promote healing.
14. **Glucosamine sulfate**—for arthritis, for joint aches and pains, for wound and injury healing.
15. **Gotu kola**—energizer; used to promote healing of minor injuries and wounds and for some skin problems.
16. **Grape seed**—antioxidant and anti-inflammatory; also used to promote healing.
17. **Hyland's Calms®**—mild, yet effective, homeopathic sleep aid; also used for calming and soothing.
18. **Lysine (amino acid)**—for cold sores, for herpes, and to aid calcium absorption.

19. **MSM**—for joint aches, inflammation and pain due to injury or illness; for arthritis, low blood sugar and allergies; for cleansing and to promote healing.
20. **Pycnogenol**—a circulation aid, antioxidant and anti-inflammatory; also used to promote healing.
21. **Selenium**—for healthy immune function and for cancer and heart problems.
22. **Tormentavena®**—for parasites; as a travel aid for diarrhea due to parasites.
23. **Traumeel®**—for stress and trauma, for healing, for accident or injury recovery.
24. **Wormwood, black walnut or other parasite remedy**—for parasites and for cleansing.

Important: You might consider other vitamins, minerals and remedies that are not mentioned here for your medicine chest, for their specific medicinal values, healing abilities and nutrients.

Herbal Teas

25. **Artichoke tea (or extract)**—for liver healing, for cleansing, to tone the digestive tract, for lowering cholesterol levels.
26. **Barberry tea**—slows heart rate and breathing; used as an intestinal aid; kills bacteria on skin when applied locally.
27. **Bilberry tea**—for eyesight problems and cataracts; for anxiety, helps stabilize blood sugar and used as a sore throat gargle.
28. **Black cohosh**—for menstrual cramps, for morning sickness; aids circulation.
29. **Buchu leaf tea**—helps balance blood sugar; for bladder, kidney and prostate problems.
30. **Comfrey leaf tea**—for internal and external healing; for insect bites and stings.
31. **Eyebright tea**—to relieve eye problems, also used as an eyewash and for some allergies, including hay fever.
32. **Fenugreek seed tea**—mild digestive aid; for eyesight and breathing problems.
33. **Hawthorn tea**—for heart problems, anemia; for circulation.

34. **Hops tea**—used as a sleep aid, for anxiety, for pain, for sexually transmitted diseases (STDs).
35. **Horsetail tea**—for strong hair and nails, strengthens heart and as an anti-inflammatory.
36. **Lobelia tea**—used in small amounts to relieve breathing difficulties and to help heal some infections. A cup or more is used to induce vomiting.
37. **Passion flower tea**—used as a sleep aid, for anxiety and hyperactivity.
38. **Saw palmetto**—for prostate problems, as a diuretic and to stimulate digestion.
39. **Taheebo tea (Pau d'Arco)**— used for Candida yeast and other infections, healing, for cancer and heart problems, and to promote healing.
40. **Yarrow leaf tea**—used for wounds and to help stop bleeding, also used as a diuretic, an anti-inflammatory, and to promote healing.

Kitchen Aids
41. **Artichokes, globe (fresh)**—used as a liver aid and an aphrodisiac.
42. **Artichokes, Jerusalem**—used to balance blood sugar and one of the best sources of FOSs.
43. **Bee pollen**—used as an energizer and an aphrodisiac; for lowering blood pressure and cholesterol.
44. **Beet powder**—used as a digestive aid, for constipation and as an anti-fungal.
45. **Horseradish**—antifungal; decongestant and cancer preventative. Food substitute for those with garlic and onion allergies.

E. Your Own Natural Medicine Chest

The suggested Natural Medicine Kit and Chests—from Basic to Master—will help you to get organized quickly and assure you have all the most important items. Or you can create your own Natural Medicine Chest by picking one or two remedies, herbal teas or kitchen aids from each of the following categories. The Fast

Fingertip Remedies (below) and the Natural Remedies Glossary (p. 164) will also help you choose the contents of your Chest.

1. Antiseptic—for burns, cuts, wounds, insect bites and stings
2. Stimulant and/or energizer
3. Relaxant, calming agent and/or sleep aid
4. Digestive aids
5. Vitamin and mineral supplements
6. Flushing agent and/or laxative
7. Diarrhea aid
8. Headache and/or pain remedy
9. Anxiety/trauma remedy
10. Yeast killer and/or parasite remedy
11. Antiviral(s)
12. Cleansing aids

FAST FINGERTIP REMEDIES

A Natural Medicine Chest can also be made up of a selection of one or two of each of the following. This list can be used as well for a quick reference guide for remedies for specific health concerns. (Not all antibacterials, anti-inflammatories and so on are included in the following lists, only the *main ones* in each category. See individual remedies and ailments for addition items.)

ANTIBACTERIALS	ANTI-INFLAMMATORIES
Aerobic oxygen	Anti-Flam®
Aloe vera	Arnica
Cayenne pepper	Barberry
Citricidal	Buchu
Garlic	Calendula
Ginger	Cat's claw
Goldenseal	Comfrey
Lemons	Echinacea
Limes	Elderberry
Myrrh	Fenugreek
Onions	Flaxseed
Rubbing alcohol (external use only)	Flammaforce®
Tea tree oil	Garlic

Ginger
Goldenseal
Grape seed
Horsetail tea
Infla-Zyme Forte®
Licorice
MSM
Myrrh
Onions
Primrose oil, evening
Pycnogenol
Silica
Slippery elm
SOD
Vitamin C
Yarrow

ANTIOXIDANTS
Beta-carotene
Bilberry tea
CoQ10
Cysteine
Ginkgo biloba
Grape seed
Green tea
Glutathione
Melatonin
Milk thistle
Pycnogenol
Selenium
SOD
Vitamin A
Vitamin C
Vitamin E
Zinc

ANTI-SPASMODICS
Black cohosh
Buchu
Catnip
Cayenne

Celery seed
Chamomile
Fennel
Lobelia
Peppermint
St. John's wort
Skullcap
Spearmint
Valerian

ANTISEPTICS
Aloe vera
Colloidal silver
Garlic
Onions
Oregano oil
Rubbing alcohol (external use only)
Tea tree oil

ANTI-VIRALS
Aloe vera
Anti-Viral Formula®
Cayenne pepper
Citricidal
Colloidal silver
Colostrum
Garlic
Ginger
Goldenseal
Lemon and lime juice
Olive leaf extract
Oregano oil
Tea tree oil
Vitamin C

APHRODISIACS
Artichokes, globe
Bee pollen
Dong quai
Energizers, all (see Energizers)

Ginseng
Royal jelly
Saw palmetto
Vitamin C
Vitamin E
Zinc

ASTRINGENTS
Aloe vera
Apple cider vinegar
Clay
Citricidal
Lemons
Limes
Oatmeal
Witch hazel
Yarrow

BLOOD SUGAR
BALANCERS
Amino acids
Artichokes, Jerusalem
Beans (brown, red and black)
Biotin
Blueberry leaf tea
Calcium and magnesium
Chromium
Dandelion greens and coffee
Garlic
Onions
Vitamin B complex

BURNS AND SUNBURN
REMEDIES
Aloe vera
Calendula cream
PABA cream
Shark oil
Tea tree oil
Vitamin C
Vitamin E

CLEANSING REMEDIES
Colloidal silver
Colostrum
Essiac ® or Flor-Essence ®
Garlic
Ginger
Lemon and lime juice
Olive leaf extract
Oregano oil
Tea tree oil

COLDS AND SORE
THROAT REMEDIES
Echinacea
Goldenseal
Ginger
Honey
Lemon and lime juice
Licorice
Myrrh
Slippery elm
Propolis
Vitamin C
Zinc

DIGESTIVE AIDS
Acidophilus
Beet juice or powder
Bile salts
Bromelain (pineapple enzymes)
Chamomile tea
Club soda
Essiac® or Flor-Essence®
Fennel seed tea
Ginger
Glutamic acid hydrochloride
Grapefruit juice
Horseradish
HCL (betaine hydrochloride)
Licorice tea
Miso soup

Papain (papaya enzymes)
Peppermint tea and oil
Plant (pancreatic) enzymes
Prunes and prune juice
Spearmint tea and oil
Swedish Bitters®
Tomato juice
Yogurt, plain

ENERGIZERS
Bee pollen
Bio Strath ®
Dong quai
Essiac ® or Flor-Essense ® (in small amounts)
Ginger
Ginkgo biloba
Ginseng
Gotu kola
Green tea (organic)
Peppermint tea or oil
Royal jelly
Vitamin C

GREEN FOOD PRODUCTS
Alfalfa
Aloe vera
Astragalus
Barley green
Blue-green algae
Chlorella
Chlorophyll
Green kamut
Spirulina
Wheat grass

HAIR AND NAIL AIDS
Calcium
Flax seeds and oil
Gelatin
Horsetail

Iron
Magnesium
Oregano oil
Shen min®
Silica
Vitamin C
Zinc

HEADACHE REMEDIES
Allergy vitamin C
Calcium and magnesium
Energizers, all (see *Energizers*)
Feverfew
Ginger
Ginseng
Peppermint
Vitamin B complex
White willow bark

IMMUNE SYSTEM BOOSTERS
Bioflavonoids
CoQ10
Echinacea
Ginseng
Grape seed extract
Pycnogenol
Royal jelly
Vitamin C

JET LAG REMEDIES
Energizers, all (see *Energizers*)
Melatonin
Vitamin B complex
Vitamin C
Vitamin E

JOINT PAIN REMEDIES
Aloe vera (externally)
Anti-Flam®
Arnica

Flammaforce®
Infla-Zyme Forte®
Glucosamine sulfate
MSM
SOD
Tea tree oil (externally)

LAXATIVES
Acidophilus
Bioxy®
Cascara sagrada
Epsom salts and warm water
Experience®
Psyllium seeds
Senna and flaxseed tea
Some digestive aids

LIVER AIDS
Beets
Black radish
Dandelion
Globe artichokes (cooked, warm)
Globe artichoke extract
Lemon juice
Milk thistle

OXYGEN BOOSTERS
Aerobic oxygen
Aloe vera
CoQ10
Garlic
Germanium
Ginseng
Onions
Shiitake mushrooms

PARASITE REMEDIES
Black walnut
Clear®
Cloves
Colloidal silver

Detoxosode D•P®
Garlic
Onions
Parasave®
Paraway®
Paragone®
Pumpkin seeds
Tormentavena ®
Wormwood

SHOCK AND TRAUMA REMEDIES
B complex
Calcium and magnesium
Hops
Rescue Remedy®
Skullcap
St. John's wort
Valerian
Traumeel®

SKIN PROBLEM REMEDIES
Aloe vera
Calendula herb or cream
Chamomile tea
Comfrey
Dandelion
Ginkgo biloba
Goldenseal
Hydrogen peroxide (use food
    grade for internal)
Oatmeal
Shark oil
Tea tree oil
Vitamin C
Vitamin E
Witch hazel
Zinc

SLEEP AIDS
Calcium and magnesium

Catnip tea
Chamomile tea
B complex
B12
Hops tea
Hylands's Calms®
Kava kava
Melatonin
Passion flower
Skullcap tea
Valerian root

TOOTHACHE REMEDIES

Clove oil
Colloidal silver
Garlic
Goldenseal and myrrh
Lemon and lime juice
Neem powder
Peelu
Propolis
Sea salt and warm water
Tea tree oil

7

HEALING AIDS— NATURAL WAYS TO SPEED HEALING

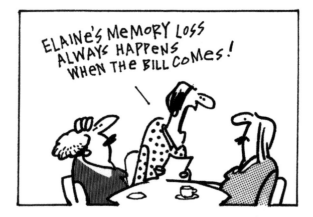

When you are not feeling your best—when your energy is low, you are ill or you require rest to speed healing—to even one small area of the body, or perhaps for the entire body, there are numerous ways to enhance healing conditions and reduce the symptoms and side effects, while you take remedies to help cure what ails you.

The body itself is the primary healer. There are however, aids that relax, cleanse, rejuvenate, soothe and assist the body in its natural healing process. Many people use drugs, but drugs may sometimes cause health problems and contribute to new health concerns when taken too frequently or unnecessarily. Hundreds of thousands of cases of drug overdose and many thousands of deaths occur annually in North America from misdiagnosis, mishandling or abusing drugs. Natural remedies, when used correctly and augmented by these simple treatments for mind, emotions and physical well being, gently aid the healing process and allow your body to use its natural abilities to achieve and maintain good health. Unlike drugs, most natural remedies do not build up in the body as toxins that can cause future damage to the body.

Ask your holistic health-care specialist, or an expert in one of the areas discussed below, to help you decide which of the following healing aids might benefit you most. There are many powerful ways to speed healing. Note the items on this list that interest you, read more about them and use some of them when needed. It is not necessary or desirable that you do everything. Simply employ whatever healing aids appeal to you and/or help you.

Acupressure

Acupressure is the non-invasive art of using the fingers and hands to apply pressure to specific points on the body to relieve pain and release energy blocks that contribute to illness and disease. Symptoms are the body's way of expressing the condition of the whole person. Acupressure practitioners employ various methods of touch to stimulate healing energy. They include pressing, rubbing, kneading and vibration, all of which stimulate the flow of blood, improve the circulation and remove blockages of life energy or "chi." Acupressure can also be self-administered.

Acupuncture

Acupuncture was developed by the Chinese and is thousands of years old. It is based on the belief that vital life energy (chi) is the basis of health. Twelve body energy pathways, called meridians, link every organ and part of the body. The acupuncturist inserts thin needles into the skin along the meridians to stimulate the chi to these meridians and allow balance and healing to take place in the body. In some techniques, larger needles are inserted more deeply into the body. Needles may stay in the body for between 3 and 30 minutes. Acupuncture is a fine art and requires an expert practitioner with proper training. Acupuncture can relieve pain, increase immune response, help headaches and migraines, assist healing sports and other injuries, ease backaches, help depression and addictions, and improve arthritis, digestive disorders and bowel problems. Sometimes as little as one treatment is required; other times a series of treatments may be needed.

Air Purifier

Unless you live in an unpolluted country area with abundant fresh air, an air purifier is a wise investment. For less than $80 you can buy one large enough to clean the air in a one-bedroom apartment. Replacement filters are only $10 to $20 per year. These compact appliances fit almost anywhere and are usually slightly smaller than a bread box. They remove some of the dust, pollen, smoke and other air pollutants. This improves your air quality and can assist healing. If you get one with an air ionizer, this adds energizing negative ions to your air supply, perfect for daytime. At night, while sleeping, turn the ionizer off. You do not want to feel energized while sleeping; it may wake you. The average air purifying unit can be kept on through the night, though it helps to prolong the life of the machine if you can find a few hours a day to turn it off and let it rest. You may notice that you feel better, day and night, when using an air purifier. Choose a high-quality model that suits the size of the area you want to purify.

Cleanliness, Household

It is essential to live in a clean living space with as little dirt, dust, and clutter as possible. Use effective, quality dish soaps and other cleaning products to reduce germs that may contribute to yeast growth. Clean all areas that have mold, mildew and grime with proper cleaning products, while wearing rubber gloves. Scrub sinks, bowls and tubs twice weekly with antibacterial cleaners. Keep your home well-vacuumed and ventilated. Air the entire place out at least once per day. Do not use strong-smelling cleaning agents that aggravate allergies or other health problems.

Cleanliness, Personal

For personal cleanliness, bathe or shower daily. Change your towels regularly (at least once or twice a week). Do not take long, hot baths, because they can weaken you and your body can absorb pollutants from the water such as chlorine, copper and bacteria that collect in water pipes, bathtubs and around bathing areas. Try a hot-cold shower or a 15-to-20-minute maximum Epsom salt bath. (For baths, make sure the tub is thoroughly clean and properly rinsed before filling.)

EPSOM SALT BATH   Pour about two cups of Epsom salts into a bathtub before you fill it with very warm or hot water. (Epsom salts do not mix well in lukewarm water). Swish the water around before getting in and then soak away. Skin toxins are purged; this bath can relieve all-over body pressure and bring soothing relief to sore body parts. After the bath, rinse off with cool water. (See *Shower Filter* for important information on filtering bath water to avoid pollutants.) Dr. Roger Rogers, a Vancouver disease expert, suggests that women not urinate before bathing or swimming; a little urine in the bladder helps prevent bacteria and pollutants in the water from entering the bladder and contributing to infections.

HOT-COLD SHOWER   This type of shower is stimulating and invigorating for daytime bathing. (Stick with a moderately hot or warm shower before bedtime.) Take a warm shower—not too hot. When ready to step out, gradually turn the water cooler and cooler until it is as cold as you can stand it. Imagine you are under a waterfall! If the change in temperature is gradual, it will not shock the body and you will feel energized and tingly all over. It can also stimulate the immune system and help circulation by sending blood to areas of the body that need it. Hot-cold baths and packs can have the same effect.

Do not just have a hot shower and expect to feel active and invigorated! Hot treatments invite sleep and slow the body down. (See *Shower Filter* for important information on filtering water to avoid pollutants.)

HOT-COLD BATH   Take a hot bath, scrubbing completely, followed by a quick cold bath—a one-minute cold plunge at least.

Cleansing
Cleansing is a rather complex issue, and it would require a huge book to cover all the possible types and methods. Some titles are listed in "Recommended Reading," though none of them is truly

complete. Look for a future book from me entitled *Complete Cleansing and Fasting Guidebook.*

Cleansing means that specific healing foods are consumed along with flushing or purging natural remedies or herbs to remove built-up toxins in the body that interfere with good health. There are full body cleanses and cleanses for the liver, colon and other specific organs. One can do a food cleanse, a toxin-purging cleanse, a parasite cleanse, an anti-viral cleanse, a cleanse for a specific disease and many more, including some with dual or multiple purposes.

Some cleanses require enemas, or colonics, but many do not. Sometimes digestive teas and/or laxatives are required and sometimes these come with package cleansing kits and the provided amounts need to be reduced for some individuals. If you use a package cleanse or specific cleansing program, *follow the directions given.* If you do not use the cleanse as recommended, digestive problems or illness could follow for even six months or a year later! Do not do more than one cleanse at a time unless your holistic doctor recommends a particular combination for your specific needs, and monitors your progress. Multiple cleanses can be dangerous, even life-threatening in some instances! Pregnant women cannot cleanse!

It is usually acceptable to eat two to three meals a day, plus snacks, and still do a very beneficial cleansing. The Phase II and Phase III diets described in my *Complete Candida Yeast Guidebook* contain particularly healthful foods suitable for most cleanses, unless you are doing a package cleanse with specific diet instructions. If you are purging too deeply during a cleanse, increase your food intake to lessen the intensity of the cleanse. If you feel you are not cleansing enough, eat less food for deeper purging of toxins.

A cleanse can last from 24 hours to 90 days, or on rare occasions (for a very mild cleanse) even longer. Most common cleanses last between 10 and 30 days. Generally, it is best to limit cleansing to a maximum of 90 days total per year except in special circumstances, such as cleansing as a cancer therapy or for specific chronic diseases.

During most cleanses, you cannot consume drugs (pleasure or medicinal), drink alcohol, or smoke anything. One drink (or cigarette) can have a tenfold effect on the body while cleansing.

Some food cleanses are described under Toxin Overload in the "Ailments and Remedies" section. For other types of cleansing, refer to the same section under Viruses or Parasites or see the "Natural Remedies Glossary." Additional information can be found in Cleansing and Fasting Books listed under "Recommended Reading." *Important:* It is safer and generally more beneficial to get advice from your holistic physician before beginning any cleanse beyond a change of diet or simple food cleanses, especially if you are sensitive or have severe health problems.

Health food stores are full of cleansing products and kits, however, it is best to get authoritative advice from your holistic doctor or a cleansing expert rather than from most salespersons. Some are quite knowledgeable while many are not and just try to sell products.

Chiropractic
This is a drugless healing art that can help to heal the body and boost energy levels through adjustment of the spinal column. Chiropractic, or spinal manipulation, is based on the principle that the major cause of disease is disturbance in the balance between "activating" and "inhibiting" nerve impulses transmitted to affected body areas. The spine and other body parts can be adjusted or manipulated to remove interference of nerve impulses that weaken the body by inhibiting the flow of natural energy currents or "life force" in the body. Regular chiropractic adjustments can increase energy levels and minimize unpleasant symptoms while healing a health problem. I highly recommend it for most individuals. Choose a chiropractor carefully: find one who meets your personal needs and whose style of adjusting works well for you. As with all professions, quality of care varies widely, as do the benefits.

An expert Vancouver chiropractor, Dr. Aaron Hoy, says, "Chiropractic health care is a branch of the natural healing arts. Its premise is based on academics, philosophy, art form and technique. Once a diagnosis is made, the treatment given can be a combination of the following: Chiropractic manipulation, soft and deep tissue techniques, exercise, ergonomic and nutritional counseling. Chiropractic stimulates the nervous system and helps direct the body's natural response to heal and maintain itself."

Colonics

Colonic irrigation is a process of flushing the colon with water and, sometimes, added herbs or other cleansing substances. This requires a colon expert who flushes water up the rectum into the colon to clean impacted fecal matter out of the body while gently massaging the abdomen. This treatment process needs to be done by an expert—a qualified colon specialist. This can be very beneficial for people with severe bowel problems. For some individuals, proper use of colonics can stimulate energy, relieve some allergies and help to clear the complexion. The practice should not be abused. The colon can be damaged by excessive use of this practice. Not everyone requires colonics. For more detailed information, see David Webster's book *Achieve Maximum Health*. Ask your holistic doctor for more information—though note that some doctors abhor the practice while others endorse it.

Deep Breathing

Breathing is essential for human life. Many people breathe too shallowly, which can lead to lower energy levels and increase health problems. Give yourself "oxygen therapy" treatments by practicing deep-breathing techniques. Everyone can practice simple breathing techniques that work wonderfully to increase energy and help reduce the side effects of allergies, cleansing, Candida and parasite treatments and other health problems. Some techniques are explained here.

PRANIC BREATHING Lie down or sit in a chair or sit cross-legged with a straight spine. Put one hand on your stomach and one on your chest so you can feel them rising and falling, until you learn how to do it correctly; then your hands can be at your sides or in your lap. Take in a deep, s-l-o-w breath through the nose; let the stomach push out a bit. Continue breathing in until you feel the chest rising, too. Take in as much air as you possibly can without straining or forcing. Breathe in very slowly and deeply, never quickly! Now reverse the process by slowly exhaling, first feeling the chest drop and then feeling the stomach area retract a little. Do a second breath the same way in and out. Continue and take at least eight slow deep breaths. Build up over time until you can do 5 or 10 minutes of pranic breathing (don't exceed 10 minutes). Practice at least once a day, or any time you are overstressed, upset, low in energy, spacy, overtired or anxious, or when you just need to relax and let go.

This technique helps you to digest food, by gently massaging your insides and moving digestive organs in a way that stimulates digestion. It will not cure indigestion, but it can help if done 30 or 60 minutes after eating. Do not do pranic breathing right after eating or before sleeping (see *Sleep-Enhancing Breathing* below).

SLEEP-ENHANCING BREATHING   Follow this technique while lying in bed, just before sleeping. Follow the directions for pranic breathing (above), but with one difference: exhale through the mouth. This can relax you and help bring on restful sleep. Take only 5 to 10 deep breaths—no more—because too much deep breathing will keep you awake. Start with five breaths until you are accustomed to this many, and then increase to 10 if it works for you. Remember to breathe slowly and deeply.

Many other types of deep breathing can be beneficial, but these methods should be taught to you personally, by a professional. Attend a beginners' Hatha yoga class, a low-key Iyengar yoga class or a yoga class that stresses gentle, easy breathing rather than fast, pushed or forced techniques. Make sure your teacher is qualified.

Dehumidifier

Damp, cold weather or damp rooms or basement apartments can contribute greatly to breathing problems, allergies, Candida and other health problems. If you live in a damp climate, buying a dehumidifier can be a wise investment in your health, as it will remove excess water from the air.

Bacteria and parasites breed in damp places. They usually perish in climates with hot dry air. This does not mean you should turn the heat on high and leave it there; that would create another set of problems and could be damaging. But try these strategies: If you are sleeping in the basement of a house, move your bedroom upstairs. Make sure towels are thoroughly dry before you use them, and the same before wearing clothes. And keep yourself warm and dry, especially when down with a cold, sore throat, flu or Candida or when experiencing other health problems.

Diet and Nutrition
A healthful diet and supplements are essential to boost the immune system and promote healing. One of the main messages of this book is to eat correctly and take proper supplements and remedies as needed. See "Recommended Reading" for information on my cookbooks and others on proper diet and recipes.

Ear Candling (Coning)
Wax, bacteria and Candida can collect in the ear canals. You would be amazed to see the amount of white, cottage cheese-like material that can clog the ears, in addition to earwax. If you want to try ear candling, find someone with experience and references to give you a treatment. A special type of hollow beeswax or paraffin candle is lit and placed in each ear in turn. The practitioner holds and trims the upper candle while it draws the aforementioned toxins out of the ear canals. When the candle burns down to a few inches it is removed and the inner contents can be examined to reveal the toxins removed. Some people advocate weekly treatments forever, but I disagree. In taking proper care of your health, one session a year (or less, as needed) should be adequate for the average person (unless your health problems are severe). Some healthy individuals may never require ear candling. Some holistic doctors discount this treatment; others think it is beneficial.

Emotional Support
As warm-blooded mammals, we humans require love and affection for optimum well-being and good health. Health problems may increase when we lose a loving relationship with a mate or family member, or if a major personal relationship in our lives alters significantly. When under the weather, it is helpful to have the love and support of a mate, family, and/or other intimate friends. It helps to have regular patterns of daily activities that allow you to keep yourself grounded and secure. Surround yourself with stable conditions, friends, and family.

Enemas
Enema/hot water bottles can be purchased at any drug store. Enemas are only recommended, on rare occasions, for some severe

bowel problems—mainly chronic constipation. Usually, other remedies for constipation are preferable. Consult your holistic doctor before considering doing an enema or wait until your doctor suggests one, if needed.

Fill the enema bag with warm (not hot) water with added herbs or special cleansing products recommended by your doctor or colon specialist, and hang it upside down with a hanger, hook or wire from a high point, usually a shower curtain rod or showerhead. Lie back in the bathtub and insert the tube tip attachment into the rectum. Open the release plug and allow the water to flow in. Hold it in for several minutes or more, as directed by your physician or internal cleansing product instructions (some advocates suggest massaging the abdomen and standing while jumping up and down a little to make the cleansing more effective), and then release it into the toilet. This process may be repeated occasionally, as required. The enema bag and tube need to be boiled between uses. It is best to boil them right after use as well as right before use, to kill bacteria that could lead to infection.

Do not overuse this practice! Enemas are not for everyone. Do not use enemas if you have a bowel disease or infection, and consult your doctor before doing an enema or more information. Other options may be preferable to enemas, such as colonics or (oral) herbal cleanses.

Exercise

Everyone requires exercise. Some people avoid exercise when they do not feel well, but this slows down the healing process. The body needs stimulation to heal effectively. Even bedridden individuals can exercise by moving different body parts slightly and tensing and relaxing them. (See *Strengthening Techniques*.)

Exercise must be done daily for optimum health. It does not have to be strenuous. At least take one 15-minute walk daily or ride a bike at a casual pace. Indoor stationary bicycles, walking machines, rowing machines and other exercise equipment are also options. It is best to exercise for at least 30 minutes; this may be broken into two 15-minute segments. If you are accustomed to more exercise, do it. Only minimums are stated here. An absolute minimum of 15 minutes per day is required for optimum health. Yoga, tai chi and swimming are other forms of easy but extremely beneficial exercise, if done in moderation. Do not remain sedentary all day and exercise at night; it may energize you so much that it keeps you awake for much of the night.

Fasting

Fasting gives the body, and especially the digestive organs, a rest from the constant work of processing foods. It increases energy and longevity and helps the body to heal.

To some people, fasting means only drinking water for 24 hours, from sun up one day to sun up—or longer, the following day. Actually, one can fast on vegetable juices, fruit juices, vegetables and/or fruits. For beginners, it is best not to fast completely on liquids. (This means that cleansing is easier for novices, because food—including regular meals—can be eaten while cleansing.) It is best to choose fruits or vegetables for a one-day (or longer) fast.

The fruit fast is easiest. One can fast on many fruits or choose just one for healing purposes. Do not make fruit salads! Chew all veggies and fruits slowly and thoroughly. Choose organic produce whenever possible. Eat two to three balanced, wholesome meals the day before a fast and the day after, and avoid meat in these meals. If you eat less than normal the day before a fast, the fast will be easier. (If you have my *Complete Candida Yeast Guidebook*, eat foods from the Phase II diet the days before and after the fast.)

One cannot smoke—at all—or drink alcohol for three days before or after a one-day fast. Avoid alcohol for longer (seven days or more before and after) for a longer fast. For more complete fasting information, see my book *For the Love of Food: The Complete Natural Foods Cookbook.*

Pleasure drugs cannot be taken by a person, at all, if they intend to fast!

Important: Prescription drugs cannot be taken while fruit fasting but can be taken with the specific vegetable fast that follows.

THE MONO FRUIT FAST

1. Drink lots of tested spring water—a minimum of eight glasses a day while fasting, and preferably more.

2. Choose one type of fruit to fast on: 1. watermelon,
   2. bananas (not too ripe, with a little green on one end),
   3. apple juice and peeled and cored apples, 4. peach juice
   and fresh peaches (in season) or 5. pear juice and fresh,
   tender pears (in season). These are the best fasting fruits.
3. Choose organic fruit and fruit juices whenever possible.
4. Drink juices at least one hour away from eating solid
   fruits. Sip juices slowly and chew fruit thoroughly!
5. You can eat as much fruit as you like, within reason, but
   limit juices to two to four glasses per day.
6. Avoid fruit juices close to bedtime. If possible, solid fruit
   should be eaten no closer than an hour or two before bed.

THE MIXED FRUIT FAST

1. Follow the main guidelines for the mono fruit fast.
2. Eat only one type of fruit (one or more pieces) at a time,
   leaving at least an hour between eating different fruits.
3. Stick to only one type of juice, if drinking juice, per day.

THE VEGETABLE FAST

(Can be done while taking prescription drugs for cancer or other
health concerns.)

1. Drink at least four to eight glasses of tested spring water
   during the day, away from meals. Drink more in hot
   weather. Sip and drink slowly.
2. For breakfast, eat a plate of steamed carrots, orange yams,
   or baked winter squash (no butter or seasonings).
   (Squash can also be boiled whole.) Or if preferred, drink
   one glass of mixed vegetable juice, including mainly
   carrots, plus add a small or medium fresh beet, and one-
   quarter to half a teaspoon of a single green food powder
   (or add a sprig of parsley, a celery stalk, a cabbage wedge,
   a handful of spinach or other green veggie instead of the
   green food). If you have bowel problems, have very
   tender cooked vegetables, not the juice.
3. For a snack, if desired, eat half a red bell pepper, a carrot
   stick, half an avocado, or grated beet with lemon juice.
   Or, if you did not have juice for breakfast, you can have

it now. If you have bowel problems, you can have the veggie juice now, or the avocado.*

4. For lunch, eat a plate of between one and three types of steamed vegetables. Include a green veggie (such as asparagus, broccoli, Brussels sprouts, cooked greens, kohlrabi or zucchini). If you are eating two or three, add an orange veggie such as carrots, yam or squash. For a third vegetable, add either another green veggie or cauliflower, turnips or parsnips. Eat a satisfying amount. For those who do not have bowel problems, a salad of grated zucchini/carrot/beet and optional peeled, grated kohlrabi may be had instead. Chew the salad to liquid before swallowing! The salad may be sprinkled with fresh lemon, lime or grapefruit juice for better digestion, nothing else! Always steam vegetables very tender.

5. Repeat the snack above, if desired.*

6. For supper, repeat lunch, but do not eat raw vegetables.

7. For a final snack, if desired, eat half an avocado, one cup or so of steamed orange vegetable or, if you have not already had two glasses of juice, you could have one now.*

8. Chew all foods to liquid. Swish juices around the mouth, and take 20 minutes to drink each glass. Drink and eat slowly.

9. Eat all the foods suggested for meals here (and hopefully snacks, too), especially if taking medication.

Important: People with bowel problems should eat no solid raw vegetables except raw avocado.

*One (only) of the snacks may be replaced by a steamed artichoke, dipped if you choose in fresh lemon, lime or grapefruit juice. Skip the juice dip if eating the artichoke at night. (See recipes.)

Foot Bath
Soak the feet and ankles in a tub of hot or very warm water with Epsom salts or a herbal tincture of one of the following: 1. chamomile, comfrey and an optional dash or two of cayenne;

2. ginger, peppermint and optional skullcap or catnip; 3. tea tree oil (several shakes or ¼–½ teaspoon). Other natural remedies or herbal astringents and soothing herbs can also be used instead. Health stores carry several natural products for foot soaking.

Fresh Air

Get country-fresh, mountain, seaside or ocean air whenever possible. Avoid polluted areas, smoky rooms, strong-smelling cleaning products, dusty or musty rooms, strong or offensive perfumes or colognes, and anything that smells offensive to you or aggravates you and interferes with your health. (See *Air Purifier*.)

Hot and Cold Packs

A hot water bottle (or well-padded heating pad) can be used on body parts that are especially sore or agitated, to relax and stimulate them. Heat treatments are even more effective if rotated with cold packs. A bag of frozen peas wrapped in a thin dish towel is the perfect ice pack. It is flexible enough to mold to different body parts and not *as freezing as a solid block of ice*. The cold pack improves circulation by forcing blood to the cold area. Apply heat first, for 5 to 15 minutes, and then alternate with cold for about the same length of time or a little less. Try two to four rotations. For severe inflammations, consult your doctor before using hot treatments. See Sprains and Strains in the "Ailments and Remedies" section.

Laughter and Play

If you want to stay (or become) healthy, learn to laugh! They say: "Laughter is the best medicine." This is definitely true. Read Norman Cousins's *Anatomy of an Illness*. He used funny movies and comedy shows to laugh his way back to health. A good belly laugh stimulates all your major organs like a wonderful massage. Laughter also helps to raise your energy levels. "Laugh and the world laughs with you," said poet Ella Wheeler Wilcox.

Play is just as essential. Go to the park or beach with your children, or borrow someone else's children. They know how to play. Roll down a grassy hill, tickle someone—just a little—or let them tickle you. Play a game, fly a kite, cuddle a teddy bear, gently and lovingly tease someone or be teased. Forget to be serious for a while.

I decree at least 15 minutes a day of pure fun and play. Choose your favorite toy and let the games begin!

Massage

A massage can help to relax you, strengthen and tone the body, enhance circulation, stimulate organ functions, and help to move poisons out of the body. Thirty to sixty minutes or more once or twice a week is ideal, however, even twice a month is much better than nothing. Make sure that the masseur or masseuse does not use overly aggressive techniques, or your body may be stimulated to release more stored poisons than it can handle removing at a time. Too many massages, or massages that are too long, can have the same result. Massage is a wonderful aid for reducing body pressures, aches and tension. Used wisely, it will help to speed healing and make a treatment process more pleasant. Avoid massages during viral infections and avoid having infected areas massaged, because it may stimulate and aggravate the infection.

Meditation

Meditation is a great way to relax and reduce stress if practiced in moderation. Meditating daily or a few times times a week, for 5 to 15 minutes a time, is ideal. There is no need to overdo it. Lengthy meditation has proved distressing to inexperienced meditators, but short periods of meditation can benefit almost anyone. There are thousands of ways to meditate. Anything that brings you a relaxed, peaceful feeling of serenity qualifies as a meditation technique, according to the foremost teachers of the art. A contented walk at sunset or a relaxing, quiet bath can be called meditating if done serenely. Or you can sit quietly in a chair or cross-legged with the spine straight and employ one of many concentration techniques. The main purpose is to lead you to that "ah" place of serenity. The "ah" state of mind is what meditation is about. It may last a few seconds or longer. Just let go. For the moment, allow nothing to affect you and feel content, serene. This is true meditation.

Try reading positive, inspiring books and then reflect on them. Repeating positive statements, like "I am healthy, happy and wonderful," is another technique. See one of the many books on the subject, especially *How to Meditate* by Lawrence LeShan, for a practical approach to meditation that almost anyone can enjoy. The main reason for meditating: It makes you feel good! And feeling good helps you maintain good health.

Oral Hygiene

See *Oral Hygiene Problems* in "Ailments and Remedies" section for how to take good care of teeth, gums and mouth.

Positive Thinking

You are what you think. To be healthy or to increase healing, you have to want to be healthy and to see yourself that way. Depression lowers healing capabilities. Keep positive and support yourself by surrounding yourself with supportive ideas and people.

Rest

Most people need seven or eight hours of sleep each night. Too much sleep makes you groggy and keeps your energy low and may interfere with the quality of sleep you get. Too little can make you hyperactive, punchy, agitated and argumentative. If you nap in the daytime, you will generally need less sleep at night. Some people who take naps have trouble sleeping at night if they are not active enough during the day.

Every hour you sleep before midnight can be more beneficial to you and this sleep is often of better quality than the sleep you get after midnight.

Each body is different; you must find your own healthful rhythm. If you are the overactive type, take time during the day to slow down, relax and do nothing—or read a book or watch TV. If you are the inactive type, make yourself take walks, work, do household chores, arts and crafts, garden or cook. If you do not sleep well, you cannot digest your food. If you do not digest your food well, you cannot sleep. This can be a vicious circle for some individuals, especially those with allergies, chronic fatigue, blood sugar problems, Candida and other health concerns. The cycle must be broken in order to heal or to maintain optimum health.

Sauna, Dry

A dry sauna helps to eliminate internal body poisons or toxins, including pesticides, preservatives and heavy metals, through the skin, and can help reduce the pressures of cleansing or healing some health concerns. A good sweat flushes and cleanses the body, speeds up the metabolism, and kills harmful bacteria and some viruses. It helps speed healing and increases immune response. Dry saunas, wet saunas or steam baths are extremely beneficial, especially if you have one between four and six times a month. A dry sauna is best if it lasts for 30 minutes or more. (See *Sauna, Wet.*)

Sauna, Wet

In a wet sauna, water is usually poured on hot rocks to create steam at self-regulated intervals. The steam helps to cleanse the body in about half the time of a dry sauna, with most of the same benefits. After either dry or wet sauna (or halfway through), it is beneficial to soap off toxins from the skin and end with a cold shower—or, if possible, a roll in the snow, as is traditional in Finland where saunas originated. No, you won't freeze! A 15-minute or longer hot sauna usually keeps your body hot, even in snow, for up to 30 minutes afterwards.

A steam bath is like a wet sauna, only the steam is continuous and not produced by pouring water on hot rocks. Temperatures vary.

Self-Burping

Babies require burping, because they are new to digesting foods. If your digestion is sluggish or hindered for any reason, you may need a kick-start with digestive aids, self-massage (see below) or self-burping. How do you burp an adult? You do not want someone else to do it for you, once you reach a certain age. This special technique makes it easy to burp yourself. With the flat palm of your hand, strike yourself quite briskly and solidly in the middle of the sternum or chest plate, one or two inches below the collarbone, just above the breast. Give yourself about seven good whacks. Repeat the seven whacks one to four times, pausing between each set. If done correctly, you will cause no hurt whatsoever and will likely find yourself giving a few healthy burps that will ease digestion and stimulate energy to the digestive tract. This technique can be used as many times daily as desired, within reason. Usually, one to three times per day is enough.

Self-Massage

When no one else is around to do it for you, self-massage is an effective release of body pressure and tensions, especially on the head or neck (to help reduce headache symptoms) and around the digestive tract, liver, gall bladder, spleen and colon (to assist digestion).

No special techniques are required. Just use your hand to knead the skin around these areas, gently at first, then more deeply as you proceed. It is a good idea to wait at least 30 minutes after a meal before doing this on the digestive tract—and do not press too hard if you have eaten within the last two hours. Knead, rub, press, stroke and jiggle with the fingertips for 2 or 3 minutes, up to 10, or until you feel some benefit and release. This is a simple, yet powerful and effective, technique for self-healing. Do it one to three times a day or as needed. As always, do not overdo it.

Shower Filter

This wonderful gadget can remove chlorine, lead, copper, asbestos, iron, algae and other contaminants from your shower water and can also be used to fill the bath. (Also, if you have soft water, it often eats away at pipes, usually made of copper and soldered with lead, adding more of these toxic metals to the water.) Pollutants can easily enter through the skin during a long, hot shower. Sensitive people may experience slight faintness or dizziness from the chlorine. Even healthy individuals are affected by chlorine and other heavy metals; although it may only be slightly, there is a build-up over time. For between $15 and $40 a small, easily installed shower filter cylinder can be purchased and will provide between 6 and 12 months of pure showers, depending on how much you use it. Shower flow decreases when the filter is old, so it's easy to know when to replace it. If you prefer to filter the entire household's water, almost all major water filter companies have small to large household units at varying prices.

Sitz Baths

This partial bath is an effective way to stimulate and increase circulation in the genital area or pelvic region. It is a good way to kill bacteria and cleanse and soothe these areas with herbal remedies. The best time for a sitz bath is during the day—do not take one too close to bedtime, as it may be too stimulating.

Fill a very large, preferably metal or enamel, bowl—or partially fill a bathtub—with enough hot water (about 103 to 110°F) to cover the hips completely. Add a healing remedy to the water. Choose one suggested for your health concern or, for healing, use several drops of 100 percent pure tea tree oil or several drops of oil of oregano; for cleansing, dissolve half a cup of Epsom salts in the water; for soothing, add to the bath half a cup chamomile herbal tea (use the dried flowers, not powdered tea or tea bags) steeped in a quart (about a litre) of water dispersed in the bath. Sit in the bath for at least 20 minutes, covering your shoulders with a towel. Add hot water as needed to keep the temperature right. Follow the bath with a hot-cold shower if possible, and rest for a while afterwards.

Skin Cleansing

While taking remedies of any kind, or while cleansing (including Candida and parasite treatment), it is imperative that poisons exit the body speedily to avoid digestive problems, constipation or blockages that will slow or impede the healing process. There are many ways to remove toxins from the skin's pores. They include saunas, steam baths, Epsom salt baths, hot-cold showers, dry brushing, wet brushing, using a loofah, and the "scrape" method. You should use one of the last four methods, even if you employ one or more of the other methods.

DRY BRUSHING Special natural bristle brushes can be purchased at health stores and some pharmacies to help brush off dead skin that may clog pores. It is best to do this all over the body (follow the instructions that come with the brush or ask a health specialist). Some people use a dry brush while walking around the house, which allows dry skin to fall all over and feed dust mites, and other microscopic bugs and bacteria. However, this method should be done standing in a bathtub before showering in the morning (not at night, or the body may get over stimulated too close to bedtime).

WET BRUSHING The same type of brush can also be used for wet brushing in the shower; however, if you want to do both, use one brush for dry use only and a separate brush for wet use.

LOOFAH CLEANSING The third way of skin brushing is by using a loofah sponge, softened by hot water in the shower or bath, to scrub away dead skin and toxins. Get one at any health food store, corner drugstore and most bath shops.

SCRAPE CLEANSING The fourth method of cleansing the skin requires only that your fingernails are not too jagged. Use the nails to scratch or "scrape" off dead skin and toxins wherever you feel a buildup (all over the body, including the face) while showering or bathing.

Using one of these four skin "scrubbing" methods regularly gives the skin a healthy, youthful glow and appearance.

Steam Bath
See *Sauna, Wet*

Strengthening Techniques (Tensing and Relaxing)
The tensing and releasing method of strengthening and relaxing muscles is often taught in yoga classes. It is a powerful yet gentle way of exercising that can be used as a way to relax and release tension. Or, if you are too tired for traditional exercise or are bedridden, this technique provides easy, beneficial stimulation for the entire body.

Lie down on a comfortable bed, sofa or mat and place the feet a foot or two apart, arms at your sides, palms slightly turned up and head centered. Start with the toes and feet: squeeze them up tightly for 5 to 10 seconds, then release and wiggle them around, and let them come to rest. Repeat the tensing-relaxing process with both legs. Then repeat with the buttocks. Next, take in a deep breath and push your stomach out like a balloon. Hold the air in for 10 to 15 seconds, then release with a big gush through your mouth. Take another deep breath and this time push out the chest, hold 10 to 15 seconds, and release in one gush through the mouth again. Next, tense the shoulders for 5 to 10 seconds, shrug them a few times and relax. Then both hands and then both arms: tense, wiggle, relax. Last, squeeze the whole face and head as if you are trying to squeeze them into a tight knot on your nose and release. Finally, roll the head, wiggle the face and relax.

Sometimes these tensing and relaxing exercises help to induce sleep. If you cannot or will not do any other kind of exercise, do this twice a day. This technique can also be done in addition to regular exercise. It helps to stimulate body organs, helps circulation, and tones the body internally and externally. It is a fantastic healing aid or beneficial technique, even for healthy individuals.

Sunshine

Even in winter, a little sunshine is a good thing. Do not overdo the sun, but when possible get at least 15 minutes of exposure a day in the summer (it is beneficial, provided you are protected so you do not burn); try to get 30 minutes or more in the winter. Even in winter you can take a walk on sunny days, or sit on a sunny porch when the weather allows. The sun is a natural healer (providing beneficial vitamin D) and an energizer when used correctly. Sun tanning may be beneficial to some and not to others. Get only as much sun as is beneficial for your body type. Consult your doctor if necessary. Avoid the sun if it harms you.

Tai Chi, Qi Gong, Yoga and Martial Arts

It is extremely beneficial to practice one of these disciplines throughout your life. The benefits of all are similar. They provide a gentle stretch of all major body parts and muscles, and they strengthen muscles in ways that most types of vigorous exercise cannot. They give the body and the senses endurance, stamina, vitality and strength. Practiced regularly, they can help to slow the aging process and keep you flexible and well toned. Any of these practices can help increase physical energy, improve mental clarity, and help create excellent muscle and skin tone. Find a class in Hatha or Iyengar yoga, tai chi, qi gong—or a variation—taught by a qualified teacher. Practicing 3 to 6 times a week for even 10 to 30 minutes brings favorable results.

RECOMMENDED READING AND BIBLIOGRAPHY

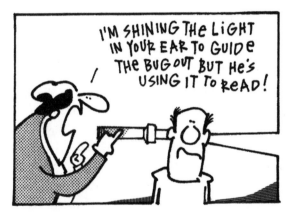

Nutrition, Supplement and Healing Books

Alternative Medicine—The Definitive Guide, compiled by the Burton
Goldberg Group, Future Medicine Publishing, Inc.
ISBN: 0-9636334-3-0

Diet and Nutrition: A Holistic Approach, Rudolph Ballentine, M.D.,
Himalayan International Institute. ISBN: 0-89389-048-0

Eat Right for Your Type, Dr. Peter J. D'Adamo with Catherine Whitney,
G.P. Putnam's Sons. ISBN: 0-399-14255-X

Encyclopedia of Natural Medicine, Michael T. Murray, N.D. and Joseph
Pizzorno, N.D., Prima Publishing. ISBN: 0-7615-1157-1

Encyclopedia of Nutritional Supplements, Michael T. Murray, N.D.,
Prima Publishing. ISBN: 0-7615-0410-9

Foods That Heal, Maureen Salaman and James F. Scheer, Statford Publishing. ISBN: 0-913087-02-5

Healthy Healing, Linda Rector Page, N.D., Healthy Healing Publications. ISBN: 0-912331-21-6

The Miracle of MSM, Stanley W. Jacob, M.D., Ronald M. Lawrence, M.D. and Martin Zucker, The Berkley Publishing Group. ISBN 0-425-17265-1

Natural First Aid Remedies From A to Z, James Kusick, Parker Publishing Co. ISBN: 0-13-063181-7

The Natural Pharmacy, Schuyler W. Lininger Jr., D.C., Alan R. Gaby, M.D., Steve Austin, N.D., Donald J. Brown, N.D., Jonathan V. Wright, M.D. and Alice Duncan, D.C., C.C.H. Prima Publishing. ISBN: 0-7615-1967-X

Nature's Virus Killers, Mark Strengler, N.D. with Arden Moore, M. Evans and Company, Inc. ISBN: 0-87131-898-9

The New Nutrition, Dr. Michael Colgan, Apple Publishing. ISBN: 0-9695272-4-1

Nutrition Almanac, Gayla J. Kirschmann and John D. Kirschmann, McGraw-Hill Publishing Co. ISBN: 0-07-034922-3

Prescription for Nutritional Healing, Phyllis A. Balch, CNC and James F. Balch, M.D., Avery Books. ISBN: 1-58333-077-1

Return to the Joy of Health, Zoltan P. Rona, M.D. and Jeanne Marie Martin, alive books. ISBN: 0-920470-62-9

Vitamin Bible, Earl Mindell, Warner Books. ISBN: 0-446-30626-6

Herb Books

Back to Eden, Jethro Kloss, Back to Eden Books. ISBN: 0-940676-001

Capsicum, Dr. John R. Christopher, Christopher Publications, P.O. Box 412, Springville, Utah 84663, U.S.A.

Chicken Soup and Other Folk Remedies, Joan Wilen and Lydia Wilen, Fawcett Columbine. ISBN: 0-449-90190-4

The Cure Is in the Cupboard, Dr. Cass Ingram, Knowledge House. ISBN: 0-911119-74-4 (book on oil of oregano)

The Essiac Report, Richard Thomas, Alternative Treatment Information Network. ISBN: 0-9639818-0-3

Feverfew, Ken Hancock, Keats Publishing. ISBN: 0-87983-798-5

Fighting Infections with Herbs, Linda Rector Page, N.D., Healthy Healing Publications. ISBN: 1-884334-29-6

Handbook of Bach Flower Remedies, Philip M. Chancellor, C. W. Daniel Company Ltd. ISBN: 0-85207-002-0

The Healing Power of Herbs, Michael T. Murray, N.D., Prima Publishing. ISBN: 1-55958-700-8

Healing Yourself, Joy Gardner, Snohomish Publishing Co. ISBN: 0-9601688-2-6

The Herb Book, John Lust, Bantam Books. ISBN: 0-553-23827-2

Herbal Aphrodisiacs, compiled by Clarence Meyer, Meyerbooks. ISBN: 0-916638-09-X

Herbal Love Potions, William H. Lee, D.Sc. and Lynn Lee, C.N., Keats Publishing, Inc. ISBN: 0-87983-544-3

The Herbalist, Joseph E. Meyer, Meyer Books. ISBN: 0-916638-00-6

Herbs to Relieve Stress, David Hoffman, Keats Publishing. ISBN: 0-87983-758-6

Indian Herbalogy of North America, Alma Hutchens, Merco, 620 Wyandotte East, Windsor, Ontario.

The New Age Herbalist, Richard Mabey, Collier Books. ISBN: 0-02-063350-5

Olive Leaf Extract, Dr. Morton Walker, Kensington Books. ISBN: 1-57566-226-4

Pau d'Arco, Immune Power from the Rain Forest, Kenneth Jones, Healing Arts Press. ISBN: 0-89281-497-7

St. John's Wort, C. M. Hawken, Woodland Publishing. ISBN: 1-58054-009-0

School of Natural Healing, Dr. John R. Christopher, BiWorld Publishers, Inc., P.O. Box 62, Provo, Utah 84601, U.S.A.

The Tea Tree Oil Bible, Doctors: Ali, Grant, Nakla, Patel, Vegotsky, Ages Publications. ISBN: 1-886508-10-1

Guides to Healing with Wholesome Foods

Colostrum—Life's First Food, Daniel G. Clark, M.D. and Kaye Wyatt, CNR Publications, 4700 South 900 East, Suite 30-257, Salt Lake City, Utah 84117, U.S.A.

Foods and Healing, Annemarie Colbin, Ballantine Books. ISBN: 0-345-30385-7

Foods That Heal, Bernard Jensen, Avery Publishing Group. ISBN: 0-89529-563-3

Fresh Food, Sylvia Rosenthal, Tree Communications.
  ISBN: 0-87690-276-X

The Guide to Natural and Healthy Eating, Renee Frappier, Les Editions
  Asclepiades Inc. ISBN: 2-9801115-3-8

The Healing Foods, Patricia Hausman and Judith Benn Hurley, Dell
  Publishing. ISBN: 0-440-21440-8

Miracle Medicine Foods, Rex Adams, Parker Publishing, Inc.
  ISBN: 0-13-58529-563-3

Natural Prozac, Dr. Joel Robertson with Tom Monte, Harper San
  Francisco. ISBN: 0-06-251354-0

Potatoes Not Prozac, Kathleen DesMaisons, Ph.D., Simon & Schuster.
  ISBN: 0-684-84953-4

The Safe Shopper's Bible, David Steinman and Samuel S. Epstein, M.D.,
  Macmillan Publishing. ISBN: 0-02-082085-2

Shopper's Guide to Natural Foods, East West Journal Editors, Avery
  Publishing Group, Inc. ISBN: 0-89529-233-5

The Wellness Encyclopedia of Food and Nutrition, Sheldon Margen, M.D.
  Random House. ISBN: 0-929661-03-6

Whole Food Facts, Evelyn Roehl, Healing Arts Press. ISBN: 0-89281-231-1

Food, Additive and Drug Guidebooks

A–Z Guide to Drug–Herb–Vitamin Interactions, Schuyler W. Lininger Jr.,
  D.C., Alan R. Gaby, M.D., Steve Austin, N.D., Forrest Batz,
  PharmD., Eric Yarnell, N.D., Donald J. Brown, N.D., George
  Constantine, R.Ph., Ph.D., Prima Publishing. ISBN: 0-7615-1599-2

Consumer's Dictionary of Food Additives, Ruth Winter, Crown
  Publishers, Inc. ISBN: 0-517-531615

Deadly Drug Interaction—The People's Pharmacy, Joe Graedon and
  Teresa Graedon, Ph.D., St. Martin's Griffin. ISBN: 0-312-15510-7

Empty Harvest, Bernard Jensen and Mark Anderson, Avery Publishing
  Group. ISBN: 0-89529-416-8

The Food and Drug Interaction Guide, Dr. Brian L.G. Morgan, Simon
  & Schuster. ISBN: 0-671-61776-1

Hard to Swallow, Doris Sarjeant and Karen Evans, alive books.
  ISBN: 0-920470-47-5

Natural Alternatives to Over-the-Counter and Prescription Drugs, Michael
  T. Murray, N.D., William Morrow & Company, Inc. ISBN: 0-
  688-12358-9

Safe Food, Michael F. Jacobson, Ph.D., Lisa Y. Lefferts and Anne Witte Garland, Living Planet Press. ISBN: 1-879326-01-9

Seasalt's Hidden Powers, Jacques de Langre, Ph.D., Happiness Press. ISBN: 0-916508-42-0

Juicing for Health
The Complete Raw Juice Therapy, Thorsons Editorial Board, Thorsons Publishing. ISBN: 0-7225-1877-3

Getting the Most Out of Your Juicer, William H. Lee, Ph.D., Keats Publishing. ISBN: 0-87983-586-9

Healing with Herbal Juices, Siegfried Gursche, alive books. ISBN: 0-920470-34-3

Chlorophyll and Green Foods
Cereal Grass—What's in It for You!, ed. Ronald L. Seibold, Wilderness Community Education Foundation. ISBN: 0-9628126-0-9

Chlorella, William Lee and Michael Rosenbaoum, Keats Publishing. ISBN: 0-87983464-1

Green Barley Essence, Yoshihide Hagiwara, M.D., Keats Publishing. ISBN: 0-87834-8-8

The Healing Power of Chlorophyll form Plant Life, Bernard Jensen, Bernard Jensen Books, Route 1, Box 52, Escondido, CA 92025, U.S.A.

Spirulina, Jack Joseph Challem, Keats Publishing. ISBN: 0-87983-262-2

The Wheatgrass Book, Ann Wigmore, Avery Publishing Group. ISBN: 0-89529-234-3

Fats And Oils
The Facts About Fats, John Finnegan, Elysian Arts Books. ISBN: 0-927425-12-2

Fats That Heal, Fats That Kill, Udo Erasmus, alive books. ISBN: 0-920470-40-8

Natural Food Cookbooks with Meat
Jeanne Marie Martin's Light Cuisine—Seafood and Poultry Recipes for Healthy Living, Harbour Publishing. ISBN: 1-55017-123-2

New York Times New Natural Foods Cookbook, Jean Hewitt, Avon Books. ISBN: 0-380-62687-X

Recipes from an Ecological Kitchen, Lorna J. Sass, William Morrow and Co., Inc. ISBN: 0-688-10051-1

Rodale's Basic Natural Foods Cookbook, Fireside Books/Simon & Schuster. ISBN: 0-671-67338-6

Vegetarian Cookbooks

For the Love of Food—The Complete Natural Food Cookbook, Jeanne Marie Martin, alive books. ISBN: 0-920470-70-X

Hearty Vegetarian Soups and Stews, Jeanne Marie Martin, Harbour Publishing. ISBN: 1-55017-050-3

Horn of the Moon Cookbook, Ginny Gallam, Harper Perennial. ISBN: 0-06-096038-8

The Moosewood Cookbook, Mollie Katzen, Ten Speed Press. ISBN: 0-89815-490-1

The New McDougall Cookbook, John A. McDougall and Mary McDougall, Dutton Books. ISBN: 0-525-93610-6

The Vegetarian Times Cookbook, The Editors of *Vegetarian Times*, Macmillan Publishing. ISBN: 0-02-010370-0

Vegan Cookbooks

(These cookbooks include recipes with no meat, dairy or animal products.)

Vegan Delights, Jeanne Marie Martin, Harbour Publishing. ISBN: 1-55017-079-1

Country Kitchen Collection, Silver Hills Guest House. ISBN: 0-88925-933-X

Simply Vegan, Deborah Wasserman and Reed Lazarus, Vegetarian Resource Group. ISBN: 093-141-105X

Vegan Vitality, Diane Hill, Thorsons Publishing. ISBN: 0-7225-1341-0

Allergy Cookbooks

All Natural Allergy Cookbook, Jeanne Marie Martin, Harbour Publishing. ISBN: 1-55017-044-9

Freedom from Allergy, Ron Greenberg, M.D. and Angela Nori, Gordon Soules Book Publishers. ISBN: 0-88925-905-4

The Self-Help Cookbook, Marjorie Hurt Jones, R.N., Rodale Press. ISBN: 0-87857-505-7

Candida Cookbooks and Information Books

Back To Health, Dennis W. Remington, M.D. and Barbara W. Higa, R.D., Vitality House International. ISBN: 0-912547-03-0

Complete Candida Yeast Guidebook, Jeanne Marie Martin and Zoltan Rona, M.D., Prima Publishing. ISBN: 0-7615-0167-3

The Yeast Connection, William G. Crook, M.D., Professional Books. ISBN: 0-933478-06-02

Men's Health

The Male Herbal, James Green, Herbalist, The Crossing Press. ISBN: 0-89594-458-8

Male Sexual Vitality, Michael T. Murray, Prima Publishing. ISBN: 1-55958-428-9

Sex for Life, The Lover's Guide to Male Sexuality, David Saul, M.D., Apple Publishing. ISBN: 1-896817-18-1

Super Nutrition for Men, Ann Louise Gittleman, M. Evans and Company, Inc. ISBN: 0-87131-793-1

Women's Health

Super Nutrition for Women, Ann Louise Gittleman, Bantam Books. ISBN: 0-553-35328-4

Take Charge of Your Body, Women's Health Advisor, Carolyn DeMarco, M.D., Well Women Press. ISBN: 0-9694766-1-2

Women's Bodies, Women's Wisdom, Christiane Northrup, M.D. ISBN: 0-553-37953-4

Books About Water

The Choice Is Clear, Dr. Allen E. Banik, Acres U.S.A. ISBN: 911-311-31-9

The Shocking Truth About Water, Paul C. Bragg, N.D., Ph.D., Health Science. ISBN: 0-87790-000-0

Water Can Undermine Your Health, Norman Walker, Ph.D., Norwalk Press. ISBN: 0-890-19-037-2

Water: Healer or Poison? Jan De Vries, Mainstream Publishers. ISBN: 1-85158-341-6

Sugar and Related Health Concerns

Breaking the Vicious Cycle (Food and the Gut Reaction), Elaine Gottshall, Kirkton. ISBN: 0-969-2768-1

Diabetes and Hypoglycemia, Michael T. Murray, N.D., Prima Publishing. ISBN: 55958-426-2

Sugar Blues, William Duffy, Warner Books. ISBN: 0-446-89288-2

Books About Intestinal Parasites

Guess What Came to Dinner, Ann Louise Gittleman, Avery Publishing Group. ISBN: 0-89529-570

Parasites—The Enemy Within, Hanna Kroeger, Ms.D., and Jerald Foote, Kroeger Products, 1122 Pearl Street, Boulder, CO 80302, U.S.A.

Cleansing and Fasting Books

Achieve Maximum Health, Colon Flora, David Webster, Hygeia Publishing. ISBN: 0-9647537-1-5

Colon Health: The Key to Vibrant Life, Norman W. Walker, Ph.D., Norwalk Press. ISBN: 0-89019-069-0

Detoxification, Linda Rector Page, N.D., Healthy Healing Publications. ISBN: 1-884334-54-7

Miracle of Fasting, Paul C. Bragg, Health Science Publishers. ISBN: 0-87790-002-7

How to Keep Slim, Healthy, and Young with Juice Fasting, Paavo Airola, Ph.D., Health Plus Publishers. ISBN: 0-932090-02-8

How to Lower Your Fat Thermostat, Dennis Remington, M.D., Garth Fisher, Ph.D. and Edward Parent, Ph.D., Vitality House International, Inc. ISBN: 0-912547-01-4

Inner Cleansing, Carson Wade, Parker Publishing Company. ISBN: 0-13-465575-3

Natural Detoxification, Jacqueline Krohn, M.D., Hartley & Marks. ISBN: 0-88179-127-X

Tissue Cleansing Through Bowel Management, Bernard Jensen and Sylvia Bell, Bernard Jensen Enterprises. ISBN: 0-960836-07-1

7-Day Detox Miracle, Peter Bennett, N.D. and Stephen Barrie, N.D., Prima Publishing. ISBN: 0-7615-1422-8

Oxygen and Ozone

O 2 Xygen Therapies / A New Way of Approaching Disease, Ed McCabe, Energy Publications. ISBN: 0-9620527-0-1

The Unmedical Miracle–Oxygen, Elizabeth Baker, Drelwood Communications. ISBN: 0-937766-12-7

Anti-Aging Books

Age Right, Karlis Ullis, M.D. with Greg Ptacek, Simon & Schuster. ISBN: 0-684-84197-5

Earl Mindell's Anti-Aging Bible, Earl Mindell, R.Ph., Ph.D., Simon & Schuster. ISBN: 0-684-81106-5

Eat Right Live Longer, Neal Barnard, N.D., Three Rivers Press. ISBN: 0-517-88778-9

Fifty & Fabulous, Zia Wesley-Hosford, Prima Publishing.
    ISBN: 0-7615-0446-X

Stop Aging Now!, Jean Carper, HarperCollins Publishers.
    ISBN: 0-06-098500-3

Homeopathic Remedy Books
The Consumer's Guide to Homeopathy, Dana Ullman, M.P.H., G.P.
    Putnam's Sons. ISBN: 0-87477-813-1

The Family Guide to Homeopathy, Dr. Andrew Lockie, Simon &
    Schuster. ISBN: 0-671-76771-2

The World Traveller's Manual of Homeopathy, Dr. Colin B. Lessell, The
    C.W. Daniel Company Limited. ISBN: 0-85207-330-5

Recommended Newsletters and Web Sites
Current Health News You Can Use, by Dr. Joseph Mercola, 1443 West
    Schaumburg, Schaumburg, Illinois, 60194, U.S.A. Phone:
    1-847-985-1777

Newsletter via e-mail: dr@mercola.com

Townsend Letter for Doctors & Patients, 911 Tyler Street, Pt. Townsend,
    Washington, 98368-6541, U.S.A. Fax: 1-360-385-0699

Web site: www.tldp.com; E-mail: tldp@olympus.net

Books by Jeanne Marie Martin are available from:
The Internet: amazon.com

In Canada from Health Management Books, Apple Publishing,
Harbour Publishing and alive books

In the U.S.A. from Nutri-Books, New Leaf Publishing Co.,
Bookpeople, Ingram Book Company, Partners West, and Integral Yoga
Distribution

Individuals can order books from their favourite bookstores or health
food stores, who can order from the above suppliers.

ABOUT THE AUTHOR

Jeanne Marie Martin, ClN, has studied herbalogy with Dr. John Christopher. She has been teaching natural cooking and nutrition in the natural health field for over 30 years. Jeanne Marie has owned and managed health food stores, worked as a wholesale herb and vitamin company sales representative, and is a clinical nutritionist who has worked with many doctors. She specializes in diets for: allergies, digestive and bowel problems, Candidiasis, parasites, chronic fatigue syndrome, viral infections, heavy metal overdose, blood sugar problems, cancer and weight problems.

In addition to nutritional consultations, Jeanne Marie currently teaches cooking and nutrition classes in British Columbia and Washington State. She has taught throughout North America, including six years for Scott Community College in the U.S., and for Langera College in Canada. Jeanne Marie is the author of over 300 magazine articles on natural cooking, nutrition and holistic lifestyles. *Your Natural Medicine Chest* is her thirteenth health book. Twelve others authored and co-authored, three written with doctors, are listed at the front of the book.

Jeanne Marie has also written one children's book and seven small poetry books. She is also a professional floral designer, gardener, published poet, singer, arts and crafts expert, meditation teacher, and qualified yoga instructor who has trained other teachers.

Write: P.O. Box 4391, Vancouver, B.C., Canada V6B 3Z8 or call 604-878-8787 for Voice Mail, to arrange international lectures or classes by Jeanne Marie Martin.

About the Cartoonist
Graham Harrop creates cartoons for the *Vancouver Sun* and a regular cartoon strip called "Backbench" for the *Globe and Mail*, both

newspapers in Canada. He has also created cartoons for travel and diet books. He lives in Vancouver, B.C., Canada.

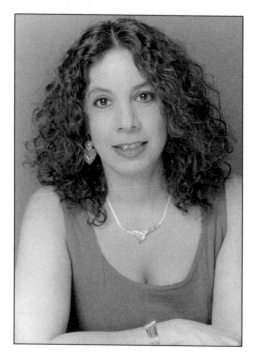

JEANNE MARIE MARTIN, CIN

NOTES